W9-CWE-857

ADVANCES IN

Surgery®

VOLUME 31

ADVANCES IN

Surgery®

VOLUMES 1 THROUGH 27 (OUT OF PRINT)

VOLUME 29

VOLUME 30

ADVANCES IN
Surgery®

VOLUME 31

Editor-in-Chief
John L. Cameron, MD
The Alfred Blalock Professor and Chairman, Department of Surgery, The Johns Hopkins University School of Medicine, Surgeon-in-Chief, The Johns Hopkins Hospital, Baltimore, Maryland

Associate Editors
Charles M. Balch, MD
President, City of Hope National Medical Center, Duarte, California

Bernard Langer, MD
Professor of Surgery, University of Toronto; Director, Hepatobiliary Program, Division of General Surgery, The Toronto Hospital and University of Toronto, Toronto, Ontario, Canada

John A. Mannick, MD
Moseley Distinguished Professor of Surgery, Harvard Medical School; Surgeon-in-Chief Emeritus, Brigham and Women's Hospital, Boston, Massachusetts

George F. Sheldon, MD
Professor and Chairman, Department of Surgery, University of North Carolina at Chapel Hill School of Medicine, Chapel Hill, North Carolina

G. Tom Shires, MD
Professor, Department of Surgery, University of Nevada School of Medicine, Las Vegas, Nevada

Ronald K. Tompkins, MD
Chief, Division of General Surgery, Professor of Surgery, University of California, Los Angeles Center for the Health Sciences, Los Angeles, California

John Wong, MD
Professor and Head, Department of Surgery, University of Hong Kong, Queen Mary Hospital, Hong Kong, China

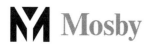

St. Louis   Baltimore   Boston   Carlsbad   Naples   New York   Philadelphia   Portland
London   Madrid   Mexico City   Singapore   Sydney   Tokyo   Toronto   Wiesbaden

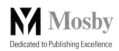
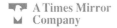

Publisher: Theresa Van Schaik
Acquisitions Editor: Cynthia Baudendistel
Developmental Editor: Susan Fox
Manager, Periodical Editing: Kirk Swearingen
Project Supervisor, Production: Joy Moore
Production Assistant: Karie House

Printed in the United States of America
Composition by The Clarinda Company
Printing/binding by The Maple-Vail Book Manufacturing Group

Mosby–Year Book, Inc.
11830 Westline Industrial Drive
St. Louis, Missouri 63146

International Standard Serial Number: 0065–3411
International Standard Book Number: 0–8151–8406–9

Contributors

Harry L. Anderson, III, M.D.
Assistant Professor of Surgery and Anesthesia, University of
Pennsylvania School of Medicine, Philadelphia, Pennsylvania

Philip S. Barie, M.D.
Associate Professor, Department of Surgery, Cornell University Medical
College, Director, Ann and Max A. Cohen Surgical Intensive Care Unit,
The New York Hospital–Cornell Medical Center, New York

Kirsten Noelle Bass, M.D.
General Surgery Resident, Duke University Medical Center, Durham,
North Carolina; Surgical Research Fellow, Johns Hopkins University
School of Medicine, Department of Surgery, Baltimore, Maryland

Michael Belkin, M.D.
Assistant Professor of Surgery, Department of Surgery, Brigham and
Women's Hospital, Harvard Medical School, Boston, Massachusetts

Ajay K. Bindal, M.D.
Staff Surgeon, Section of Neurosurgery, Saint Joseph's Hospital,
Houston, Texas

Rajesh K. Bindal, M.D.
Department Resident/Neurological Surgery, Indiana University School of
Medicine, Indianapolis, Indiana

Murray F. Brennan, M.D.
Professor, Chairman, Department of Surgery, Memorial Sloan-Kettering
Cancer Center, New York, New York

Gregory B. Bulkley, M.D.
Professor of Surgery, Johns Hopkins University School of Medicine,
Baltimore, Maryland

Benjamin B. Chang, M.D.
Assistant Professor of Surgery, Department of Vascular Surgery, Albany
Medical College, Albany, New York

Edward M. Copeland III, M.D.
Professor and Chairman, Department of Surgery, University of Florida,
Gainesville, Florida

R. Clement Darling, III, M.D.
Associate Professor of Surgery, Department of Vascular Surgery, Albany Medical College, Albany, New York

Magruder C. Donaldson, M.D.
Associate Professor of Surgery, Department of Surgery, Brigham and Women's Hospital, Harvard Medical School, Boston, Massachusetts

Timothy J. Eberlein, M.D.
Chief, Division of Surgical Oncology, Brigham and Women's Hospital, Boston, Massachusetts; Richard E. Wilson Professor of Surgery, Harvard Medical School, Boston, Massachusetts

Jose P. Garcia, M.D.
Cardiothoracic Resident, Division of Thoracic Surgery, Brigham and Women's Hospital, Harvard Medical School, Boston, Massachusetts

A.G. Greenburg, M.D., Ph.D.
Department of Surgery, The Miriam Hospital and Brown University, Providence, Rhode Island

Linda Sanders Haigh, M.D., Ph.D.
Assistant Professor, Department of Surgery, University of Florida, Gainesville, Florida

Lawrence E. Harrison, M.D.
Assistant Professor of Surgery, Department of Surgery, University of Medicine and Dentistry of New Jersey/New Jersey Medical School, Newark, New Jersey

Bronwyn Jones, M.D.
Professor of Radiology, Johns Hopkins University School of Medicine, Baltimore, Maryland

H.W. Kim, Ph.D.
Department of Surgery, The Miriam Hospital and Brown University, Providence, Rhode Island

Brock K. King, M.D.
Resident in Surgery and Nutrition Research, The University of Tennessee, Memphis, Tennessee

Kenneth A. Kudsk, M.D.
Professor of Surgery, Director of Surgical Research, The University of Tennessee, Memphis, Tennessee

Shimon Kusne, M.D.
Associate Professor of Medicine and Surgery, Division of Transplantation Medicine, Thomas E. Starzl Transplantation Institute, Division of Infectious Diseases, University of Pittsburgh, Pittsburgh, Pennsylvania

Bernard Langer, M.D., F.R.C.S.(C)
Professor of Surgery, University of Toronto; Director, Hepatobiliary
Program, Division of General Surgery, The Toronto Hospital and
University of Toronto, Toronto, Ontario, Canada

Robert P. Leather, M.D.
Professor of Surgery, Department of Vascular Surgery, Albany Medical
College, Albany, New York

John A. Mannick, M.D.
Moseley Distinguished Professor of Surgery, Department of Surgery,
Brigham and Women's Hospital, Harvard Medical School, Boston,
Massachusetts

Joseph P. Minei, M.D.
Associate Professor, Department of Surgery, The University of
Texas–Southwestern Medical Center, Director of Trauma and Surgical
Critical Care, Parkland Health and Hospital Systems, Dallas, Texas

Jeffrey A. Norton, M.D.
Professor of Surgery, University of California, San Francisco

Philip S.K. Paty, M.D.
Assistant Professor of Surgery, Department of Vascular Surgery, Albany
Medical College, Albany, New York

Douglas Reintgen, M.D.
Program Leader, Cutaneous Oncology, Moffit Cancer Center, Tampa,
Florida; Professor of Surgery, University of South Florida, Tampa,
Florida

William G. Richards, Ph.D.
Research Associate, Division of Thoracic Surgery, Brigham and Women's
Hospital, Harvard Medical School, Boston, Massachusetts

Alexander S. Rosemurgy, M.D.
Professor and Chief, Division of General Surgery, University of South
Florida, Tampa, Florida

Raymond Sawaya, M.D.
Chairman, Department of Neurosurgery, M.D. Anderson Cancer Center,
Houston, Texas

Scott R. Schell, M.D., Ph.D.
Chief Resident, Department of Surgery, School of Medicine, Johns
Hopkins University, Baltimore, Maryland

Dhiraj M. Shah, M.D.
Professor of Surgery, Department of Vascular Surgery, Albany Medical
College, Albany, New York

Ron Shapiro, M.D.
Associate Professor of Surgery, Director, Renal Transplantation, Thomas E. Starzl Transplantation Institute, University of Pittsburgh, Pittsburgh, Pennsylvania

Samuel Singer, M.D.
Surgical Director, Sarcoma Program, Dana Farber Cancer Institute, Boston, Massachusetts Surgeon, Brigham and Women's Hospital, Boston, Massachusetts; Assistant Professor of Surgery, Harvard Medical School, Boston, Massachusetts

David J. Sugarbaker, M.D.
Chief, Division of Thoracic Surgery, Brigham and Women's Hospital, Harvard Medical School, Boston, Massachusetts

Mark A. Talamini, M.D.
Associate Professor and Director of Minimally Invasive Surgery, Department of Surgery, School of Medicine, Johns Hopkins University, Baltimore, Maryland

Kenneth K. Tanabe, M.D.
Surgical Director, Pigmented Lesion Clinic and Melanoma Center, Massachusetts General Hospital, Boston, Massachusetts; Assistant Professor of Surgery, Harvard Medical School, Boston, Massachusetts

Bryce R. Taylor, M.D., F.R.C.S.(C.)
Professor of Surgery, University of Toronto; Chairman, Division of General Surgery; Associate Chair, Department of Surgery, University of Toronto; Head, Division of General Surgery, The Toronto Hospital, Toronto, Canada

Robert Udelsman, M.D.
Associate Professor and Director of Endocrine and Oncologic Surgery, Department of Surgery, School of Medicine, Johns Hopkins University, Baltimore, Maryland

Anthony D. Whittemore, M.D.
Chief, Professor of Surgery, Department of Surgery, Brigham and Women's Hospital, Harvard Medical School, Boston, Massachusetts

Emmanuel E. Zervos, M.D.
Fellow, Digestive Disorders Center, Department of Surgery, University of South Florida, Tampa, Florida

Contents

Flank vs. Abdominal Approach for Abdominal Aortic Surgery: The Flank Approach.
By R. Clement Darling III, Robert P. Leather, Philip S.K. Paty, Benjamin B. Chang, and Dhiraj M. Shah

Extrapleural Pneumonectomy for Malignant Mesothelioma.
By David J. Sugarbaker, William G. Richards, and Jose P. Garcia

CHAPTER 1

Current Management of Small-Bowel Obstruction

Kirsten Noelle Bass, M.D.

General Surgery Resident, Duke University Medical Center, Durham, North Carolina; Surgical Research Fellow, Johns Hopkins University School of Medicine, Department of Surgery, Baltimore, Maryland

Bronwyn Jones, M.D.

Professor of Radiology, Johns Hopkins University School of Medicine, Baltimore, Maryland

Gregory B. Bulkley, M.D.

Professor of Surgery, Johns Hopkins University School of Medicine, Baltimore, Maryland

HISTORICAL PERSPECTIVE

> [The] pain of the intestines was intense, sometimes it constricted the intestines like a bandage; sometimes it concentrated its force. . . . At times the pain remitted; at times it came in paroxysms . . . then the vomiting became more frequent, and the constipation more obstinate . . . [resulting] in a total inversion of peristaltic motion and ileus . . . . I regulate my practice by the pain, and repeat the narcotic until it either ceases or grows mild . . . . The disease, however, was only palliated, not cured.
>
> Thomas Sydenham, 1670

Sydenham's eloquent description[1] of "bilious colic" accurately reflects the signs and symptoms of small-bowel obstruction. Not surprisingly, Sydenham and many of his contemporaries in the 17th century advocated nonoperative approaches for the treatment of bowel obstruction. He would bleed his patients to rid the body of bad humors and then proceed with the administration of cathartics while attempting to keep the patient comfortable during the purge by administering large amounts of laudanum. Even in his day, however, he realized that these techniques usually provided only temporary relief at best, not a resolution of the obstruction.

According to Wangensteen, Praxagoras, in the third or fourth century B.C., was one of the first to report a surgical operation for strangulated hernia. He described making an incision over the swollen area, freeing the intestine, and establishing an "artificial anus" from the large bowel. Not surprisingly, however, it took many centuries for operative intervention to become an accepted treatment for the management of bowel obstruction. Along with Sydenham, many physicians turned to treatments other than surgery. During the 18th and 19th centuries, it was popular to feed the patient many pounds of mercury or other heavy metals such as lead in the hope that the heavy metal would force its way through the occluding lesion and eventually be evacuated in the stool.[2]

Over the centuries, operative intervention was carried out sporadically, but with only moderate success. With the acceptance of antisepsis and then aseptic surgical technique, operative intervention in bowel obstruction became more acceptable. In 1885, Greves reported a case of a patient who suffered for 5 days from complete bowel obstruction. An operation was performed under antiseptic precautions, during which division of a constrictive band around the ileum resulted in full recovery of the patient.[3] This report stimulated the interest of the London surgical community in the operative treatment of intestinal obstruction. By 1899, things had clearly changed: Frederick Treves of the London Hospital stated that "It is less dangerous to leap from the Clifton Suspension Bridge than to suffer from acute intestinal obstruction and decline operation."[2] This reminds us of the more modern adage to "never let the sun rise and set on a patient with (complete) bowel obstruction."

Just as our surgical predecessors, the surgeon of today relies most heavily on the history and physical examination when diagnosing small-bowel obstruction. Recently, however, advances in diagnostic and especially imaging techniques have assisted in more accurate characterization, particularly with regard to the critical distinction between partial and complete obstruction. Moreover, a number of clinical trials have also been conducted to address the question of appropriate timing of surgical intervention in patients with partial small-bowel obstruction. More recently, research efforts have focused on the prevention of adhesion formation, the leading cause of small-bowel obstruction in the industrialized world. Although modern surgeons have the advantage of centuries of experience with small-bowel obstruction, some aspects of its management remain quite controversial.

PATHOGENESIS

Small-bowel obstruction may be caused by a variety of intrinsic or extrinsic lesions (Table 1). In technologically advanced countries, the predominant cause is adhesions from a prior laparotomy (50% to 80% of the cases in many centers),[4, 5] although in less developed nations, advanced hernias, volvuli, and intussusception are the predominant causes.[6, 7]

Adhesions are responsible for approximately 60% of all cases of intestinal obstruction in the United States. In a retrospective analysis of 144 cases of small-bowel obstruction from adhesions, Cox et al. found that the most common reasons for previous laparotomy associated with obstruction were appendectomy (23%), colorectal resection (21%), gynecologic procedures (12%), and upper gastrointestinal (gastric, biliary, splenic) (9%) and small-bowel surgery (8%). The remaining 24% of the patients had had multiple laparotomies, the most common combination being appendectomy and one or more gynecologic procedures (10%). Thus a total of 80% had had a prior operation in the pelvis. They also confirmed the widely held clinical impression that single-band adhesions were most commonly found in cases of strangulating obstruction and that multiple, matted adhesions were found more often in cases of simple (nonstrangulating) obstruction. Significantly, band adhesions were found most commonly after prior appendectomy, colorectal surgery, and gynecologic resection.[8] In a retrospective study of 567 patients undergoing the aforementioned procedures at Yale-New Haven Hospital, the overall incidence of small-bowel obstruction within 5 years after laparotomy was reported to be 11% after appendectomy and 6% after cholecystectomy.[9] These and many other studies indicate that lower abdominal and pelvic operations

---

TABLE 1.

Etiology of Small-Bowel Obstruction

Etiology	Approximate Incidence, %
Adhesions	60
Malignant tumor	20
Hernia	10
Inflammatory bowel disease	5
Volvulus	3
Miscellaneous	2

are more likely than upper gastrointestinal tract procedures to be associated with the development of subsequent small-bowel obstruction. One explanation is that the bowel is normally tethered more cephalad at the root of the mesentery and is therefore more mobile caudad in the pelvis. Adhesions forming in the pelvis, where the intestine is normally more mobile, appear to be more likely to produce an obstructing torsion.

Malignant tumors account for approximately 20% of cases of small-bowel obstruction, with few being primary small-bowel neoplasms and most being secondary malignant foci.[5] Several mechanisms of malignant spread can produce obstruction. Direct intraabdominal extension of tumor from a colonic, gastric, pancreatic, or ovarian cancer may produce lesions that extrinsically compress the bowel lumen or obstruct by direct invasion. Spread to lymph nodes only occasionally produces masses large enough and in the right location to impinge on adjacent bowel. Perhaps the most common cause of small-bowel obstruction from malignancy is secondary peritoneal implants that have spread transcoelomically from an intra-abdominal primary tumor, typically ovarian, pancreatic, gastric, or colonic. Less often, malignant cells from distant sites may spread hematogenously and subsequently transcoelomically within the abdomen. For example, breast or lung cancer may metastasize hematogenously to the ovary or adrenal and then spread transcoelomically to produce peritoneal carcinomatosis with subsequent bowel obstruction.

Hernias account for about 10% of all cases of small-bowel obstruction but are more often than adhesions associated with strangulation.[10, 11] These hernias include ventral, inguinal, and internal hernias, as might occur if the mesentery is not adequately reapproximated after bowel resection or colostomy. Femoral hernias must not be overlooked, especially in obese females. Often misdiagnosed is an obturator hernia, which is uncommon but not rare in certain populations. For example, obturator hernias account for 1% of all hernia repairs and 1.6% of cases of small-bowel obstruction at the Queen Mary Hospital in Hong Kong. The most common patient population affected is elderly, emaciated women with multiple chronic diseases.[12] With an increasingly aging population with chronic disease, obturator hernias may become more prevalent.

Inflammatory bowel disease (Crohn's disease) accounts for approximately 5% of all cases of small-bowel obstruction. This subclass of patients often has a chronic, subacute, or intermittent form of partial obstruction that is usually approached differently from other forms of small-bowel obstruction (see later).

Miscellaneous causes represent only 2% to 3% of cases of small-bowel obstruction, but it is nevertheless important to recognize uncommon causes. For example, gallstone ileus is rare in the general population but more common in the elderly.[13] Small-bowel obstruction is also uncommon during pregnancy, but it has been reported with an incidence of 1 in 16,709 deliveries. Most of these women had undergone previous surgery, and 50% had had a previous appendectomy. Obstruction most commonly occurs during the first pregnancy after surgery. Fetal mortality is reported to be as high as 38%.[14] In the pediatric population, congenital intestinal atresia, pyloric stenosis, and intussusception are commonly encountered. Other causes in adult patients include phytobezoar in patients with a history of previous gastric outlet surgery[15] and familial Mediterranean fever, a disease characterized by recurring, self-limiting attacks of febrile inflammation of the peritoneum, pleura, and synovium, where small-bowel obstruction has been found to be the most frequent complication.[16]

An important cause of small-bowel obstruction, especially partial obstruction, that is rarely listed in most clinical series is a localized intra-abdominal abscess from any cause, but commonly from a ruptured appendix or diverticulum or an anastomotic leak. At surgery, these patients do not exhibit actual mechanical occlusion of the bowel lumen; rather, it appears that their clinical obstruction is caused by an intense *local* ileus in the bowel directly adjacent to the abscess that simulates the clinical manifestation of obstruction.

PATHOPHYSIOLOGY

Mechanical small-bowel obstruction is accompanied first by the development of mild proximal intestinal distension that results from the accumulation of normal gastrointestinal secretions and gas above the obstructed segment. Initially this distension physiologically stimulates peristalsis above *and below* the point of obstruction. This distal peristalsis accounts for the frequent loose bowel movements that may accompany partial and even complete small-bowel obstruction in the early hours after its onset. This distension also stimulates the physiologic secretion of fluid, electrolytes, and succus entericus into the bowel lumen.[17, 18] One may imagine that the bowel initially "thinks" that it is being fed. (Indeed, the gut nervous system coordinates that physiologic response.) Because of the secretory and peristaltic response, increased distension occurs and a positive-feedback loop between secretion, peristalsis, and distension is established.

As more severe distension occurs, the intraluminal hydrostatic pressure increases to the point (only a few centimeters of water) where compression of the intestinal mucosal villus lymphatics, the lacteals, results in obstruction of the normally substantial level of lymphatic flow and the subsequent development of bowel wall lymphedema. The accumulation of fluid in the bowel wall and subsequently in the lumen further increases intraluminal hydrostatic pressure. Consequent compression of the precapillary venules eventually results in elevated hydrostatic pressure at the venous end of the capillary; this increased hydrostatic pressure disrupts the Starling relationship of capillary fluid exchange, and the net filtration of fluid, electrolytes, and protein across the capillary bed into the bowel wall and lumen is increased. This "third space" loss of extracellular fluid from the intravascular space results in dehydration and hypovolemia that can sometimes be massive. If the obstruction is proximal, the dehydration may be accompanied by hypochloremic, hypokalemic, metabolic alkalosis secondary to vomiting. Prolonged dehydration may result in oliguria, azotemia, and hemoconcentration. Eventually, hypotension and hypovolemic shock ensue. Increasing abdominal distension may also lead to increased intra-abdominal pressure, which may impair ventilation by diaphragmatic elevation and further reduce venous return from the lower extremities by caval compression, thereby potentiating the effects of hypovolemia.

Venous hypertension and ischemia may occasionally progress directly to arterial occlusion and subsequent frank ischemia at the microvascular level. However, it is more common for the loop of distended bowel to further twist upon itself and its associated mesentery and result in *macrovascular* arterial occlusion of the mesenteric vascular branches at the root of the mesentery. Bowel ischemia and necrosis then progress rapidly and, if left untreated, may eventually lead to bowel perforation, peritonitis, and death from sepsis.

Normally, the mucosa of the gastrointestinal tract acts as a barrier to the systemic circulation of bacteria that normally reside within the gut lumen. However, the gastrointestinal tract may suffer failure of its immunologic gut barrier function under certain conditions.[19, 20] Normally, the proximal segment of intestine contains relatively few bacteria. However, during periods of intestinal stasis, these bacteria proliferate rapidly. Many studies have found that indigenous bacteria colonizing the gastrointestinal tract can cross the mucosal epithelium to infect mesenteric lymph nodes and even systemic organs.[21, 22] This process has been referred to as *bac-*

terial translocation. Simple intestinal obstruction is associated with increased bacterial translocation to mesenteric lymph nodes even in patients without an intra-abdominal infection. In one series, 59% of the patients undergoing laparotomy for simple small-bowel obstruction had bacteria cultured from the mesenteric lymph nodes as compared with only 4% of the patients operated on intra-abdominally for other reasons. *Escherichia coli* was the most common species.[23] If this occurs so often in simple small-bowel obstruction, it seems likely that this process would be greatly facilitated in cases of strangulation, especially just after detorsion (reperfusion). Nevertheless, it remains unclear whether antibiotics have a role in the preoperative management of simple (nonstrangulating) small-bowel obstruction.

CLINICAL PRESENTATION

The diagnostic and therapeutic approach to small-bowel obstruction should be systematic and lends itself to classification into four phases: (1) recognizing mechanical obstruction, (2) distinguishing partial from complete obstruction, (3) distinguishing simple from strangulating obstruction, and (4) identifying the underlying etiology. This illustrates that the initial approach to bowel obstruction is generic, with attention to the underlying cause usually a secondary consideration.

RECOGNIZING SMALL-BOWEL OBSTRUCTION

In most cases, identification of a patient with small-bowel obstruction is straightforward and based on the characteristic symptoms, physical signs, and supine and upright plain abdominal radiographs. The patient's history is usually remarkable for previous abdominal surgery, often pelvic. The patient typically has a variable period of abdominal pain (usually colicky, especially in the early period), nausea, vomiting, obstipation, or perhaps "diarrhea," i.e., the passage of several small loose stools (from distal to the point of obstruction). The nature of the pain may be helpful because colicky pain is said to be encountered most frequently in cases of simple obstruction whereas constant pain has been attributed to late or strangulating obstruction. Diarrhea, if present, is secondary to the increased peristalsis distal to an early complete or most partial obstructions. Patients who come to the emergency room with crampy abdominal pain, nausea, vomiting, and diarrhea with hyperactive bowel sounds may have gastroenteritis misdiagnosed if a complete evaluation, including supine and upright plain abdominal films, is not undertaken.

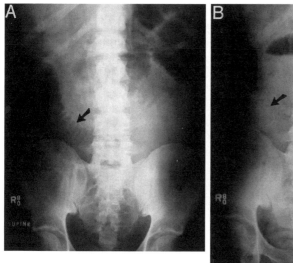

FIGURE 1.

Supine and upright plain abdominal radiographs in a patient with small-bowel obstruction. **A,** supine film showing characteristic dilated loops of small bowel *(arrow)* and a paucity of colonic air. **B,** upright film revealing air-fluid levels *(small arrow)* and the "string of pearls" sign *(large arrow)* in the right lower quadrant.

On physical examination, the patient will have abdominal distension, the degree often varying with the level of obstruction. Duodenal or high proximal small-bowel obstruction may occur with little evident distension. Bowel sounds may be either hyperactive early or hypoactive if the patient is seen late in the course of simple obstruction or has a strangulating lesion. Mild abdominal tenderness may be present with or without a palpable mass. The presence of peritoneal signs may again point toward late or strangulating obstruction. The importance of careful examination to rule out an obvious incarcerated hernia in the groin, the femoral triangles, or the obturator foramina (palpable on digital rectal examination) cannot be overemphasized. Rectal examination should also be performed to screen for intraluminal masses and to check for the presence of gross or occult blood.

On initial plain-film examination, the findings of distended loops of small bowel with air-fluid levels (on upright views) and a paucity of colonic air are characteristic (Fig 1). However, plain films may be diagnostic only 46% to 80% of the time.[24, 25] For example, a patient may have a gasless abdomen on plain films in the presence of complete obstruction. This may be caused by a closed-loop obstruction that precludes the accumulation of gas within the obstructed loop. Closer evaluation of such a film may reveal a "ground glass" haziness in the midabdomen or displacement of adjacent bowel by the "invisible" dilated, closed loop[25] (Fig 2). In such situations, if there is any question on the plain films as to whether an obstruction is present, further evaluation with other radiologic modalities is indicated.

Computed tomography (CT) has recently been applied to patients with small-bowel obstruction. The CT diagnosis of bowel obstruction and its discrimination from an adynamic ileus are based on the detection of fluid and/or air-filled loops of bowel proximal to the obstruction, the presence of a definite localized transition zone, and the presence of collapsed loops of small bowel or colon distal to the obstruction. The exact point of obstruction can sometimes be visualized as a beaklike narrowing in patients with adhesions as the etiology. One advantage of CT is that extrinsic causes such as hematoma, abscess, inflammation, and extraluminal tu-

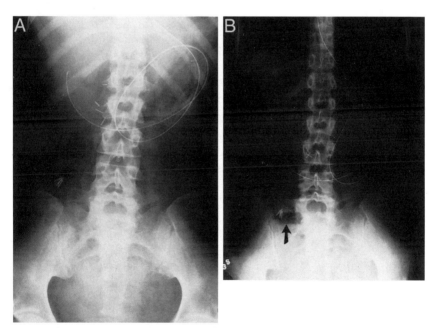

FIGURE 2.

Supine and upright plain abdominal radiographs in a patient with a closed-loop small-bowel obstruction. **A,** supine film showing a relatively "gasless" abdomen and the "ground glass" appearance of the midportion of the abdomen. **B,** upright film revealing only a few air-fluid levels *(arrow)* in the right lower quadrant.

mors, which cannot be directly visualized on plain-film or conventional contrast studies, are often well visualized on CT.[26] The use of intravenous (IV) contrast is recommended so that the bowel wall can be examined in more detail. Although oral contrast is not absolutely essential for the identification of obstruction because fluid and air can easily be distinguished in the bowel loops,[27] it is quite helpful in discriminating partial from complete obstruction and in localizing the level of obstruction. Certain limitations to the use of CT in the setting of small-bowel obstruction include the location of an obstructing lesion at the ileocecal valve with residual feces in the colon, which may incorrectly lead to the diagnosis of an ileus.[26]

Two other approaches to imaging have been used. In a world where cost must be carefully monitored, ultrasound (US) may become an increasingly valuable diagnostic tool as compared with more expensive modalities like CT or magnetic resonance imaging (MRI). A retrospective study suggested that US correctly diagnosed small-bowel obstruction 89% of the time when the US findings were compared with the diagnosis made at the time of surgery. Sonographic indicators of obstruction included small-bowel loops dilated more than 3 cm, dilated bowel segments larger than 10 cm in length, active peristalsis of the dilated segment, and colon collapse[28] (Fig 3). Ultrasound has been reported to be particularly useful in pregnant patients, where radiation exposure is a concern. Magnetic resonance imaging has also been suggested as an adjunct to evaluate small-bowel obstruction when used in combination with retrograde bowel insufflation after scopolamine has been administered to relax the ileocecal valve.[29]

DISCRIMINATING PARTIAL FROM COMPLETE OBSTRUCTION

Because the management of complete obstruction is often operative and that of partial small-bowel obstruction is, at least initially, almost always nonoperative, distinction between the two is important. The patient's history may provide a clue inasmuch as the continued passage of flatus or stool, especially 6 to 12 hours after onset, is more consistent with a partial obstruction. However, even a complete small-bowel obstruction can be accompanied early by loose stools secondary to peristalsis distal to the obstruction. On plain film, the persistence of residual colonic gas after 6 to 12 hours is also suggestive of partial obstruction. It is important to note that rectal examination of supine patients does not introduce significant rectal air whereas sigmoidoscopy, flexible or rigid, may well do so.

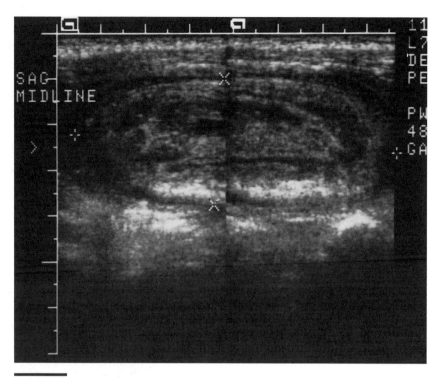

FIGURE 3.

Ultrasonogram of a pediatric patient with an ileal intussusception. (Courtesy of Sheila Sheth, M.D.)

Despite the foregoing, many patients present a real diagnostic challenge because early complete obstruction can be difficult to distinguish from partial, high-grade obstruction on plain films. In these cases, it is useful to give 50 mL of undiluted thin barium sulfate via the nasogastric tube after the initial plain abdominal films have been obtained. The tube is then clamped for about an hour, or even less if the patient cannot tolerate it without vomiting. Flat and upright abdominal films are obtained, and then nasoenteric suction is resumed. Sequential films are taken over the ensuing 12- to 24-hour period of resuscitation, and the degree of obstruction is almost always evident: patients with partial obstruction will almost invariably have barium in the cecum or beyond. Barium should not be used if the presence of colonic obstruction is suspected. The barium may become inspissated and cause an impaction that may convert a partial to a complete colonic obstruction. (Contrary to popular misconception, this is not a risk in the small intestine.) In equivocal cases, a barium enema should be performed to first rule out colonic obstruction.

An alternative approach is to use one of the water-soluble contrast media, either nonionic low-osmolar (e.g., iopamidol or io-hexol) or hyperosmolar (e.g., sodium diatrizoate [Gastrografin]). A randomized trial comparing barium sulfate with iopamidol reported that iopamidol was a useful alternative to barium for small-bowel contrast radiology.[30] However, as has been found previously, barium provides better mucosal coating that allows for more detailed examinations (because water-soluble contrast becomes more dilute the more distal it travels). Therefore, barium is still the agent of choice for elective examinations, especially enteroclysis (see later).[30] Meglumine diatrizoate (Gastrografin) has also been shown to be a safe and effective contrast agent that can be used in the diagnosis of small-bowel obstruction.[31] Because it is hyperosmolar, it promotes intestinal peristalsis and has been used as a therapeutic agent (see later), although it can cause severe colic as well. This can constitute inhumane treatment inasmuch as most experienced clinicians appropriately eschew narcotics in their patients until after surgery. Moreover, unlike barium, hyperosmolar contrast media present a very serious risk of pulmonary injury in the event of aspiration, a not uncommon event in an elderly, distended patient who is vomiting. They also potentiate the shift of intravascular fluid into the bowel lumen, thus necessitating close monitoring and aggressive IV fluid repletion.

Computed tomography may prove useful for discriminating complete from partial obstruction by determining the degree of collapse and the amount of residual air and fluid in the collapsed (distal) intestinal segment.[26] One of the limitations of using CT to evaluate partial obstruction is that a mild partial obstruction may not reveal a clear transition zone on CT, which could lead to a misdiagnosis of ileus[26] if there is not a close correlation with the history and physical findings.

DISCRIMINATING SIMPLE FROM STRANGULATING OBSTRUCTION

Early recognition of strangulation in patients with mechanical small-bowel obstruction has always been controversial. This issue has been greatly confused by the indiscriminate mixing of patients with partial and complete obstruction in many series. Except for the rare patient with a strangulated Richter's hernia that has gone undetected on physical examination, patients with partial obstruction can be considered to be at minimal risk of strangulation.

On the other hand, patients with complete obstruction are at substantial risk of strangulation. In operative series, this risk has been consistently reported to be 20% to 40%.[4, 5, 10] The "five classic signs" of strangulation obstruction have been variously cited to include continuous (vs. colicky) abdominal pain, fever, tachycardia, peritoneal signs, leukocytosis, acidosis, the presence of a painful mass, the absence of bowel sounds, and blood in the stool. However, it has been found in both retrospective[5, 11, 25, 32] and prospective[10] studies that these signs are neither sensitive, specific, nor accurately predictive of strangulation. Elevated serum levels of amylase, potassium, phosphate, alkaline phosphatase, aspartate aminotransferase, alanine aminotransferase, lactate dehydrogenase, and creatinine phosphokinase are also not practically useful in diagnosing strangulation.[10] Furthermore, no combination of these signs can accurately predict vascular compromise.[10, 25] Moreover, despite frequent assurances to the contrary by surgeons convinced of their own diagnostic acumen, the senior operating surgeon's ability to prospectively recognize strangulation in operative cases of small-bowel obstruction was no better than chance alone.[10] In addition, only one of the six patients with early *reversible* ischemia in that series was detected preoperatively. The reason for this is clearly evident: all the signs that have been used to indicate strangulation are actually signs of the body's inflammatory response to (irreversible) tissue necrosis. Although most surgeons can correctly identify advanced ischemic bowel in a septic patient with a rigid abdomen, early, *reversible* ischemia is simply not discernible. These factors contribute to the high mortality of patients with a strangulated bowel. Indeed, nearly half of all deaths from small-bowel obstruction occur secondary to strangulation and its complications,[25] and in most series the presence of strangulation doubles the mortality[4, 11] (from about 10% to 20%) associated with small-bowel obstruction. The morbidity of strangulation is also as high as 42%, with wound infections and urinary and pulmonary complications being the most frequent.[11]

Recently, CT has been reported to be useful in the diagnosis of strangulation (Fig 4). Intravenous contrast is recommended because the pattern of bowel wall enhancement can be useful in recognizing edema secondary to ischemia. The CT signs of strangulation include thickening of the bowel wall (Fig 4,A), with or without a "target sign"; pneumatosis intestinalis (Fig 4,B and 4C); portal venous gas (Fig 4,D); mesenteric haziness, fluid, or hemorrhage and ascites; a serrated beak sign[33]; and nonenhancement (or rarely increased bowel wall enhancement due to prolonged washout of intravascular contrast material) after an IV contrast bolus.[26] Once again, however, these signs (e.g., pneumatosis intestinalis) usually indicate irreversible necrosis rather than reversible ischemia.

Ultrasound has been reported to be 90% sensitive and 93% specific for the recognition of strangulation in one prospective study of 231 patients with adhesive small-bowel obstruction. However, the positive predictive value for strangulation was only 73%. The criteria for strangulation included the presence of an akinetic dilated loop, the presence of increased peristaltic activity proximal to the akinetic loop, and rapid accumulation of peritoneal fluid after the onset of obstruction.[34] However, without independent confirmation in a study that discriminates *reversible* from *irreversible* strangulation and that is controlled for the number of "tough calls" by another diagnostic modality, it is unlikely that US can be truly discriminant.

Finally, Stordahl et al. have reported that in cases of strangulation in which the gastrointestinal mucosa becomes permeable,

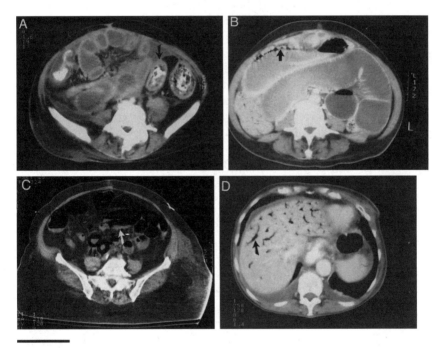

FIGURE 4.

Computed tomography in a patient with signs of strangulation. **A,** note the massively thickened bowel wall from edema *(arrow).* **B** and **C,** note the areas of pneumatosis intestinalis *(single arrows),* a late sign of ischemic necrosis. Note the "bull's eye" *(double arrows)* on the sagittal view indicative of the massive amounts of air within the bowel wall. **D,** note extensive portal venous gas within the liver *(arrow),* a very late sign of advanced intestinal ischemia. (Courtesy of Elliot Fishman, M.D.)

opacification of the urinary bladder may occur when water-soluble contrast is used in a small-bowel series.[35, 36] Once again, however, this implies de facto, probably *irreversible* tissue damage.

In summary, given the present state of the art, no clinical indicator, combination of indicators, diagnostic test, or "experienced clinical judgment" can reliably discriminate *reversible* strangulating obstruction from simple obstruction. In the only prospective study of overall diagnostic capability, the (often confident) diagnosis of "nonstrangulating obstruction" was wrong 31% ±15% of the time.[10]

IDENTIFYING THE UNDERLYING CAUSE OF OBSTRUCTION

In most situations, management decisions, including surgery, are made on the basis of the aforementioned factors regardless of the suspected cause of the obstruction. Several situations, however, warrant special attention and possible modification of this approach. These include patients with small-bowel obstruction secondary to an incarcerated hernia, recurrent malignant tumor, inflammatory bowel disease, intra-abdominal abscess, radiation enteritis, *acute* postoperative obstruction, and multiple recurrent small-bowel obstruction, each of which will be discussed in more detail later. Although the most important clues to this particular component of the diagnosis are the history and physical examination, often an enteroclysis study can be helpful in this regard. In most cases, however, identification of the underlying cause is made at surgery, with little disadvantage to the patient.

MANAGEMENT

SYSTEMIC RESUSCITATION

Patients with small-bowel obstruction are usually intravascularly depleted, often massively, because of decreased oral intake, vomiting, and the sequestration of fluid from the intravascular space within the bowel wall and lumen. This requires aggressive replacement with an IV isotonic saline solution such as Ringer's lactate. Routine laboratory measurements of serum sodium, potassium, chloride, bicarbonate, and creatinine should be monitored. Serial measurements of the hematocrit, white blood cell count, and serum electrolytes are monitored closely to assess the adequacy of fluid repletion and as a possible indication of late tissue necrosis. Because of their large fluid requirements, many patients will need either central venous pressure monitoring or the placement of a pulmonary artery catheter. Almost all patients will need the placement of a Foley catheter so that hourly urine output may be monitored. Broad-spectrum antibiotics are also sometimes given pro-phylactically in light of the evidence of bacterial translocation occurring in even simple obstruction, or they are given as prophylaxis for resection or inadvertent enterotomy at surgery. However, this is a practice that varies greatly and has not been subjected to rigorous study.

MANAGEMENT OF OBSTRUCTION

Virtually all patients with small-bowel obstruction benefit from the use of nasoenteric suction, whether it be via a nasogastric or long intestinal tube such as a Cantor or Baker tube. This provides almost immediate symptomatic relief from the nausea and vomiting and, often to a significant degree, the abdominal pain. It allows the administration of contrast material to these nauseated patients. It also helps prevent aspiration at the time of induction of anesthesia. In some situations, a long tube may provide a postoperative splint to prevent recurrent obstruction. Sometimes it provides definitive treatment in lieu of surgery. However, the decision to use a nasoenteric tube must be made without regard to whether or when surgery is to be performed.

A prospective, randomized trial of short (nasogastric) vs. long (nasointestinal) tubes detected no significant difference with regard to the decompression achieved, the success of nonoperative treatment, or the morbidity after surgical intervention.[37] Other studies also report similar success with nonoperative treatment regardless of whether short or long tubes are used.[4] The primary advantages of a nasogastric tube include easy placement and rapid, more effective gastric decompression, which is especially essential in the setting of anesthetic induction, where the risk of aspiration is increased. Use of the nasogastric tube is not associated with some of the rare complications of long tubes, including perforation and the very rare possibility of mercury intoxication in the event of reservoir rupture.[38, 39] The rare fatalities and morbidities from mercury are associated with pulmonary aspiration of it after inadvertent rupture of the reservoir tip of the tube during removal through the nasopharynx. Spillage of small amounts of mercury into the gastrointestinal tract are, on the other hand, usually accompanied by harmless passage of the mercury into the stool without evident complications. Intussusception of the small bowel either over the tube while it is in place or over adjacent bowel on removal of the tube[40, 41] is occasionally associated with the use of long tubes.

The use of long tubes also has several advantages. Some surgeons believe that the weighted tip of the Cantor tube will open obstructed loops of bowel as it passes more distally, but there is no evidence to support this. A long tube also provides suction close to the area of obstruction when positioned correctly.[37] The presence of a long intestinal tube also greatly enhances bowel decompression at surgery, often facilitating primary closure of the abdominal wall without the need for enterotomy.[37] The alternative method of decompression at surgery is retrograde stripping of the small-bowel contents into the stomach with subsequent nasogastric suction. (Enterotomy is usually contraindicated.) In rats, manipulation of the bowel either by stripping or enterotomy significantly increased the incidence of *E. coli* bacteremia.[42] Therefore, effective preoperative decompression with a long tube may decrease the amount of bowel manipulation required in the operating room. Unfortunately, the U.S. Food and Drug Administration (FDA) has recently prohibited use of the Cantor tube because of the presence of mercury in its weighted tip, a decision that protects the FDA, not the patient.

The most controversial aspect of this disease is the role of early surgery vs. a trial of nonoperative management in patients with small-bowel obstruction. On the one hand, there is no way to clinically discriminate patients with early reversible strangulation. On the other hand, a number of large retrospective series report success with nonoperative management in patients without signs of strangulation, followed by surgery only in selected patients. For example, in a retrospective analysis of 123 admissions with adhesive small-bowel obstruction, the obstruction resolved in 85 patients without surgery. In 88% of *these* patients, the obstruction resolved within 48 hours. Resolution of the obstruction in the remaining patients occurred within 72 hours.[43] These authors reported no untoward effects in patients who required surgery after initially being treated nonoperatively. Another retrospective series reported a 73% rate of resolution of adhesive obstruction without a significant increase in mortality or the rate of strangulated bowel when compared with outcomes in other series. In this series, a trial of tube decompression for more than 5 days was ineffective.[44] These authors argue that a trial of 2 to 3 days, even up to 5 days in selected patients, of nonoperative nasoenteric decompression is reasonable in most patients without evidence of strangulation. The problem with these and similar studies is that they include a large, undefined population of patients with small-bowel obstruction, usually mixing patients with both complete and partial obstruction. (Indeed, there is little controversy that *partial* obstruction should be managed initially nonoperatively.) They therefore fail to definitely resolve the controversy as to the management of complete small-bowel obstruction (see later), but they do indicate that such an approach is safe in patients with partial obstruction.

If initial nonoperative management fails, several operative approaches are available via conventional laparotomy. Often, the obstruction is caused by the presence of one or more constricting adhesive bands, and the obstruction is relieved through simple lysis of the adhesions and detorsion. An obstructing lesion may also be present and require local bowel resection with primary reanastomosis. An intestinal bypass procedure or, rarely, the placement of enterocutaneous stomata may be the appropriate management of malignant obstructing lesions or radiation enteritis.

Advances in laparoscopic surgery have modified the approach to many general surgical problems, and laparoscopic management of acute small-bowel obstruction is also being addressed. Franklin et al. reported 23 patients with acute obstruction evaluated initially with laparoscopy (after an initial trial of failed conservative management). Twenty patients had successful laparoscopic resolution of their obstruction whereas 3 required laparotomy. The 3 patients who were converted to laparotomy had severe adhesions, anatomy that precluded complete examination of the entire length of the bowel, and suspected ischemic necrosis, respectively. The authors emphasized the importance of using nontraumatic bowel clamps when manipulating the dilated, friable bowel during laparoscopy to avoid injury.[45]

During exploration, whether by laparotomy or laparoscopy, it is sometimes difficult to evaluate bowel viability after the release of strangulation. The conventional clinical criteria generally used include the presence of normal color, peristalsis, and arterial pulsations. A prospective, controlled trial comparing standard clinical judgment with the use of a Doppler probe and with fluorescein for the intraoperative discrimination of viability found that the Doppler ultrasonic flow probe adds little to the conventional clinical judgment of the surgeon, which is usually correct if thought to be so. On the other hand, the pattern of fluorescein fluorescence was significantly more reliable than clinical judgment alone or the use of Doppler US in assessing intestinal viability. In difficult, borderline viability bowel segments, this is the only method of viability assessment that has been formally evaluated in a prospective, controlled clinical trial. Because clinical judgment is usually accurate in this assessment, the use of fluorescein is recommended in those cases in which borderline bowel segments are difficult to evaluate clinically.[46]

Another approach to the assessment of bowel viability is a "second-look" laparotomy or laparoscopy 18 to 48 hours after the initial procedure. Most advocates of these techniques suggest that the decision to perform a second-look laparotomy be made before closure, at the time of the initial procedure.[47] However, carefully controlled, well-documented studies in animals have found that fluorescein, when used correctly, identifies those segments of bowel that will ultimately survive.[48, 49] However, a recent study (which looked at a small number of patients in an inconsistently controlled, incompletely defined fashion) reported that fluorescein fluorescence, pulse palpation, and Doppler analysis during initial laparotomy were not accurate predictors of bowel viability in their hands when compared with findings (in a few patients) at second-look laparotomy.[50] Unfortunately, no details of the viability assessment techniques are given; if they were as superficial as described in this report, they would not represent a fair assessment of the state of the art of these techniques. In the absence of controlled clinical trials, it remains unclear whether or when a second-look laparotomy significantly enhances the assessment of intestinal viability. It is evident, however, that a second-look laparotomy is clearly indicated in a patient whose systemic condition deteriorates *after* the initial assessment because of the intestine's particular vulnerability of the vasoconstrictive, hemodynamic response to shock, sepsis, and severe physiologic stress.[51, 52]

Almost all patients, except those in frank septic shock, benefit from a period of 12 to 24 hours of nasoenteric suction, fluid and electrolyte resuscitation, and often the administration of antibiotics. This allows not only resuscitation but also completion of the diagnostic studies described earlier, including, in almost all cases, definitive discrimination of partial from complete obstruction. At this point, the role of early (i.e., after the initial 12 to 24 hours) surgery vs. a trial of nonoperative management remains extremely controversial. Much of the controversy, however, may be avoided if one discriminates the subsequent management of partial from complete bowel obstruction.

MANAGEMENT OF PARTIAL OBSTRUCTION

While the role of early surgery vs. expectant management of complete obstruction remains controversial in some circles, there is little controversy with respect to partial obstruction. Most of these patients benefit from an extension of the initial 12- to 24-hour period of nonoperative management for several days. A number of studies indicate that 60% to 85% of these patients will ultimately

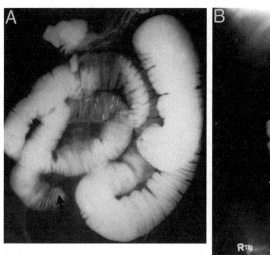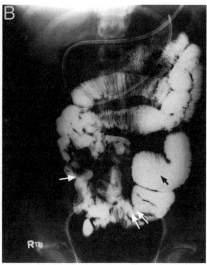

FIGURE 5.

Small-bowel enteroclysis study. **A,** enteroclysis study in a patient with *complete* obstruction. Note the area in the right lower quadrant where contrast material fails to pass beyond a point of *complete* obstruction *(arrow).* **B,** enteroclysis study in a patient with *partial* obstruction caused by an adhesive band. Note the dilated bowel loops proximal to the point of obstruction *(small arrow),* the transition zone at the point of obstruction *(double arrows),* and collapsed bowel loops filled with contrast distal to the point of *partial* obstruction *(large arrow).*

resolve their obstruction and be discharged without the need for surgery.[53–55] Even those who do not respond are better prepared for surgery because of better mechanical bowel decompression, often even an antibiotic bowel preparation, a long period of resuscitation to allow better intercompartmental fluid and electrolyte equilibration, and usually the benefits of planned surgery by a fresh operative team during daylight hours. Sometimes a more definite idea about the underlying cause can be obtained. If the total period without intake is prolonged more than a few days, parenteral nutrition should be provided. In summary, there are many benefits and few disadvantages from an initial trial of nonoperative management of most patients with *partial* small-bowel obstruction.

A substantial adjuvant to the management of partial small-bowel obstruction is the enteroclysis study (Fig 5) whereby graded volumes of dilute barium are given through a long tube localized either by peristalsis or direct fluoroscopic positioning in the small bowel just proximal to the site of the obstruction. This study, in the hands of an experienced radiologist, can often help define the degree of obstruction, its location, and its progression (improvement or lack thereof) over time. This is quite useful in deciding whether to intervene surgically or to wait longer for resolution. Sometimes the underlying cause can be inferred (e.g., allowing the discrimination of an adhesion from a neoplasm).[56]

To help resolve partial small-bowel obstruction nonoperatively, some groups have advocated the use of hyperosmolar water-soluble gastrointestinal contrast agents as therapeutic as well as diagnostic modalities. In a prospective randomized trial looking at the effect of Gastrografin in the nonoperative management of partial small-bowel obstruction, among the patients successfully managed nonoperatively, those who received 100 mL of Gastrografin had a significant reduction in the number of days until the first stool and in the length of overall hospital stay, from approximately 4 to 2 days. However, this trial found no significant difference in the proportion of patients who eventually required surgical intervention.[57] Stordahl et al. have also reported water-soluble contrast agents to be useful as therapeutic agents; however, there was no control group treated with nasogastric suction alone.[36] Others have reported that although administration of the hyperosmolar contrast materials was safe in patients with partial small-bowel obstruction, no advantage over conventional nonoperative management of partial small-bowel obstruction was found.[58]

MANAGEMENT OF COMPLETE OBSTRUCTION

Few other issues in surgery have generated such heated controversy for such a long period as the question of primary operative vs. primary nonoperative treatment of patients with small-bowel obstruction. Despite a preponderance of good evidence (but still not a randomized, prospective trial), experienced surgeons often express strongly polarized opinions. The conventional argument of those who advocate primary nonoperative management is that it is often successful and that by careful monitoring and "experienced clinical judgment" they can recognize those patients with early strangulation in time to operate on them before the bowel becomes nonviable. The 60% to 85% success rates cited in several large series are undeniable, but as mentioned before, these series contain predominately patients with partial obstruction—patients who rarely manifest strangulation. As discussed earlier, patients with partial obstruction should *usually* be treated nonoperatively, at least initially, and there is little controversy about this. Patients with complete obstruction are another matter. The incidence of strangulation in these groups varies from 20% to 40% (admittedly in operative series that necessarily exclude patients successfully managed nonoperatively). Moreover, prospective and retrospective studies are *unequivocally* clear in indicating that early irreversible strangulation is simply not discernible. Therefore, the risk of deciding to manage a patient nonoperatively based on a clinical assessment of "simple (nonstrangulating) obstruction" necessarily entails the substantial (about 30%) risk that one is delaying the treatment of intestinal strangulation until *after* that injury becomes irreversible. It is therefore reasonable to weigh the benefits and risks of each approach as we do in every clinical decision. However, one of the risks of primary nonoperative management that *must* be taken into account is the risk of strangulation. In an acutely unstable patient, such as someone with an acute myocardial infarction, treatable arrhythmia, hypovolemia, or shock, this risk is a reasonable one in return for the benefits of improved systemic stability in the nonoperative period, even if it proves to be a preoperative period. On the other hand, a patient with chronic, irreversible risk factors mandates a *correct,* not necessarily a nonoperative decision. In these situations and in conventional patients with complete small-bowel obstruction, the substantial risk of unrecognized (or unrecognizable) strangulation mandates primary operative management after the initial 12 to 24 hours of resuscitation. Indeed, although several retrospective studies report that a 12- to 24-hour delay of surgery in patients with *complete* small-bowel obstruction is safe,[53, 59] the incidence of strangulation and other complications significantly increases after longer periods of nonoperative management.[59]

MANAGEMENT OF SPECIFIC LESIONS

ADHESIONS

The pathophysiology of adhesion formation has been studied extensively, and the process is clearly initiated by the formation of a fibrin clot (from transudated fibrinogen activated by tissue factor, regardless of bleeding). Peritoneal trauma is a well-known cause.[60] The peritoneum (mesothelium) has been found to possess fibrinolytic activity via plasminogen activation.[61] Ischemia, a known stimulus of adhesion formation, causes a marked reduction in plasminogen activator activity levels through the release of plasminogen activator inhibitors.[62, 63] This pathway for adhesion formation lends support to the use of fibrinolytics in the prevention of adhesions. In the past, streptokinase and urokinase have been used with various degrees of success in animal models.[64, 65] Their use in humans has been avoided for this purpose for fear of bleeding complications, especially in those patients after extensive dissection who are at greatest risk of adhesion formation. Nonsteroidal antiinflammatory agents, including ketorolac tromethamine, have also been found to be useful in inhibiting adhesion formation in pigs.[66] Once again, however, steroids and antimetabolites, although effective in animal models, are not usually used in patients for fear of inhibiting wound healing, especially after extensive dissection and in the presence of distension.

Hyaluronic acid, a product of a strain of *Streptococcus,* is highly lubricious and nonimmunogenic and can coat and protect serosal surfaces. It seems to be effective in keeping traumatized surfaces separate, thus hindering the formation of connecting fibrous bands.[67] Recently, Becker et al. have conducted the first prospective study of postoperative abdominal adhesion formation by using standardized direct peritoneal visualization. In this study, 183 patients with ulcerative colitis or familial polyposis who underwent colectomy and ileal pouch–anal anastmosis with diverting loop ileostomy were randomized to receive or not receive a bioresorbable membrane of hyaluronic acid and carboxymethylcellulose placed directly beneath the midline abdominal incision. At the subsequent ileostomy closure, laparoscopy revealed that the number of patients who had adhesions was reduced by more than 50% in those treated with the bioresorbable membrane. The extent and severity of these adhesions as well were significantly reduced in the treatment group.[68] Although the implications of this study are limited by the fact that the worst obstructing adhesions do not usually form at the old incision site but within the pelvis, the feasible extension of this technology to serosal surfaces could represent a significant advance.

Independent of adjuvant therapy for the prevention of adhesion formation, several operative steps should be taken at any laparotomy, *especially lysis of adhesions,* to help minimize the extent of future adhesion formation. These include gentle handling of the bowel to reduce serosal trauma, avoidance of unnecessary dissection, exclusion of foreign material from the peritoneal cavity (i.e., the use of absorbable suture material when possible, the avoidance of excessive use of gauze sponges, and the removal of starch from gloves), adequate irrigation and removal of infectious and ischemic debris, preservation and use of the omentum around the site of surgery or in the denuded pelvis, and avoidance of lysis of adhesions that do not involve the small bowel.[69]

Patients who are initially seen with acute small-bowel obstruction from adhesions usually benefit from early operative lysis. Generally, a technically simple laparotomy (or laparoscopy) is all that is required. Except under unusual circumstances, enterotomy should be avoided if possible.

INCARCERATED HERNIA

When an incarcerated abdominal wall hernia is the cause of obstruction, the obstruction can often be managed initially by simple manual reduction. However, the patient should always be admitted for close observation. During this hospitalization, elective hernia repair should be performed in an attempt to prevent recurrent incarceration and the possibility of strangulation. An acutely incarcerated, irreducible hernia is a clear indication for primary early operative management.

MALIGNANT TUMOR

Small-intestinal obstruction caused by a primary malignant tumor is rare; it is much more often caused by a neoplasm from another organ such as the colon or ovary. These patients are managed the same as patients with simple small-bowel obstruction from adhesions, combined with resection of the obstructing tumor whenever feasible.

More challenging from a therapeutic standpoint are patients with intestinal obstruction who have been previously treated for cancer or who have known peritoneal carcinomatosis. In a retrospective analysis of 81 episodes of small-bowel obstruction in 61 patients with previously treated malignancy, 69 episodes involved the small bowel, and 24 of these were diagnosed as complete obstructions. Eight percent of these patients had concurrent small- and large-bowel obstruction. In 59 cases the etiology was established: 61% of these obstructions were due to metastatic tumor and 39% were due to benign causes (adhesion, radiation, stricture). Forty-five percent of the cases of partial obstruction that were managed conservatively resolved without surgery. On the other hand, only 4% of the cases of complete obstruction were successfully managed without operative intervention.[70] One of the most important lessons from this study is that patients with a history of cancer who have an obstruction should not be assumed to have carcinomatosis as the etiology of their obstruction. At surgery the entire bowel must be examined to rule out multiple lesions. The surgeon should not necessarily avoid operating on a patient with obstruction from carcinomatosis, although the management of such patients must be individualized, with the desires of the patient taken into account. Of course, not every terminally ill patient is an operative candidate, and parenteral nutrition combined with percutaneous endoscopic gastrostomy offers the advantage of terminal care at home for those patients who either have obstruction not amenable to surgery or have chosen not to undergo surgery.[70]

INFLAMMATORY BOWEL DISEASE

Patients with Crohn's disease of the small intestine can have either complete, partial, or intermittent small-bowel obstruction. The obstruction may be secondary to the primary inflammatory process itself or to the gradual development of a fibrotic stricture as a sequela to previous episodes of inflammation and healing, with or without treatment. These patients, often with partial obstruction, can frequently be initially managed nonoperatively with tube decompression[4] in combination with pharmacologic treatment of the inflammatory process, for example, with high-dose steroids. Parenteral nutrition should be provided because the period of required bowel rest may be prolonged. On the other hand, if fibrotic strictures are the primary cause of the obstruction, primary bowel resection may be necessary to relieve the obstruction. This does not imply that a nonoperative trial should not be attempted; the obstruction related to the strictures may prove to be partial as the associated inflammation resolves. Recently there have been a number of reports of success of operative strictureplasty, with or without concomitant bowel resection in other areas, for multiple, short strictured segments in patients with Crohn's disease.[71]

INTRA-ABDOMINAL ABSCESS

Often, an acute intra-abdominal abscess may produce a clinical scenario that is practically indistinguishable from complete, mechanical small-bowel obstruction. This is often not due to intraluminal obstruction, nor even to external compression of the bowel lumen, but to a severe localized ileus secondary to local inflammation and edema. Drainage of the abscess is often sufficient to relieve the obstruction. This does not necessarily require laparotomy because the abscess may be accessible by using US- or CT-guided percutaneous drainage. However, if the obstruction persists, laparotomy should be undertaken without delay.

RADIATION ENTERITIS

Of importance in the current management of malignancies of many types is the concomitant use of radiotherapy. In a retrospective analysis of patients at UCLA undergoing radical hysterectomy, a 5% incidence of small-bowel obstruction was reported in those undergoing surgery alone as compared with a 20% incidence in patients receiving adjuvant radiation therapy.[72] Small-bowel obstruction is a recognized late complication of radiation therapy instituted for the treatment of rectosigmoid and rectal cancer after low anterior resection and abdominoperineal resection. The rate has been reported to be as high as 30% in patients treated with daily extended-field radiotherapy, 21% in those receiving single pelvic-field radiotherapy, and 9% in those with multiple pelvic fields in a retrospective review of 224 patients at M.D. Anderson Cancer Center. In this study, patients with small-bowel exclusion achieved by using the open table top device technique had an incidence of obstruction of only 3%. The incidence of recurrent small-bowel obstruction was also significantly correlated with the incidence of postsurgical small-bowel obstruction in these patients.[73] Another technique for small-bowel exclusion that has been explored is the use of intraperitoneal saline-filled tissue expanders[74] to keep the bowel out of a specific radiation field such as the pelvis during radiotherapy.

Despite these precautions, however, cases of acute and chronic radiation enteritis do occur and are sometimes accompanied by bowel obstruction. If obstruction occurs within a few weeks of radiotherapy, it is often useful to treat it nonoperatively with tube decompression and steroids. However, complications from irradiation may not appear for many years after the completion of therapy and are usually progressive thereafter. When the obstruction occurs in this chronic setting, nonoperative management is rarely effective and laparotomy is usually required. The surgeon may choose to either locally resect the irradiated bowel or bypass the affected area. Whether one resects or bypasses, it is essential to avoid anastomosis of irradiated bowel.

ACUTE POSTOPERATIVE OBSTRUCTION

Small-bowel obstruction that occurs in the immediate postoperative period presents a challenge for both diagnosis and treatment. Diagnosis is often difficult because the primary symptoms of abdominal pain and vomiting may often be masked and/or attributed to incisional pain and postoperative ileus. A careful history may reveal pain that is colicky in nature, as opposed to pain that is dull and constant.

Abdominal plain films may be helpful in distinguishing ileus from obstruction, but they are often not diagnostic. Computed tomography has been shown to be especially useful in distinguishing postoperative ileus from obstruction. In fact, Frager et al. reported 100% sensitivity and specificity when CT was used to distinguish early (within 10 days of laparotomy) postoperative ileus from small-bowel obstruction.[75] Furthermore, some common causes of postoperative obstruction such as intra-abdominal abscesses are easily visualized on CT scan. Upper gastrointestinal series with water-soluble contrast may also be quite useful in revealing not only the presence but also the level of obstruction. Barium contrast may also be used, but only if there is little danger of perforation or anastomotic leakage.

Once the diagnosis of obstruction has been established, it should be managed like obstruction that occurs late in the postoperative period. Specifically, partial obstruction may be afforded a trial of tube decompression. In fact, in this situation the opportunity to temporarily stabilize the patient and delay surgery a while longer into the postoperative period may be an advantage. Complete obstruction is a relatively clear indication for early exploration. However, in the postoperative setting it is not uncommon for the surgeon to prefer an initial trial of nonoperative management. Caution must be taken, however, because several series have reported a potentially high rate of missed strangulation in patients with postoperative obstruction.[25] Moreover, an initial delay can move the timing of surgery to 10 to 14 days postoperatively, a time at which new, vascularized, dense adhesion formation can make the operative dissection difficult and dangerous.

RECURRENT OBSTRUCTION

Patients with multiple recurrent adhesive obstructions represent a difficult management problem. (Various studies report recurrence rates of approximately 10% to 30%.)[5, 76] Recurrent obstruction appears to be a particular problem for patients with extensive, dense intraperitoneal adhesions. An initial nonoperative trial is usually desirable and often safe. However, a retrospective study found that recurrence occurred sooner and more frequently in patients managed conservatively than in patients managed operatively after their second episode of recurrence.[77] This does not mean that every patient with recurrent obstruction should be managed operatively. Each patient must be fully evaluated as an individual, and their previous responses to particular interventions must be taken into account when their management plan is formulated.

Bowel fixation procedures have been used at surgery in an attempt to splint the bowel in a nonobstructive configuration while the inevitable adhesions form. There are two categories of bowel fixation, external and internal. External plication procedures include the Noble[78] and Childs-Phillips[79] procedures and other variations of these techniques whereby the small intestine or its mesentery is sutured in large, gently curving loops. Variable success in preventing recurrent obstruction has been reported when these techniques are used.[78–81] Common complications are the development of enteroenteric, enterocolic, and enterocutaneous fistulas, gross leakage, peritonitis, and death.[78–81] For this reason and because of the low overall success rate, these procedures have largely been abandoned. Internal fixation or stenting procedures use a long intestinal tube inserted via the nose, a gastrostomy, or even a jejunostomy to splint the bowel in gentle, unobstructing curves. The intestinal tube is then left in place for at least 1 week postoperatively, even after nasoenteric suction has been discontinued. The hope is that adhesions will form in such a manner that future torsion of loops about band adhesions is less likely. Several series have reported moderate success with the use of this approach.[82–85] Complications associated with the use of internal stenting tubes include prolonged drainage of bowel contents from the tube insertion site after removal of the tube, intussusception of bowel either over the tube while it is in place or after tube removal, and difficult removal of the tube, which may require surgical reexploration.[82–86] Close and Christensen have looked at the late recurrence of obstruction in patients undergoing Childs-Phillips plication or Baker tube stenting vs. enterolysis alone in a retrospective series. They found that the recurrence rate of obstruction was relatively low after all three interventions, with the highest recurrence occurring after enterolysis alone (6.5%). These authors recommend that for single-band or few adhesions, enterolysis alone is adequate intervention. In cases of severe, multiple adhesions, they suggest that either Childs-Phillips plication or Baker tube stenting be performed. They further specify that in cases of massive bowel distension, the Baker tube should be used because of its ability to decompress the bowel as well as a means of providing plication. Moreover, they recommend that in cases in which peritonitis is encountered, Baker tube stenting is preferred over external plication because the transmesenteric sutures may provide a nidus of infection.[87]

SUMMARY

In conclusion, most of the recent advances in the management of small bowel obstruction consist of developments in the imaging modalities available to assist in the diagnosis itself, particularly with regard to the distinction between partial and complete obstruction. Unfortunately, little progress has been made to enable physicians to detect *early, reversible* strangulation, and therefore the surgical management of small-bowel obstruction has changed very little over the past 10 years. Because of the inability to detect reversible ischemia, there is a substantial risk of progression to *irreversible* ischemia (and an inherent rise in morbidity and mortality) when surgery is delayed for an extended period of time, especially in the setting of suspected complete obstruction. However, almost all patients do benefit from an initial 12 to 24 hours of resuscitation and decompression in cases of complete obstruction; resuscitation and decompression can usually be extended for a longer period of time in those patients with partial obstruction who exhibit no signs of progression (Fig 6).

It is encouraging, however, that some advances have been made in understanding the pathophysiology and prevention of adhesion

Management of Small Bowel Obstruction

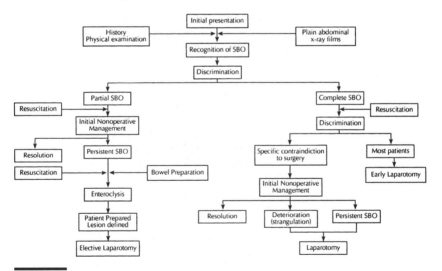

FIGURE 6.

Algorithm for the management of patients with small-bowel obstruction *(SBO)*. Note that after the diagnosis of small-bowel obstruction, most of the management decisions are based on the distinction between partial and complete obstruction. (Modified from Bulkley GB: Intestinal obstruction, in Bayless T [ed]: *Current Therapy in Gastroenterology and Liver Disease.* Philadelphia, BC Decker, 1986, pp 232–239.)

formation. Research efforts in the future should continue to focus on these issues as well as on the development of methods to better recognize *early* signs of strangulation.

REFERENCES

1. Sydenham T: The works of Thomas Sydenham translated from the Latin edition of Dr. Greenhill with a life of the author by R.G. Latham, vol. 1, London, 1848, pp 193–198.
2. Wangensteen OH: Historical aspects of the management of acute intestinal obstruction. *Surgery* 65:363–383, 1969.
3. Greves EH: On a case of acute intestinal obstruction in a boy, with remarks upon the treatment of acute obstruction. *Liverpool M-Chir J* 5:118–130, 1885.
4. Bizer LS, Liebling RW, Delany HM, et al: Small bowel obstruction. The role of nonoperative treatment in simple intestinal obstruction and predictive criteria for strangulation obstruction. *Surgery* 89:407–413, 1981.
5. Mucha P Jr: Small intestinal obstruction. *Surg Clin North Am* 67:597–620, 1987.
6. Chiedozi LC, Aboh IO, Piserchia NE: Mechanical bowel obstruction. Review of 316 cases in Benin City. *Am J Surg* 139:389–393, 1980.
7. Holcombe C: Surgical emergencies in tropical gastroenterology. *Gut* 36:9–11, 1995.
8. Cox MR, Gunn IF, Eastman MC, et al: The operative aetiology and types of adhesions causing small bowel obstruction. *Aust N Z J Med* 63:848–852, 1993.
9. Zbar RIS, Crede WB, McKhann CF, et al: The postoperative incidence of small bowel obstruction following standard, open appendectomy and cholecystectomy: A six-year retrospective cohort study at Yale–New Haven Hospital. *Conn Med* 57:123–127, 1993.
10. Sarr MG, Bulkley GB, Zuidema GD: Preoperative recognition of intestinal strangulation obstruction. Prospective evaluation of diagnostic capability. *Am J Surg* 145:176–182, 1983.
11. Shatila AH, Chamberlain BE, Webb WR: Current status of diagnosis and management of strangulation obstruction of the small bowel. *Am J Surg* 132:299–303, 1976.
12. Lo CY, Lorentz TG, Lau PWK: Obturator hernia presenting as small bowel obstruction. *Am J Surg* 167;396–398, 1994.
13. Reisner RM, Cohen JR: Gallstone ileus: A review of 1001 reported cases. *Am Surg* 60:441–446, 1994.
14. Meyerson S, Holtz T, Ehrinpreis M, et al: Small bowel obstruction in pregnancy. *Am J Gastroenterol* 90:299–302, 1995.
15. Lo CY, Lau PWK: Small bowel phytobezoars: An uncommon cause of small bowel obstruction. *Aust N Z J Med* 64:187–189, 1994.
16. Ciftci AO, Tanyel FC, Büyükpamukçu N, et al: Adhesive small bowel obstruction caused by familial Mediterranean fever: The incidence and outcome. *J Pediatr Sur* 30:577–579, 1995.

17. Shields R: The absorption and secretion of fluid and electrolytes by the obstructed bowel. *Br J Surg* 52:774–779, 1965.
18. Wright HK, O'Brien JJ, Tilson MD: Water absorption in experimental closed segment obstruction of the ileum in man. *Am J Surg* 121:96–99, 1971.
19. Alexander JW, Boyce ST, Babcock GF, et al: The process of microbial translocation. *Ann Surg* 212:496–510, 1990.
20. Wells CL, Maddaus MA, Simmons RL: Proposed mechanisms for the translocation of intestinal bacteria. *Rev Infect Dis* 10:958–979, 1988.
21. Berg RD, Garlington AW: Translocation of certain indigenous bacteria from the gastrointestinal tract to the mesenteric lymph nodes and other organs in a gnotobiotic mouse model. *Infect Immun* 23:403–411, 1979.
22. Reed LL, Martin M, Manglano R, et al: Bacterial translocation following abdominal trauma in humans. *Circ Shock* 42:1–6, 1994.
23. Deitch EA: Simple intestinal obstruction causes bacterial translocation in man. *Arch Surg* 124:699–701, 1989.
24. Frager DH, Baer JW: Role of CT in evaluating patients with small-bowel obstruction. *Semin Ultrasound CT MR* 16:127–140, 1995.
25. Silen W, Hein MF, Goldman L: Strangulation obstruction of the small intestine. *Arch Surg* 85:121–129, 1962.
26. Balthazar EJ: CT of small-bowel obstruction. *AJR Am J Roentgenol* 162:255–261, 1994.
27. Blake MP, Mendelson RM: Computed tomography in acute small bowel obstruction. *Australas Radiol* 38:298–302, 1994.
28. Ko YT, Lim JH, Lee DH, et al: Small bowel obstruction: Sonographic evaluation. *Radiology* 188:649–653, 1993.
29. Chou C-K, Liu G-C, Chen L-T, et al: The use of MRI in bowel obstruction. *Abdom Imaging* 18:131–135, 1993.
30. Sandikcioglu TG, Torp-Madsen S, Pedersen IK, et al: Contrast radiography in small bowel obstruction. A randomized trial of barium sulfate and a nonionic low-osmolar contrast medium. *Acta Radiol* 35:62–64, 1994.
31. Joyce WP, Delaney PV, Gorey TF, et al: The value of water-soluble contrast radiology in the management of acute small bowel obstruction. *Ann R Coll Surg Engl* 74:422–425, 1992.
32. Snyder EN Jr, McCranie D: Closed loop obstruction of the small bowel. *Am J Surg* 111:398–402., 1966.
33. Ha HK, Park CH, Kim SK, et al: CT analysis of intestinal obstruction due to adhesions: Early detection of strangulation. *J Comput Assist Tomogr* 17:386–389, 1993.
34. Ogata M, Imai S, Hosotani R, et al: Abdominal ultrasonography for the diagnosis of strangulation in small bowel obstruction. *Br J Surg* 81:421–424, 1994.
35. Stordahl A, Laerum F: Water-soluble contrast media compared with barium in enteric follow-through. Urinary excretion and radiographic efficacy in rates with intestinal ischemia. *Invest Radiol* 23:471–477, 1988.

36. Stordahl A, Laerum F, Gjølberg T, et al: Water-soluble contrast media in radiography of small bowel obstruction. Comparison of ionic and non-ionic contrast media. *Acta Radiol* 29:53–56, 1988.
37. Fleshner PR, Siegman MG, Slater GI, et al: A prospective, randomized trial of short versus long tubes in adhesive small-bowel obstruction. *Am J Surg* 170:366–370, 1995.
38. Zimmerman JE: Fatality following metallic mercury aspiration during removal of a long intestinal tube. *JAMA* 208:2158–2160, 1969.
39. Dzau VJ, Szabo S, Chang YC: Aspiration of metallic mercury. A 22-year follow-up. *JAMA* 238:1531–1532, 1977.
40. Sower N, Wratten GP: Intussusception due to intestinal tubes. Case reports and review of literature. *Am J Surg* 110:441–444, 1965.
41. Hunter TB, Fon GR, Silverstein ME: Complications of intestinal tubes. *Am J Gastroenterol* 76:256–261, 1981.
42. Merrett ND, Jorgenson J, Schwartz P, et al: Bacteremia associated with operative decompression of a small bowel obstruction. *J Am Coll Surg* 179:33–37, 1994.
43. Cox MR, Gunn IF, Eastman MC, et al: The safety and duration of non-operative treatment for adhesive small bowel obstruction. *Aust N Z J Med* 63:367–371, 1993.
44. Seror D, Feigin E, Szold A, et al: How conservatively can postoperative small bowel obstruction be treated? *Am J Surg* 165:121–126, 1993.
45. Franklin ME Jr, Dorman JP, Pharand D: Laparoscopic surgery in acute small bowel obstruction. *Surg Laparosc Endosc* 4:289–296, 1994.
46. Bulkley GB, Zuidema GD, Hamilton SR, et al: Intraoperative determination of small intestinal viability following ischemic injury. A prospective, controlled trial of two adjuvant methods (Doppler and fluorescein) compared with standard clinical judgment. *Ann Surg* 193:628–637, 1981.
47. Schneider TA, Longo WE, Ure T, et al: Mesenteric ischemia. Acute arterial syndromes. *Dis Colon Rectum* 37:1163–1174, 1994.
48. Gorey TF: The recovery of intestine after ischemic injury. *Br J Surg* 67:699–702, 1980.
49. Bulkley GB, Wheaton LG, Strandberg JD, et al: Assessment of small intestinal recovery from ischemic injury after segmental, arterial, venous, and arteriovenous occlusion. *Surg Forum* 30:210–213, 1979.
50. Ballard JL, Stone WM, Hallett JW, et al: A critical analysis of adjuvant techniques used to assess bowel viability in acute mesenteric ischemia. *Am Surg* 59:309–311, 1993.
51. Bastidas JA, Reilly PM, Bulkley GB: Mesenteric vascular insufficiency, in Yamada T (ed): *Textbook of Gastroenterology*. Philadelphia, JB Lippincott, 1995, pp 2490–2523.
52. Reilly PM, Peters JH, Merine DS: Vascular Insufficiency, in Yamada T (ed): *Atlas of Gastroenterology*. Philadelphia, JB Lippincott, 1992, pp 415–430.
53. Peetz DJ Jr, Gamelli RL, Pilcher DB: Intestinal intubation in acute, mechanical small-bowel obstruction. *Arch Surg* 117:334–336, 1982.
54. Brolin RE: The role of gastrointestinal tube decompression in the

treatment of mechanical intestinal obstruction. *Am Surg* 49:131–137, 1983.

55. Wolfson PJ, Bauer JJ, Gelernt IM, et al: Use of the long tube in the management of patients with small-intestinal obstruction due to adhesions. *Arch Surg* 120:1001–1006, 1985.

56. Shrake PD, Rex DK, Lappas JC, et al: Radiographic evaluation of suspected small bowel obstruction. *Am J Gastroenterol* 86:175–178, 1991.

57. Assalia A, Schein M, Kopelman D, et al: Therapeutic effect of oral Gastrografin in adhesive, partial small-bowel obstruction: A prospective randomized trial. *Surgery* 115:433–437, 1994.

58. Feigin E, Seror D, Szold A, et al: Water-soluble contrast material has no therapeutic effect on postoperative small-bowel obstruction: Results of a prospective, randomized clinical trial. *Am J Surg* 171:227–229, 1996.

59. Sosa J, Gardner B: Management of patients diagnosed as acute intestinal obstruction secondary to adhesions. *Am Surg* 59:125–128, 1993.

60. Ellis H: The aetiology of post-operative abdominal adhesion. An experimental study. *Br J Surg* 50:10–16, 1962.

61. Porter JM, McGregor FH Jr, Mullen DC, et al: Fibrinolytic activity of mesothelial surfaces. *Surg Forum* 20:80–82, 1969.

62. Buckman RF, Woods M, Sargent L, et al: A unifying pathogenetic mechanism in the etiology of intraperitoneal adhesions. *J Surg Res* 20:1–5, 1976.

63. Buckman RF Jr, Buckman PD, Hufnagel HV, et al: A physiologic basis for the adhesion-free healing of deperitonealized surfaces. *J Surg Res* 21:67–76, 1976.

64. Gervin AS, Puckett CL, Silver D: Serosal hypofibrinolysis. A cause of postoperative adhesions. *Am J Surg* 125:80–88, 1973.

65. James DCO, Ellis H, Hugh TB: The effect of streptokinase on experimental intraperitoneal adhesion formation. *J Pathol Bacteriol* 90:279–287, 1965.

66. Montz FJ, Monk BJ, Lacy SM, et al: Ketorolac tromethamine, a nonsteroidal anti-inflammatory drug: Ability to inhibit post–radical pelvic surgery adhesions in a porcine model. *Gynecol Oncol* 48:76–79, 1993.

67. Holzman S, Connolly RJ, Schwaitzberg SD: Effect of hyaluronic acid solution on healing of bowel anastomoses. *J Invest Surg* 7:431–437, 1994.

68. Becker JM, Dayton MT, Fazio VW, et al: Prevention of postoperative abdominal adhesions by a sodium hyaluronate–based bioresorbable membrane: A prospective, randomized, double-blind multicenter study. *J Am Coll Surg* 183:297–306, 1996.

69. Menzies D: Postoperative adhesions: Their treatment and relevance in clinical practice. *Ann R Coll Surg Engl* 75:147–153, 1993.

70. Tang E, Davis J, Silberman H: Bowel obstruction in cancer patients. *Arch Surg* 130:832–837, 1995.

71. Tjandra JJ, Fazio VW: Strictureplasty without concomitant resection for small bowel obstruction in Crohn's disease. *Br J Surg* 81:561–563, 1994.

72. Montz FJ, Holschneider CH, Solh S, et al: Small bowel obstruction following radical hysterectomy: Risk factors, incidence, and operative findings. *Gynecol Oncol* 53:114–120, 1994.

73. Mak AC, Rich TA, Schultheiss TE, et al: Late complications of postoperative radiation therapy for cancer of the rectum and rectosigmoid. *Int J Radiat Oncol Biol* Phys 28:597–603, 1994.

74. Hoffman JP, Lanciano R, Carp NZ, et al: Morbidity after intraperitoneal insertion of saline-filled tissue expanders for small bowel exclusion from radiotherapy treatment fields: A prospective four year experience with 34 patients. *Am Surg* 60:473–483, 1994.

75. Frager DH, Baer JW, Rothpearl A, et al: Distinction between postoperative ileus and mechanical small-bowel obstruction: Value of CT compared with clinical and other radiographic findings. *AJR Am J Roentgenol* 164:891–894, 1995.

76. Landercasper J, Cogbill TH, Merry WH, et al: Long-term outcome after hospitalization for small-bowel obstruction. *Arch Surg* 128:765–770, 1993.

77. Barkan H, Webster S, Ozeran S: Factors predicting the recurrence of adhesive small-bowel obstruction. *Am J Surg* 170:361–365, 1995.

78. Noble TB Jr: Plication of small intestine as prophylaxis against adhesions. *Am J Surg* 35:41–44, 1937.

79. Childs WA, Phillips RB: Experience with intestinal plication and a proposed modification. *Ann Surg* 152:258–265, 1960.

80. McCarthy JD: Further experience with the Childs-Phillips plication operation. *Am J Surg* 130:15–19, 1975.

81. Ferguson AT, Reihmer VA, Gaspar MR: Transmesenteric plication for small intestinal obstruction. *Am J Surg* 114:203–208, 1967.

82. Baker JW: A long jejunostomy tube for decompressing intestinal obstruction. *Surg Gynecol Obstet* 109:519–520, 1959.

83. Baker JW, Ritter KJ: Complete surgical decompression for late obstruction of the small intestine, with reference to a method. *Ann Surg* 157:759–769, 1963.

84. Ramsey-Stewart G, Shun A: Nasogastrointestinal intraluminal tube stenting in the prevention of recurrent small bowel obstruction. *Aust N Z J Surg* 53:7–11, 1983.

85. Weigelt JA, Snyder WH III, Norman JL: Complications and results of 160 Baker tube plications. *Am J Surg* 140:810–815, 1980.

86. Kieffer RW, Neshat AA, Perez LM, et al: Indications for internal stenting in intestinal obstruction. *Milit Med* 158:478–479, 1993.

87. Close MB, Christensen NM: Transmesenteric small bowel plication or intraluminal tube stenting. Indications and contraindications. *Am J Surg* 138:89–96, 1979.

88. Bulkley GB: Intestinal obstruction, in Bayless T (ed): *Current Therapy in Gastroenterology and Liver Disease*. Philadelphia, BC Decker, 1986, pp 232–239.

CHAPTER 2

Management of Minimal Breast Cancer

Linda Sanders Haigh, M.D., Ph.D.
Assistant Professor, Department of Surgery, University of Florida, Gainesville, Florida.

Edward M. Copeland III, M.D.
Professor and Chairman, Department of Surgery, University of Florida, Gainesville, Florida.

B reast cancer is the most common malignancy of American women, and the incidence of breast cancer in this population has risen dramatically since 1982. Based on data collected by the Surveillance Epidemiology and End Results Program of the National Cancer Institute, the steepest increase lies in the rates of in situ and localized invasive tumors of the breast, whereas the rates of breast cancers with regional and distant metastases have remained relatively stable.

Because the prognosis of a patient with breast carcinoma depends to a large extent on the stage of disease at the time of diagnosis, early detection and screening for breast cancer have been emphasized. Heightened awareness of breast disease among physicians and women in general has led more than one in two women to consult her physician for a breast complaint. Of these, more than one in four will undergo core or surgical biopsy.

The combined effects of an increasing incidence of breast cancer over the last decade, identification of risk factors, and improved detection of small tumors have resulted in a number of minimally invasive and in situ carcinomas for which increased survival can be expected with appropriate management.[1] The potential for improved survival from early breast cancer detection makes it imperative for general surgeons to comprehend current management issues. This review therefore addresses the surgical evaluation of minimal breast cancer.

The term *minimal breast cancer* defines three breast diseases that have been found to have different biological behaviors. Included in the minimal breast cancer category are lobular carcinoma in situ (LCIS), ductal carcinoma in situ (DCIS), and early invasive carcinoma.[2–6] Contemporary wisdom suggests that invasive breast cancer is preceded by a period in which normal epithelial cells undergo malignant transformation. This relatively long indolent period may be represented clinically by the diagnosis of LCIS or DCIS. As malignant cells pile up within the breast ducts, the clinical recognition of DCIS becomes evident. Finally, as malignant cells penetrate the basement membrane of the duct, infiltrating or invasive carcinoma is diagnosed histologically. In LCIS, the risk of breast cancer subsequently developing is about 15% if the incidence of multiple series is averaged. The risk of subsequent invasive breast cancer if DCIS is left untreated is at least 50% and would approach 100% if affected patients were to live long enough.[7, 8] It is clear, then, that the main impact that general surgeons will have on improved survival of patients with breast cancer is in the management of patients with minimal breast cancer to prevent in situ disease from becoming malignant.

This review examines the incidence, features, and management of minimal breast cancer. General surgeons are confronted with a number of biopsy reports for minimal breast cancer for which treatment algorithms vary according to the specific disease encountered. Management of LCIS is expectant, management of invasive disease is definitive, and management of DCIS is somewhere in between these two, depending on its manifestation. Finally, the problem of axillary node metastasis in early breast cancer is reviewed. Always a subject of controversy, management of the axilla has regained importance in prognosis and therapeutic decision making in early carcinoma of the breast.

LOBULAR CARCINOMA IN SITU

Lobular carcinoma in situ is a risk factor for the subsequent development of breast cancer rather than a premalignant lesion. Because it has no distinctive mammographic or clinical findings, the true incidence of LCIS is unknown. The typical histologic features of LCIS—distension of the terminal duct with bland homogeneous cells and an absence of mitosis and necrosis—are found in 1% to 8% of all breast biopsy specimens.[9] It is usually an incidental finding.

Lobular carcinoma in situ is noted to be more common in premenopausal women, with the average age at diagnosis being 44 to

47. The fact that this age range is 10 to 15 years younger than that of women in whom invasive carcinoma is diagnosed tends to support the transition theory of breast cancer development. However, LCIS is a marker rather than an anatomical precursor of subsequent invasive breast cancer. Most of the cancers found 15 or more years after the diagnosis of LCIS have an invasive ductal rather than lobular histology, and the relative risk is equal in each breast.[10] The probability of future malignancy ranges from 10% to 37%, and the incidence of simultaneous foci of invasive carcinoma at the time of LCIS diagnosis in either breast is around 5%.[11, 12] The amount of LCIS present in a biopsy specimen or multifocal LCIS does not predict the behavior or the incidence of future carcinomas.

Based on this information, treatment options for a woman with LCIS include close follow-up or bilateral simple mastectomy.[13] Careful observation with biannual physical examination and yearly mammography is a logical management plan, as it is for any woman with increased breast cancer risk because of previous contralateral breast cancer or a positive family history. It is not necessary to obtain histologically negative margins on biopsy because LCIS is a diffuse lesion. Contralateral or "mirror-image" biopsy of the opposite, otherwise normal breast is not necessary and would not change management decisions.[14]

For women unwilling to accept the 10% to 37% risk of subsequent invasive carcinoma, surgical treatment of LCIS must be directed at both breasts. Treatment of one breast with simple mastectomy and contralateral biopsy is illogical because the risk of subsequent breast cancer is bilateral regardless of the original biopsy site. Prophylactic bilateral mastectomy with or without reconstruction may be chosen by a patient with high anxiety or concurrent risk factors such as multiple first-degree relatives with breast cancer, a prior contralateral breast cancer, and possibly in the future, a positive screen for *BRCA-1* or *BRCA-2* genes in a family member with breast cancer.[15] In this case, all breast tissue, including the nipple-areolar complex, is removed.[15] No axillary dissection is done because the risk of axillary node metastases for pure LCIS is 2%. Were axillary lymph nodes to be involved, the metastases would be from unsuspected occult microinvasive disease.[14]

Adjuvant chemotherapy and radiation therapy have no role in the treatment of LCIS. However, patients with LCIS are candidates for the National Surgical Adjuvant Breast and Bowel Project (NSABP) tamoxifen trial and can be included in other chemoprevention trials.

DUCTAL CARCINOMA IN SITU

Ductal carcinoma in situ is a heterogeneous disease that requires a variety of treatment approaches. The challenge is to use available clinical prognostic and pathologic data to select appropriate therapy for each patient. Clinical guidelines have been confusing in the past because a number of variables must be considered. The incidence, natural history, histologic features, and presence of biological markers of aggressiveness all contribute to treatment planning for DCIS, as do tumor size, location, and multifocality.

Ductal carcinoma in situ represents approximately 13% of all newly diagnosed breast cancers in the United States.[16] The disease may be manifested as a clinically palpable mass or be seen only on a mammogram. The typical mammographic appearance of DCIS is radiologically dense breast tissue with multiple punctate calcifications. Recent studies show that the incidence of DCIS increased from 1983 to 1992, coincident with the widespread use of mammographic screening.[17] At screening centers relying on mammography, up to 40% of new breast cancer are DCIS. Annually, 50,000 new cases of DCIS are diagnosed.

The evidence that DCIS is a true precursor of invasive carcinoma comes from multiple observations. First, the age at diagnosis is 47 to 63 years,[18] which is the same age as those women with confirmed invasive carcinoma. The probability of subsequent invasive carcinoma after biopsy-proven but untreated DCIS is 25% to 50%, and the invasive disease is virtually always in the same breast quadrant as the biopsy site. The histology of the invasive disease is ductal carcinoma. The size and extent of DCIS are directly related to the incidence of multifocal disease and synchronous invasive foci. The recurrence rate of DCIS after treatment is proportional to the presence of microscopically positive surgical margins and the diffuseness of the original disease[19, 20] (Table 1).

The histologic appearance of DCIS has been correlated with the incidence of progression to invasive disease. Ductal carcinoma in situ is characterized microscopically by proliferation of the inner cuboidal layer of ductal epithelium to form papillary ingrowths into the duct lumen. These ingrowths may crowd the lumen until the rounded spaces between papillary stalks produce a cribriform pattern. As this solid pattern further distends the ducts, anaplastic and mitotic cells become prominent. The comedo pattern develops as the central cells far from the epithelial capillary become anoxic and necrotic. Hence in the continuum from normal duct epithelium to invasive ductal carcinoma, the more aggressive sub-

TABLE 1.
Characteristics of Ductal and Lobular Carcinoma In Situ of the Breast

Characteristic	LCIS	DCIS
Age, average yr	44–47	47–63
Incidence, %	2.5	2–3
Clinical signs	None	Mass, nipple discharge
Mammographic signs	None	Microcalcifications
Premenopausal	2/3	1/3
Incidence of synchronous invasive carcinoma	5	18
Multicentricity, %	60–90	40–80
Bilaterality, %	50–70	10–20
Axillary metastases, %	1	2–3
Subsequent carcinomas		
Incidence, %	25–35	25–50
Laterality	Bilateral	Ipsilateral
Interval to diagnosis, yr	15–20	5–10
Histology	Ductal	Ductal

Abbreviations: LCIS, lobular carcinoma in situ; *DCIS,* ductal carcinoma in situ.
(Modified from Frykberg ER, Ames FC, Bland KI: Current concepts for management of early [in situ and occult invasive] breast carcinoma, in Bland KI, Copeland EM [eds]: *The Breast: Comprehensive Management of Benign and Malignant Diseases.* Philadelphia, WB Saunders, 1991.)

types, cribriform and comedo DCIS, contain more calcification, anaplasia, and possible microinvasion. Pure papillary DCIS has a more orderly appearance and nonaggressive behavior. The cribriform subtype is less aggressive then comedo, and more recent classifications divide DCIS into comedo and noncomedo subtypes.

In addition to histology, pathologic diagnosis of DCIS includes an estimate of nuclear grade as a means of quantifying the biological aggressiveness of the tumor. It is thought that lesions with high S-phase and aneuploid DNA patterns may be further along the biological path to invasive carcinoma than those with lower nuclear grade, low S-phase, and diploid DNA patterns.[19] These high-grade lesions are more likely to be associated with an occult invasive breast cancer.[20] Because the distinction between comedo and noncomedo is sometimes difficult, nuclear grade is becoming as important as the comedo feature in stratifying DCIS.

As in invasive tumors, the size of a DCIS lesion will direct therapeutic considerations. Mammography can detect tiny foci of DCIS less than 1 cm in diameter. Larger size portends a more difficult surgical excision, greater tumor aggressiveness, and multicentricity.[21] Hormone receptor status is also a factor. In an aggressive tumor, many of these histologic indices overlap so that approximately 80% of comedo lesions are aneuploid and estrogen receptor (ER)-negative. The remaining 20% of ER-positive lesions are less likely to contain microinvasive disease and recur after appropriate therapy. Just as with invasive tumors, DCIS with a high rate of mitosis translates into a higher recurrence rate often approaching 20%.[22]

Surgical management of the various guises of DCIS must consider both eradication of tumor and cosmetic result. Because DCIS is a true precursor of invasive disease, consideration must be given to treating the entire breast either by mastectomy or by radiation therapy. Routine axillary node dissection is not indicated because axillary node metastases are found in fewer than 2% to 3% of patients. As with LCIS, pure DCIS does not metastasize, and any positive lymph nodes result from occult invasive carcinoma. Treatment options for DCIS include wide excision alone, wide excision with breast irradiation, and total mastectomy.[23, 24]

Controversy arises concerning DCIS therapy because of the paucity of prospective randomized studies. The ideal width of the surgical excision margin for DCIS is unknown. Residual disease is found in up to 50% of all specimens re-excised for "close margins." However, data suggest that recurrence after wide excision alone (without radiation therapy) approaches zero for small cribriform tumors without necrosis and for micropapillary histologic variants of DCIS when margins are negative pathologically.[23] Thus in some cases, excisional biopsy alone is all that is required for the occasional microscopic focus of DCIS found incidentally at biopsy for an otherwise benign lesion, assuming that the lesion is totally excised and the mammogram and physical examination are otherwise normal.

The NSABP B-17 study examined the role of radiation in the treatment of DCIS. Although the initial report did not stratify DCIS lesions according to size and histology, the addition of radiation therapy to wide excision reduced the recurrence rate at 4 years from 16.4% with wide excision alone to 7.0% with wide excision and radiation therapy. Although long-term survival is unknown, this report suggests that the addition of radiation therapy may reduce the incidence of invasive recurrences. In other studies, recurrence is higher after breast-conserving surgery for DCIS when the lesions are large (greater than 2.5 cm in size) and the histologic pattern is cribriform or comedo with necrosis.[22] In these situations, wide excision and radiation therapy can still be used with caution, provided that no mammographic or physical evidence of multicentricity exists and margins of the resected specimen are free of DCIS. The risk of local recurrence is greater after breast conservation therapy for DCIS than for mastectomy, but it should be remembered that the likelihood of metastatic disease is small because most recurrences are DCIS. Thus wide excision to microscopically clear margins followed by radiation therapy has become an accepted alternative to total mastectomy.

Mastectomy is indicated for DCIS when the tumors are large, multifocal, and biologically aggressive. The favorable prognosis of DCIS as compared with other forms of breast cancer may have been influenced by the uniform mastectomy treatment in the older data.[20] In these retrospective studies, survival rates approached 100%. Chest wall recurrence after mastectomy for DCIS is also low (3%).[21] Current practice favors mastectomy over breast conservation therapy when the mammogram shows diffuse microcalcifications or multiple areas of microcalcifications, when pathologic margins show diffuse involvement with DCIS, and when other risk factors such as family history or previous contralateral breast cancer are associated with the disease. Until data are available from ongoing randomized prospective trials, mastectomy is a reasonable choice for lesions with high nuclear grade, aneuploid DNA patterns, high S phase, and extensive necrosis. In fact, a level I node dissection or sentinel node biopsy should also be considered because these lesions are more likely to be associated with an occult invasive breast cancer.[25] Many surgeons find that dissection must be carried into the lower portion of the axilla to ensure that the entire axillary tail of the breast is removed with the specimen.

The best treatment for DCIS with microinvasion is controversial. Wide excision with radiation therapy and no axillary dissection is probably adequate treatment, yet lymph node metastases have been reported in as many as 10% of dissected axillary specimens.[26] The argument for breast-conserving therapy in these borderline cases is that salvage mastectomy may be done in the event of recurrence. Reconstruction after mastectomy in an irradiated patient is, however, more complex, For this reason, many surgeons prefer mastectomy with immediate reconstruction. Again, the aggressiveness of the lesion histologically should be used to dictate whether axillary dissection, mastectomy, or both should be performed. Small, well-differentiated, nonnecrotic lesions with an occasional focus of microinvasion are no doubt very different lesions from those displaying cellular anaplasia, multiple areas of central necrosis, and widespread microinvasion.

General surgeons frequently encounter women with DCIS who are otherwise candidates for hormone replacement therapy. The concern is whether estrogen increases the risk of local or even distant recurrence of the breast cancer. The issue is an active area of investigation, but the relative risk is unknown. Many women in the perimenopausal or early postmenopausal stage are given hormone replacement therapy to prevent osteoporosis or reduce their risk of cardiovascular disease. For this reason, some surgeons have recommended total mastectomy over breast conservation therapy in breast cancer patients who require estrogen supplementation. This recommendation would remove one breast from the estrogen effect, but the hormone may still pose a risk to the other breast. If the benefits of hormone therapy are significant enough to warrant treatment for an individual patient, the type of surgical procedure the patient either has or will have should not make any difference in the recommendation to undergo hormone replacement therapy.

EARLY INVASIVE CARCINOMA

As a result of clinical trials in the last decade, it is now known that long-term survival with treatment either by lumpectomy, axillary dissection, and irradiation or by modified radical mastectomy is the same for stages I and II breast cancer.[27–29] Local recurrence rates average 5% to 10% after breast conservation therapy.

Most women with early invasive breast cancer are candidates for breast conservation therapy. Because the factors influencing prognosis and outcome for each patient are multiple, a team approach to breast cancer treatment has been advocated at several centers. The breast cancer therapy team consists of the surgeon, radiation therapist, medical oncologist, and plastic surgeon. The surgeon and radiation therapist are primarily involved in local control of disease, whereas the medical oncologist evaluates and manages systemic disease. The patient herself must be an active participant in the decision analysis. It is both her privilege and her burden to help make management decisions in the treatment of her disease.

Lymph node metastases in patients with all stages of breast cancer strongly correlate with overall survival. Most early invasive carcinomas are small and have no axillary node involvement. But several biological features of these tumors may influence prognosis including DNA ploidy, S-phase fractions, nuclear grade, hormone receptor status, and stromal lymphatic and blood vessel invasion.[30, 31]

Treatment options for early invasive carcinoma are aimed at surgical ablation of disease. Because these lesions are usually small, breast conservation surgery followed by radiation therapy is often indicated. For lesions less than 2 cm in size with negative axillary lymph nodes, cytotoxic chemotherapy or hormonal therapy is dictated by evaluation of the biological markers for tumor aggressiveness. Patients with lesions greater than 2 cm in size are usually candidates for adjuvant therapy based on size alone. Despite progress made over the past few years in radiation and chemotherapeutic management of breast cancer, surgery remains the primary modality of treatment. Any compromise in surgical excision is accompanied by compromise in local control and perhaps in survival; any residual tumor diminishes the effect of adjuvant therapy.[4] With these concepts in mind, wide local excision alone is rarely indicated in the treatment of early invasive carcinoma because of the high rate of local recurrence. Radiation therapy successfully supplements surgical excision, presumably by destruction of multicentric foci of occult malignancy that probably lead to recurrence.[32] Patients with subareolar lesions should not be eliminated as candidates for breast conservation but will require loss of the nipple-areolar complex to achieve an adequate lumpectomy.[16] Because obtaining clear margins is probably the most critical factor in decreasing the risk of local recurrence, the suspicion of diffuse multifocal or multicentric disease may warrant mastectomy, as does multiple primary cancers in the same breast and an extensive intraductal component.[33] Relative indications for mastectomy are lymphatic and/or vascular invasion, especially if associated with anaplasia, aneuploidy, or a high S phase (Table 2).

Distant disease still develops in some patients with early breast cancer in spite of surgical and radiation treatments. Chemotherapy and hormone therapy now have active roles in the management of both measurable and occult metastases. Combination chemotherapy is clearly superior to single-agent treatment.[34] Adjuvant chemotherapy is administered when no evidence of metastases is present but the size and biological characteristics of the primary tumor indicate that microscopic systemic spread may have occurred. Until recently, most women given adjuvant chemotherapy had positive axillary nodes but no other apparent disease. In the premenopausal, node-positive population, adjuvant chemotherapy was more effective than hormonal therapy in decreasing the incidence of recurrence. In postmenopausal node-positive women,

TABLE 2.
Indications for Mastectomy for Stage I Breast Cancer

Diffuse disease, either intraductal or invasive
Multiple primary lesions
Primary greater than 5 cm in size
Inadequate cosmesis after local excision
Collagen vascular disease
Patient preference
Logistic difficulty in radiation treatment
Recurrence after radiation therapy

however, hormone therapy was as effective as chemotherapy and less morbid.[35, 36] This approach changed in 1988 when adjuvant therapy for even node-negative breast cancer patients was recommended by the National Cancer Institute.[37] Several studies have shown a decreased incidence of recurrence when node-negative women are given adjuvant chemotherapy. In node-negative premenopausal women, this decrease in recurrence rate has translated into a 20% to 30% survival advantage.[38] Postmenopausal node-negative patients may have a similar benefit from adjuvant tamoxifen.

AXILLA

After distant metastases, the most powerful prognostic factor for survival in breast cancer is the presence or absence of lymph node metastases.[39] Variables such as tumor size, ER status, and ploidy may add to the prognostic model, but only after nodal status is considered. The current standard of care includes at least a level I and II lymph node dissection for both modified radical mastectomy and breast conservation procedures in the management of invasive breast carcinoma. Dissecting the axilla in patients with breast cancer provides pivotal information for prognosis and planning of adjuvant therapy and reduces the rate of axillary recurrence.[40]

The hypothesis that microscopic metastases may be present in the regional lymph nodes without systemic disease has led to the rationale for routine axillary lymph node dissection (ALND) in the management of early-stage breast cancers. In support of this hypothesis are a number of studies that demonstrate an increased survival in patients who underwent ALND in addition to mastectomy when compared with simple mastectomy alone.[26, 41-44] Controversy arises over the extent of axillary dissection for staging purposes. The NSABP studies indicate that 10 to 12 axillary lymph nodes are needed to ensure an accurate sampling. The possibility of "skip metastasis" has been evaluated by several authors. When only a level I dissection is done, the probability of positive nodes remaining in levels II and III ranges from 2% to 29%. The probability of missed positive nodes in level III after a level I and II dissection is only 1% to 3%.[45]

Axillary lymph node dissection is not without risk, however. Significant morbidity is commonly seen after routine ALND, including postoperative paresthesia and lymphedema of the arm, postmastectomy pain syndrome, axillary seroma, lymphocele, infection, and skin necrosis.[46] Dissection of the axilla also requires general anesthesia, usually hospital admission, and arrangements for nursing and drain care.

A number of strategies have been evaluated in identifying those breast cancer patients who would profit most from ALND, thereby sparing morbidity for women with negative nodes. Clinical examination by palpation of the axilla is unfortunately inaccurate at best, with false negative rates of 30% to 40% and false positive results as high as 67%.[45] Noninvasive techniques such as mammography, US, CT, or MRI do not reliably predict lymph node involvement in breast cancer. Radionuclide and positron emission tomographic scans are similarly disappointing. When blind random biopsy of axillary lymph nodes is performed, the false negative rate is about 40%.[45]

Some authors have questioned the need for ALND because most patients with invasive breast cancers today are treated with some form of adjuvant therapy regardless of their lymph node status. Thus the current challenge is to identify patients with early breast cancer who might benefit from adjuvant therapy and distinguish them from patients with in situ or minimal carcinomas that can be controlled by surgical excision and radiotherapy alone.

Recently, a sentinel lymph node mapping technique has been described for the management of intermediate-stage melanoma.[47] In this technique, blue dye is injected intradermally at the melanoma site and is used to trace the drainage basin of that skin segment. The sentinel lymph node is the node that receives primary lymphatic drainage of the melanoma site. Sentinel lymph node mapping has high predictive value for metastatic melanoma, and a similar technique has now been used to evaluate the lymph node status of early-stage breast cancer.[48–50] Preliminary results suggest that a sentinel lymph node can be demonstrated in breast cancer when the peritumor tissue or biopsy site is injected with blue dye or radiotracer and followed into the axilla.

Several features of melanoma sentinel node mapping may be applicable to lymphatic mapping in breast cancer. First, melanoma metastatic to the sentinel lymph node was an indicator of more extensive disease within the lymphatic basin.[48] On the other hand, a negative sentinel lymph node was highly predictive of a lymphatic basin free of disease. In contrast to the random biopsy technique, evidence of skip metastases is found less than 1% of the time. Location of the sentinel lymph node may vary in patients even when tumors are in the same quadrant of the breast. The sentinel lymph node is not necessarily the node closest to the site, which may explain the finding of "skip metastases" in breast cancer.[51]

Recent evidence demonstrates a direct correlation between tumor size and axillary lymph node involvement in patients with carcinomas of the breast (Table 3). In a study of 259 patients, T_{1a} tumors (5 mm or less) were associated with a 10% incidence of positive nodes, T_{1b} tumors (5 to 10 mm) with a 15% incidence, and T_{1c}

TABLE 3.
Predictors of Lymph Node Metastases in Patients With T_1 Carcinoma of the Breast

Predictor	*P* Value
Tumor size	0.0001
ER/PR status	1.000
S phase	0.293
Ploidy	1.000
Age, yr	0.370
Histology	0.077
Presence of DCIS	0.156

Abbreviations: ER, estrogen receptor; *PR,* progesterone receptor; *DCIS,* ductal carcinoma in situ. (Adapted from Giuliano AE, Barth AM, Spirack B, et al: Incidence and predictors of axillary metastases in T_1 carcinoma of the breast. *J Am Coll Surg* 183:185–189, 1996. By permission of the *Journal of the American College of Surgeons.*)

TABLE 4.
Lymph Node Involvement as a Function
of Tumor Size

Tumor Size, mm	Lymph Node–Positive Patients	Percent
≤5	2/20	10
5–10	9/68	13
10–20	51/171	30
≤10	11/88	13
>10	51/171	30

(Adapted from Giuliano AE, Barth AM, Spirack B, et al: Incidence and predictors of axillary metastases in T_1 carcinoma of the breast. *J Am Coll Surg* 183:185–189, 1996. By permission of the *Journal of the American College of Surgeons*.)

tumors (10 to 20 mm) with a 30% incidence of axillary metastasis (Table 4). Further, if the sentinel node contained no tumor, then 98% of the patients were tumor free when the rest of the nodes from ALND were examined.[52, 53]

Data from sentinel lymph node mapping studies demonstrate two very important findings for future management of early breast cancer. First, axillary lymph node metastases are present even in very small cancers—15% in tumors under 1 cm.[54–59] Second, most patients (85%) may be spared the morbidity of ALND if the sentinel lymph node is negative. The true incidence of node metastases in small breast cancers may turn out to be somewhat higher when small numbers of nodes (one or two) are subjected to serial sectioning or immunohistochemical staining rather than examination of single sections of many nodes in an ALND sample. These node-positive women can then be selected for adjuvant therapy. Sentinel node biopsy enhanced by radiochemical or immunochemical staining to increase accuracy may eventually replace routine ALND in the management of early-stage breast cancers. Those investigators most familiar with sentinel lymph node biopsy point out the steep learning curve associated with this technique. Classic axillary dissection should not be abandoned until experience in multiple institutions has proved the efficacy of the technique and the surgeon has developed competency with it.

REFERENCES

1. Henderson IC: Risk factors for breast cancer development. *Cancer* 71:2127S, 1993.
2. Gallagher HS, Martin JE: An orientation to the concept of minimal breast cancer. *Cancer* 28:1505–1507, 1971.
3. Frazier TG, Copeland EM, Gallagher HS, et al: Prognosis and treatment in minimal breast cancer. *Am J Surg* 133:697–701, 1977.
4. Frykberg ER, Bland KI, Copeland EM: The detection and treatment of early breast cancer, in Thompkins RK (ed): *Advances in Surgery,* vol 23. St Louis, Mosby, 1990, pp 285–301.
5. Hartmann WJ: Minimal breast cancer: An update. *Cancer* 53:681–684, 1984.
6. Rosen PP, Saigo PE, Braun DW, et al: Predictors of recurrence in stage I ($T_1N_0M_0$) breast carcinoma. *Ann Surg* 193:15–25, 1981.
7. Page DL, Jensen RA: Evaluation and management of high risk and premalignant lesions of the breast. *World J Surg* 18:32, 1994.
8. Frykberg ER, Bland KI: Management of in situ and minimally invasive breast carcinoma. *World J Surg* 18:45, 1994.
9. Frykberg ER, Santiago F, Betsill WL Jr, et al: Lobular carcinoma in situ of the breast. *Surg Gynecol Obstet* 164:285–301, 1987.
10. Davis N, Baird RM: Breast cancer in association with lobular carcinoma in situ: Clinicopathologic review and treatment recommendation. *Am J Surg* 147:641–645, 1984.
11. Gallagher HS: Minimal breast cancer: Results of treatment and long term follow up, in Feig SA, McLeilard R (eds): *Breast Carcinoma: Current Diagnosis and Treatment.* New York, Mason, 1983, pp 291–294.
12. Hutter RVP: The management of patients with lobular carcinoma in situ of the breast. *Cancer* 53:798–802, 1984.
13. Kinne D: Clinical management of lobular carcinoma in situ, in Harris JR, Hellman S, Henderson IC, et al (eds): *Breast Diseases.* Philadelphia, JB Lippincott, 1991, pp 239–245.
14. Frykberg ER, Ames FC, Bland KI: Current concepts for management of early (in situ and occult invasive) breast carcinoma in Bland KI, Copeland EM (eds): *The Breast: Comprehensive Management of Benign and Malignant Diseases.* Philadelphia, WB Saunders, 1991, pp 731–751.
15. Narod SA, Feunteum J, Lynch HT, et al: Familial breast-ovarian cancer locus on chromosome 17q21–q23. *Lancet* 338:82–89, 1991.
16. Morrow M: Precancerous breast lesions: Implications for breast cancer prevention trials. *Int J Radiat Oncol Biol Phys* 23:1071–1078, 1992.
17. Radford DM, Cromack DT, Troop BR, et al: Pathology and treatment of impalpable breast lesions. *Am J Surg* 164:427–432, 1992.
18. Westbrook FC, Gallagher HS: Intraductal carcinoma of the breast: A comparative study. *Am J Surg* 130:667–670, 1975.
19. Fisher ER: Prognostic and therapeutic significance of pathological features of breast cancer. *Natl Cancer Inst Monogr* 1:29, 1986.

20. Laigos MD, Mangolin FR, Westdahl PR, et al: Mammographically detected duct carcinoma in situ: Frequency of local recurrence following tylectomy and prognostic effect of nuclear grade or local recurrence. *Cancer* 63:618–623, 1989.
21. Laigos MD, Westdahl PR, Margolin FR, et al: Duct carcinoma in situ: Relationship of extent of non-invasive disease to the frequency of occult invasion, multicentricity lymph node metastases and short term treatment failures. *Cancer* 50:1309–1314, 1982.
22. Silverstein MJ, Waisman JR, Gamagami P, et al: Intraductal carcinoma of the breast (208 cases): Clinical factors influencing treatment choice. *Cancer* 55:102–108, 1990.
23. Fisher B, Constantino J, Redmond C, et al: Lumpectomy compared with lumpectomy and radiation therapy for the treatment of intraductal breast cancer. *N Engl J Med* 328:1581–1584, 1993.
24. Lichter AS, Lippman ME, Danforth DN, et al: Mastectomy versus breast-conserving therapy in the treatment of stage I and II carcinoma of the breast. *J Clin Oncol* 10:976–982, 1992.
25. Copeland EM III: Malignant breast disease, in Levine BA, Copeland EM, Howard RJ, et al (eds): *Current Practice of Breast Skin and Soft Tissue Surgery.* New York, Churchill Livingstone, 1994, pp 2–42.
26. Cabones PA, Salmon RJ, Vilcoy JR, et al: Value of axillary dissection in addition to lumpectomy and radiotherapy in early breast cancer. *Lancet* 339:1245–1248, 1992.
27. Veronesill U, Barfi A, DelVecchio M, et al: Comparison of Halstead mastectomy with quadrantectomy, axillary dissection and radiotherapy in early breast cancer: Long term results. *Eur J Cancer Clin Oncol* 22:1085–1095, 1986.
28. Fisher B, Bauer M, Margolese R, et al: Five-year results of a randomized clinical trial comparing total mastectomy and segmental mastectomy with or without radiation in the treatment of breast cancer. *N Engl J Med* 312:665–671, 1985.
29. Fisher B, Redmond C, Poisson R, et al: Eight year results of a randomized clinical trial comparing total mastectomy and lumpectomy with or without radiation in the treatment of breast cancer. *N Engl J Med* 320:822–825, 1989.
30. Contesso JC, Delance J, Mouriesse H, et al: Correlation between hormone receptors and histologic characters in human breast tumors. *Pathol Biol* 31:747–754, 1983.
31. Rosis DF, Bell DA, Flotle TJ, et al: Pathologic predictors of recurrence in stage I ($T_1N_0M_0$) breast cancer. *Am J Clin Pathol* 78:817–822, 1982.
32. Recht A, Danoff BS, Solin LJ, et al: Intraductal carcinoma of the breast: Results of treatment with excisional biopsy and radiation. *J Clin Oncol* 3:1339–1343, 1985.
33. Holland R, Connolly JL, Gelman R, et al: The presence of an extensive intraductal component following a limited excision correlates with prominent residual disease in the remainder of the breast. *J Clin Oncol* 8:113–115, 1990.

34. Fisher B, Redmond C, Fisher E, et al: Systemic adjuvant therapy in treatment of primary operable breast cancer: NSABP experience. *Monogr Natl Cancer Inst* 1:35–51, 1986.
35. Consensus conference: Adjuvant chemotherapy for breast cancer. *JAMA* 254:3461–3472, 1985.
36. Fisher B, Constantino J, Redmond C, et al: A randomized trial evaluating tamoxifen in the treatment of patients with node negative breast cancer who have estrogen receptor positive tumors. *N Engl J Med* 320:473–486, 1989.
37. Clinical Alert from the National Cancer Institute, May 16, 1988.
38. Early Breast Cancer Trialists Collaborative Group: Systemic treatment of early breast cancer by hormonal, cytotoxic, or immune therapy: 133 randomized trials involving 31,000 recurrences and 24,000 deaths among 75,000 women. *Lancet* 339:71–85, 1992.
39. Lin PP, Allison DC, Wainstock J, et al: Impact of axillary lymph node dissection on the therapy of breast cancer patients. *J Clin Oncol* 11:1536–1544, 1993.
40. Henderson IC, Canellos GP: Cancer of the breast, the last decade. *N Engl J Med* 202:17–25, 1980.
41. Moffat FL, Senofsky GM, Davis K, et al: Axillary node dissection for early breast cancer: Some is good but all is better. *J Surg Oncol* 51:8–13, 1992.
42. Siegel BM, Maysel KA, Love SM: Level I and II axillary dissection in the treatment of early stage breast cancer. *Arch Surg* 125:1144–1147, 1990.
43. Silverstein MJ, Rosser RJ, Gierson ED, et al: Axillary lymph node dissection for intraductal carcinoma: Is it indicated? *Cancer* 59:1819–1824, 1987.
44. Harris JR, Osteen RT: Patients with early breast cancer benefit from effective axillary treatment. *Breast Cancer Res Treat* 5:17–21, 1985.
45. Davies G, Millis R, Hayward J: Assessment of axillary lymph node status. *Ann Surg* 192:148–151, 1980.
46. Larson D, Weinstein M, Goldberg I, et al: Edema of the arm as a function of the extent of axillary surgery in patients with stage I–II carcinoma of the breast treated with primary radiotherapy. *Int J Radiat Oncol Biol Phys* 12:1572–1582, 1986.
47. Morton DL, Wer DR, Wong JH, et al: Technical details of intraoperative lymphatic mapping for early stage melanoma. *Arch Surg* 127:392–399, 1992.
48. Reintgen DS, Cruse CW, Berman C, et al: An orderly progression of melanoma nodal metastases. *Ann Surg* 220:759–767, 1994.
49. Krag DN, Miegis SJ, Weaver DL, et al: Minimal access surgery for staging of malignant melanoma. *Arch Surg* 130:654–658, 1995.
50. Guiliano AE, Kingan DM, Guenther MD, et al: Lymphatic mapping and sentinel lymphadenectomy for breast cancer. *Ann Surg* 220:391–401, 1994.

51. Carter CL, Allen C, Henson D: Relation of tumor size, lymph node status, and survival in 24,740 breast cancer cases. *Cancer* 63:181–187, 1989.
52. Guiliano AE, Barth AM, Spivack B, et al: Incidence and predictors of axillary metastases in T$_1$ carcinoma of the breast. *J Am Coll Surg* 183:185–189, 1986.
53. Guiliano AE: Sentinel lymphadenectomy: A new axillary staging procedure for primary breast carcinoma. *Breast Dis* 7:16–17, 1996.
54. Walls L, Boggis CRM, Wilson M, et al: Treatment of the axilla in patients with screen detected breast cancer. *Br J Surg* 80:436, 1993.
55. Rosen PP, Grosten S: Factors influencing survival and prognosis in early breast carcinoma. *Surg Clin North Am* 70:937–960, 1990.
56. Chada M, Chjabon AB, Friedman P, et al: Predictors of axillary lymph node metastases in patients with T$_1$ breast cancer. *Cancer* 73:350–353, 1994.
57. Silverstein MJ, Gierson ED, Waisman JR, et al: Axillary lymph node dissection for T$_{1a}$ breast carcinoma: Is it indicated? *Cancer* 73:664–667, 1994.
58. Cady B: The need to reexamine axillary lymph node dissection in invasive breast cancer. *Cancer* 73:505–508, 1994.
59. Hainsworth PJ, Tjardra JJ, Stillwell RG, et al: Detection and significance of occult metastases in node-negative breast cancer. *Br J Surg* 80:459–463, 1993.

CHAPTER 3

Can an Enteral Diet Decrease Sepsis After Trauma?

Brock K. King, M.D.

Resident in Surgery and Nutrition Research, The University of Tennessee, Memphis, Tennessee

Kenneth A. Kudsk, M.D.

Professor of Surgery, Director of Surgical Research, The University of Tennessee, Memphis, Tennessee

I nfection and sepsis account for the majority of late deaths after trauma. Challenged with multiple violations of natural host defenses, trauma patients must mount an immunologic response with humoral and cellular immunity, heal wounds induced by injury and/or therapy, and generate nutrient substrates to support cellular function. Over the last century, principles of tissue management, fluid and electrolyte therapy, blood transfusions, ventilator management, and the selective of antibiotic therapy have been refined. One of the most recent principles being adapted into the management of trauma patients is the use of early enteral nutrition to augment host defenses.

Traumatic injury generates a hypercatabolic and hypermetabolic state that, if unchecked, produces depletion of protein and fat stores.[1, 2] As the protein compartment decreases, the vigor to withstand subsequent challenges appears to be impaired, and susceptibility to complications and mortality increase as significant protein malnutrition develops. Fortunately, the majority of trauma patients are usually well nourished and can withstand these metabolic challenges at least over the short term. In the first 10 days after injury, these patients have an increased risk of pneumonia and intra-abdominal abscess, which can lead to a more chronic state of malnutrition and subsequent wound problems. Because most infections would seem to occur before the onset of "malnutrition," other factors than just protein-calorie deficits are implicated. Enteral feeding appears to reduce the risk of these early infections through mechanisms that are just now being defined.

THE GASTROINTESTINAL TRACT

A common factor among the plethora of traumatic injuries has been the temporary loss of gastrointestinal function secondary to injury, atony, and sepsis. The splanchnic bed appears to be an intricate regulator of cytokine response, protein production, and the immunologic barrier in the postinjury state of hypercatabolism and metabolism. Gastrointestinal tract "starvation" in animal models produces mucosal atrophy,[3] bacterial overgrowth, increased intestinal permeability,[4] loss of mucosal defenses against translocation of bacteria or toxins,[5, 6] and atrophy of the gut-associated lymphoid tissue.[7] It has been well demonstrated that injury is associated with an increase in permeability of the gut in many patients[8–10] and translocation of bacteria under certain circumstances.[11] Although these observations may not be related to the development of pneumonia or intra-abdominal abscess, it is becoming increasingly clear that the early delivery of nutrients via the gastrointestinal tract significantly reduces the incidence of extraintestinal infections when compared with either parenteral nutrition or nothing but IV dextrose (Table 1).[12–19] Nutrition support begins at the operating table, and given a situation in which septic complications are likely to develop, it is becoming a basic principle that access into the small intestine be obtained beyond the ligament of Treitz to gain these benefits of enteral nutrition.

CLINICAL STUDIES IN BLUNT AND PENETRATING TRAUMA

SUPPORTIVE STUDIES OF ENTERAL NUTRITION

The first experimental evidence that the route of nutrition was important in maintaining host defense came from the laboratory of Dr. Sheldon in the early 1980s. In models of malnourished[20] and well-nourished animals[21] randomized to either IV total parenteral nutrition (TPN) or enteral TPN, mortality was significantly reduced after a septic challenge in animals fed via the gastrointestinal tract. Moore and Jones[12] first confirmed this observation in a randomized, prospective study of 75 trauma patients. At the time of surgery, patients at increased risk of infectious complications were identified by the Abdominal Trauma Index (ATI).[22] The ATI correlates the number of intra-abdominal injuries and the severity of these individual injuries with the subsequent development of sep-

TABLE 1.
Nutritional Supplementation in Blunt and Penetrating Trauma

Author	Route/Timing	Patient Characteristics	Findings	Comments
Moore,[12] 1986	Early enteral vs. IV fluids; delayed TPN if necessary	ATI, 16–40	Significantly less abscess formation in early enteral group	Late group fasted Exclusion of severely injured patients Less septic morbidity with early enteral feeds
Adams[13] 1986	TPN vs. enteral	Injury to 2 or more body systems	No significant difference in pneumonia or abscess between groups	Enteral group had more head and severe chest injuries, pelvic fractures, and soft tissue injuries Calorie/nitrogen ratio different between groups
Moore,[14] 1989	Early TPN vs. early enteral	ATI >15 < 40 Exclusion for excessive blood loss/transfusions and early reoperations Severe pelvic fractures	Significantly less pneumonia and abscess formation in early enteral group	Exclusion of most severely injured patients Less septic morbidity with enteral feeds
Kudsk,[15] 1992	Early TPN vs. early enteral	ATI, 15 or greater No exclusion for ATI of >40, excessive blood loss/transfusion, or early reoperation	Significantly fewer pneumonias, abscesses, line sepsis, infections per patient, infections per infected patient in early enteral group	Inclusion of most severely injured patients Benefits regarding sepsis in severely injured patients only Less septic morbidity with early enteral feeds

(continued)

TABLE 1. (continued)

Author	Route/Timing	Patient Characteristics	Findings	Comments
Moore,[16] 1992	Early TPN vs. early enteral	Same as Moore, 1989 General surgical and trauma patients	Significantly fewer pneumonias and abscesses in enteral group	Meta-analysis of multiple individual studies Exclusion of most severely injured patients Less septic morbidity with early enteral feeds
Eyer,[17] 1993	Early enteral vs. late enteral	ISS, >13	Total infections significantly greater in early group	Total infections include UTIs, sinusitis, eye infection, and wound infection Diets and prescriptions changed during study
Moore,[18] 1994	Early enteral with immune-enhancing formula vs. early enteral with standard formula	ATI, 18–40 ISS, 16–45 GCS, <8 *Excluded:* Pelvic fracture requiring >6 U of blood, 24-hr transfusion requirement of >20 U of blood, or planned early reoperation	Significantly higher levels of T lymphocytes in immune-enhancing group Significantly fewer abscesses in immune-enhancing group	Standard diet contained much less nitrogen Less septic morbidity with early immune-enhancing enteral feeds

(continued)

TABLE 1. (continued)

Author	Route/Timing	Patient Characteristics	Findings	Comments
Kudsk,[19] 1996	Early enteral with immune-enhancing formula vs. early enteral with standard formula vs. unfed group (no enteral access)	ATI, >25/ISS, >20	Significantly fewer abscesses in immune-enhancing than standard enteral and unfed groups Required significantly fewer days of antibiotics and significantly fewer days of hospitalization in immune-enhancing group as compared with standard enteral and control group	Unfed group had significantly more colon injuries and less blood loss than other groups Unfed patients consistently had longest hospital stay, most antibiotic days, and highest infection rate Complications after severe colon injuries fewer with immune-enhancing diet Less septic morbidity with early immune-enhancing enteral feeds

Abbreviations: TPN, total parenteral nutrition; *ATI,* Abdominal Trauma Index; *ISS,* Injury Severity Score; *UTI,* urinary tract infection; *GCS,* Glasgow Coma Scale score.

sis. Because their previous work[23] demonstrated that patients with an ATI greater than 40 had increased gastrointestinal intolerance to rapid progression of enteral feeding—and the desire to reach calculated nutrient goals within 72 hours—selection of patients was limited to those with an ATI between 16 and 40. Patients were randomized at surgery to receive either an elemental diet by needle catheter jejunostomy placed at that surgery or no supplemental nutrition postoperatively until the fifth postoperative day and then only if necessary. Approximately 25% of the patients required IV nutrition at that time. Both groups were similar in ATI, mechanism of injury, baseline acute-phase proteins, nutritional parameters, and injuries. Although the authors did notice a significantly improved nitrogen balance in the early-fed group, the most significant finding was a reduction in intra-abdominal abscesses in the early-fed group as compared with the fasted patients.

Subsequently, the Denver group conducted a similar study but used the same entry criteria as the first study to randomize patients to either early enteral feeding with a defined formula diet or early IV nutrition.[14] In addition to limitation by the ATI, patients were also excluded for total blood loss of more than 25 U in the first 24 hours, repeat laparotomy within the first 72 hours, or severe pelvic fractures requiring more than 5 U of blood. Intravenous nutrition or enteral feedings were begun within 12 hours of surgery. Although no significant differences were noted in age, gender, mechanism of injury, ATI, or baseline nutritional parameters, significantly fewer major infectious complications—in particular, pneumonia—developed in the enteral group than in patients randomized to IV nutrition. Analysis of multiple risk factors for pneumonia identified TPN as the significant risk factor. The authors speculated that bacterial translocation could be responsible for the increase in pneumonia noted in the TPN group, consistent with animal work demonstrating that IV nutrition significantly increases bacterial translocation to mesenteric lymph nodes.

Our group also investigated the effect of nutrient support on the recovery of 98 blunt and penetrating trauma patients in a prospective, randomized study.[15] All patients entered in the study had intra-abdominal injuries requiring laparotomy and an ATI of 15 or greater, but patients were not excluded because of early relaparotomy, an ATI greater than 40, pelvic fractures with blood loss, or more than 25 U of blood lost during the first 24 hours. All patients had enteral access to the small bowel with a jejunostomy but were subsequently randomized to receive either enteral feeding with a defined formula diet or IV feeding via central venous catheters by the nutrition support service. Enteral and IV feedings were nutritionally equivalent and begun within 24 hours of injury.

No significant differences were found between groups with respect to age, ATI, Injury Severity Score (ISS), mechanism of injury, blood requirements, or nitrogen balance. Patients randomized to IV nutrition received significantly more calories and protein per kilogram per day than did patients randomized to enteral feeding, thus reflecting the need for slower progression of enteral feeding in trauma patients. Despite this lower nutritional intake, enteral patients had a significantly lower incidence of pneumonia, intra-abdominal abscess, and line sepsis than did patients randomized to parenteral nutrition, as well as significantly fewer infections per patient and fewer infections per infected patient.

The severity of injury was an important cofactor, with no significant differences between groups in patients with an ATI of 24 or less or an ISS less than 20. All benefits were noted in the most severely injured patients, i.e., those with an ISS greater than 20 or an ATI greater than 24 or a subgroup of patients with both a high ISS and a high ATI. If these subpopulations were randomized to TPN, their risk of significant infection increased by 6.3, 7.3, and 11.3 times, respectively. Although the reduced frequency of infections in enterally fed, blunt trauma patients approached statistical significance, significance was reached in enteral patients sustaining penetrating trauma. After stratification according to individual injuries, enterally fed patients with upper abdominal injuries appeared to benefit the most.

In a meta-analysis of combined data from eight prospective, randomized trials of early enteral and parenteral feeding of high-risk surgical patients, Moore et al. noted significantly fewer septic complications in patients randomized to early enteral feeding with a defined formula diet than in patients randomized to parenteral nutrition.[16] Although the most dramatic improvement was noted in patients sustaining blunt or penetrating trauma, septic complications tended to also be lower in patients undergoing general surgical procedures such as gastrectomy, complex biliary procedures, pancreatectomies, and colectomies. In this meta-analysis, the authors also noted that enteral feeding was more challenging than parenteral feeding. Enterally fed patients experienced significantly more abdominal distension and diarrhea than did IV-fed patients, which somewhat limited the advancement of patients on an enteral diet. However, it was clear that although less nutrition was delivered by the gastrointestinal tract, patients sustained significantly fewer pneumonias and intra-abdominal abscesses when fed by this route.

CONFLICTING STUDIES

Not all authors have noted significant improvements with enteral feeding. In one of the earliest studies comparing enteral with parenteral nutrition, Adams et al.[13] randomized trauma patients with major injuries to two or more body systems to either IV TPN or enteral nutrition via needle catheter jejunostomy. Nutrition was advanced as tolerated in both groups. Although there were no significant differences in age, ISS, or nutritional status as measured by the Prognostic Nutritional Index, they noted a similar rate of infectious complications—in particular, pneumonia—between the two groups and observed that it was more difficult to provide adequate nutrition via the gastrointestinal tract, usually because repeated operations necessitated discontinuation of tube feedings before and during the procedures.

Although this study tends to be at odds with the studies noted earlier, several problems in design, patient population, and diagnosis of infectious complications must be addressed. When compared with the TPN group, enteral patients sustained twice as many head injuries, three times as many severe chest injuries, and three times as many pelvic fractures, as well as six times as many major soft tissue injuries. In particular, the increased incidence of severe chest injuries in the enteral group rendered the diagnosis of pneumonia questionable because at the time of publication, infectious studies commonly used fever, leukocytosis, and a new or changing radiographic infiltrate as the primary criteria to diagnose pneumonia. With these criteria, pneumonia is overdiagnosed in two thirds to three quarters of patients.[24] With the increased incidence of thoracic injury in the enterally fed group, one must be suspicious that pulmonary contusions, atelectasis, and pleural effusions might have been misdiagnosed as pneumonia in many of these patients. In addition, this study was never designed to evaluate the interaction between route of nutrition and infectious outcome. The enteral and parenteral nutrients were not well matched from the onset. The IV nutritional formula had a calorie:nitrogen ratio of 157:1, whereas enteral patients received a nutrient solution with a calorie:nitrogen ratio of 170:1. After the study had been partially completed, the enteral formula was changed to a solution containing a calorie:nitrogen ratio of 116:1. Thus although the authors concluded that enteral feeding did not appear to provide any additional significant benefit when compared with IV nutrition, the groups did not appear to be well matched by injury or nutritional formula, the nutrient formula was altered significantly during the study, and the diagnosis of infectious complications appeared to be unreliable.

A second study questioning the benefits of enteral feeding was conducted by Eyer et al.,[17] who randomized 52 patients admitted to the ICU with an ISS greater than 13 to either earlier (<24 hours) or late (>72 hours) enteral feeding. Patients with acute spinal cord injuries were excluded from this study, whereas patients with closed-head injury were not. In an evaluation of the hospital course of these patients, total infectious complications, ranging from pneumonia to an eye infection, were significantly greater in the group randomized to early enteral feeding, with significantly more pneumonias and urinary tract infections in the early-fed group.

Although this study would also tend to run counter to the Denver and Tennessee studies, critical data were not provided to assess the patient populations. Even though the ISS scores were similar between the two groups, it is unclear what injuries were sustained by the patients in the two patient populations. There appeared to be more severe chest injuries in the blunt trauma patients randomized to early enteral nutrition because patients in this group had significantly more severe lung injury as measured by depressed Pao_2/Fio_2 ratios. Eleven of 19 patients in the early group had a Pao_2/Fio_2 ratio of less than 150, whereas only 4 of 19 patients reflected such severe ventilation-perfusion mismatch. Because pneumonia was again diagnosed by fever, leukocytosis, and new or changing infiltrates on the chest radiograph, as well as "significant growth on sputum cultures," one would suspect an overdiagnosis of pneumonia. If one assumes all pneumonias to be real, however, it could be explained by the increased chest trauma in the early-fed group. The urinary tract, wound, sinus, and eye infections noted to be frequent in the enteral group are unlikely to be affected by the route of nutrition support but rather by Foley catheter placement, transnasal tubes, and inappropriate closure of contaminated wounds. Unfortunately, data are unavailable in the manuscript to analyze these important issues.

SPECIALTY DIETS

Over the past two decades there has been increased interest in the use of specific nutrients to upregulate the immune system and eliminate the well-recognized immunosuppression after severe trauma.[25] Nutrients such as glutamine, arginine, ω-3 fatty acids, nucleotides, and β-carotene have all been demonstrated in experimental models to be less immunosuppressive, to be immunostimulatory, or to serve as specific fuels for lymphocytes, macrophages, and the gastrointestinal mucosa.[26–29] Currently, two randomized, prospective studies are evaluating these formulas in blunt and penetrating trauma patients.[18, 19]

Moore et al.[18] randomized patients sustaining major chest and abdominal trauma to receive enteral nutrition with either an immune-enhancing diet containing glutamine, arginine, ω-3 fatty acids, and nucleotides or a defined formula diet that they had used in earlier studies. In the design of this study, patients with an ATI between 18 and 40 or an ISS between 16 and 45 were considered eligible unless they had a head injury with a Glasgow Coma Scale (GCS) score less than 8, a pelvic fracture requiring more than 6 U of blood in the first 12 hours, a 24-hour transfusion requirement of more than 20 U of blood, or a planned repeat laparotomy within 72 hours. Of the 98 evaluable patients, both groups had comparable age, weight, and GCS, ISS, and ATI values and were well matched for chest and intra-abdominal injuries.

The two enteral formulas were not well matched, however, for nitrogen load. Many of the early studies using these immune-enhancing diets considered the supplemental amino acids to be pharmacologic agents rather than specific nutrients and did not include the arginine and/or glutamine within the overall nitrogen calculation.[30–32] In this study, as in those, nitrogen administration to the patients receiving the immune-enhancing diet was significantly higher (approximately double in this study), although total calories per kilogram were very similar.

After 7 days of feeding, patients receiving the immune-enhancing diet had significant improvement in T-lymphocyte and T-helper cell numbers, as well as total lymphocyte count. More importantly, the patients receiving the immune-enhancing diet had significantly fewer intra-abdominal abscesses and less multiple organ dysfunction than did groups receiving the hyponitrogenous control diet. Ventilator days, ICU days, and hospital days were consistently fewer in the individuals randomized to the immune-enhancing diet but failed to reach statistical significance. Consistent with early enteral studies, the incidence of pneumonia was quite low in both enterally fed groups (8%).

Because of concern over the nonisonitrogenous nature of the control diet (and the observation in burn patients that a protein-supplemented diet improved morbidity and mortality rates in pediatric burn patients), severely injured patients at our institution with early enteral access at the time of initial laparotomy for trauma were randomized to either the immune-enhancing diet containing glutamine, arginine, ω-3 fatty acids, and nucleotides or an isonitrogenous/isocaloric diet.[19] Because of our earlier work that showed benefits of nutrition only in the most severely injured patients, only patients with an ATI greater than 25 and/or an ISS greater than 20 were entered into the study. In addition, because of criticism that most of the nutritional studies do not have an unfed "placebo" control population,[33] we prospectively analyzed the postoperative course of patients eligible for the study by severity of injury but in whom enteral access had not been obtained. There were no significant differences in ATI, GCS, or ISS among the three groups; however, several other differences were noted. Patients in the prospective, unfed group sustained significantly more colon injuries but had significantly less blood loss—two important predictors of infectious complications—than did patients who received access beyond the ligament of Treitz. Seven of the 13 unfed control patients with a colon injury were considered to have very severe injuries (grade 4 or grade 5), and 5 of the 6 patients randomized to the immune-enhancing diet sustained severe colon injuries, which allowed these two groups to be compared for abscess formation after severe colon injury.

No significant differences were found in nitrogen intake, caloric intake, or days of diet in the two fed groups, but significant differences were noted in outcome. Intra-abdominal abscesses and major septic complications were significantly less frequent in the group receiving an immune-enhancing diet than in either the isonitrogenous control group or the unfed placebo population. Although there were no significant differences in prophylactic or empirical antibiotic use between the three groups, patients randomized to the immune-enhancing diet required significantly fewer days of therapeutic antibiotics than did either the fed or nonfed control group. Hospital stay was significantly shorter in the group that received an immune-enhancing diet. Consistently, the unfed population sustained the highest incidence of abscess, pneumonia, and bacteremia; received the most therapeutic antibiotics; and had the highest hospital charges.

SUMMARY

When all the studies of blunt and penetrating trauma are considered, it appears that delivery of nutrients via the gastrointestinal tract significantly reduces infectious complications when compared with IV nutrition or dextrose solutions alone.[12, 14–16] When enteral access has been obtained in severely injured patients, an immune-enhancing diet appears to give additional benefits not found with standard enteral formulas.[18, 19] The severity of injury plays an important role because severely injured trauma patients will gain the most benefit from nutrition support. These, of course, are the patients who spend prolonged periods of time in ICU, and use significant amounts of hospital resources.

These data provide compelling evidence that the gastrointestinal tract plays an important role in the reduction of infectious complications and that obtaining access beyond the ligament of Treitz, either by jejunostomy, transgastric jejunostomy, or nasoenteric tube at the time of surgery, will allow the delivery of nutrients directly into the small intestine. Access beyond the ligament of Treitz is important because intragastric feeding is usually unsuccessful in these patients because of associated gastroparesis present for at least the first 5 postinjury days or longer if septic complications subsequently develop.[34]

THERMAL TRAUMA

ENTERAL VS. PARENTERAL NUTRITION

Two studies, both from the Shriners Burn Institute in Galveston, Texas, have examined the effect of route of nutrition in severely burned trauma patients (Table 2). In the first study,[35] 28 burn patients were prospectively randomized into groups receiving either IV TPN supplementation or no parenteral supplementation for the first 10 days after the burn injury. In addition, patients from both groups received continuous enteral feeding with a commercial enteral product or milk after the return of bowel function. All patients suffered greater than 50% total burn surface area (TBSA), but there were no differences in age, TBSA, or percentage of third-degree burns between groups. Patients supplemented with TPN received significantly more calories during the first 7 postburn days. Natural killer cell function was higher in TPN-supplemented patients, but this failed to reach statistical significance. OKT4/OKT8 ratios were significantly lower in the IV-supplemented group through postburn day 10. Although no correlations were noted between these immunologic functions and septic morbidity, the data suggested increased immunologic suppression in association with TPN.

In a follow-up, prospective study[36] of 39 burn patients with greater than 50% TBSA from the same institution, patients were randomized to receive either parenteral nutrition supplementation in addition to enteral feedings or enteral feedings alone. Enteral feedings were started after the return of postburn bowel function. There were no significant differences in age, TBSA, third-degree burn, or inhalation injuries between the two groups. Mortality was significantly higher in the parenterally supplemented group than

TABLE 2.
Nutritional Supplementation in Thermal Trauma

Author	Route/Timing	Patient Characteristics	Findings	Comments
Herndon,[35] 1987	TPN supplementation to enteral vs. no TPN supplementation to enteral	>50% TBSA	OKT4/OKT8 ratio significantly depressed in TPN group No difference in mortality between groups	Low number of study patients Septic morbidity not observed
Herndon,[36] 1989	Same as 1987	Same as 1987	OKT4/OKT8 ratio significantly depressed in TPN-supplemented group Mortality significantly higher in TPN-supplemented group	Suggests relationship between parenteral nutrition, immune dysfunction, and increased mortality Septic morbidity not observed
Chiarelli,[37] 1990	Early enteral vs. late enteral	No inhalation injuries TBSA, 25%–60%	Urinary catecholamine levels significantly higher in late group Insulin levels significantly higher in early group Glucagon levels significantly lower in early group	Early enteral feedings blunt hypercatabolism and hypermetabolism in burn patients by blunting catecholamine stress response

(continued)

TABLE 2. (continued)

Author	Route/Timing	Patient Characteristics	Findings	Comments
Alexander,[38] 1980	Standard enteral vs. protein-supplemented standard enteral	TBSA, 60%	Significantly fewer bacteremic days and higher survival in protein-supplemented group	Standard-diet group received significantly more TPN supplementation
Gottschlich,[39] 1990	Immune-enhanced diet vs. standard enteral diet	Pediatric burns	Significantly fewer wound infections in immune-enhanced diet group Significantly reduced hospital stay per percent body burn in immune-enhanced diet group	Diets with ω-3 fatty acids and arginine supplements improve septic morbidity
Saffle,[40] 1996	Immune-enhanced diet vs. standard enteral diet	Adult burns	No significant differences in hospital stay or wound infections	Standard enteral diet was high in protein, possibly blunting differences between groups

Abbreviations: TPN, total parenteral nutrition; *TBSA,* total burn surface area.

the enterally fed group, and survivors from either the enteral or the parenteral groups received significantly more enteral calories than did nonsurvivors. Although both groups had decreases in natural killer cell activity when compared with controls throughout the experiment, the CD4/CD8 ratio remained significantly depressed at days 7 and 14 only with parenteral supplementation. Septic morbidity was not defined in this study, but parenteral supplementation was clearly associated with increased mortality. These immunologic data in association with the clinical outcome strongly suggest an association between parenteral nutrition, immune dysfunction, and increased mortality.

TIMING AND PROTEIN CONTENT

Chiarelli et al.[37] investigated the metabolic response of 20 thermally injured patients randomized to receive enteral feedings started immediately after admission to the burn unit or feedings started 48 hours after admission. No patient sustained an inhalation injury, but each had a TBSA between 25% and 60%. Consistent with earlier work showing a blunted hypermetabolic response in burned guinea pigs receiving early enteral nutrition, Chiarelli and associates noted that urinary catecholamines remained within the normal range throughout the 28-day study period with early enteral feeding but were significantly higher in the delayed enteral group by day 12 and fell to normal by day 16. Although no significant differences were noted in blood sugar, the early-fed group had plasma insulin levels that were significantly higher on day 8 and plasma glucagon levels that were significantly lower on days 8, 12, and 20 than did patients fed later. The authors concluded that consistent with experimental laboratory studies, early enteral feeding blunted the hypermetabolic and hypercatabolic response to burn injury by blunting the catecholamine stress response and the elevation in serum glucagon levels. As a result of the depressed catecholamine secretion, insulin was not suppressed in the early-fed group.

After burns, the protein load influences outcome. Alexander et al.[38] first noted this in pediatric burn patients randomized to a protein-supplemented or standard enteral diet. Patients with burns averaging 60% TBSA were randomized to receive either 16% of their calories from protein or 23% of their calories from protein by supplementation with milk whey protein. Although the normal-protein group had higher caloric intake, various parameters of nutritional status, including transferrin, serum protein, serum levels of C3, and IgG, were significantly lower. Most importantly, the protein-supplemented patients sustained significantly fewer bacteremic days and had a higher survival rate than did patients fed the low-protein diet. The single confounding variable in this study, however, is that the patients receiving the low-protein diet received significantly more IV nutritional supplementation than did the patients receiving the high-protein diet, which might explain the improved outcome.

SPECIALTY DIETS

Specialty nutrients have shown clinical benefits in certain burn populations. In a study[39] of pediatric burn victims randomized to a high-protein, ω-3–enriched, low-fat diet with supplemental arginine and cysteine, there were significantly fewer wound infections and a significantly reduced length of stay per percent body burn when compared with patients receiving a standard enteral diet with whey, casein, and soy and with 40% of the fat as corn oil and 10% as soybean oil. A third group received a diet enriched with casein, soybean oil, and medium-chain triglyceride oil. Although there were no significant differences in age, percentage of third-degree burn, number of days of tube feeding, or incidence of inhalation injury, wound infection was significantly lower in patients receiving the ω-3–enriched diet with supplemental arginine. There were also fewer infectious episodes and a lower incidence of pneumonia, which approached statistical significance. In pediatric burn patients, this immune-enhancing formula appeared to be effective. In a recently presented study[40] of *adult* burn patients randomized to receive either a commercial immune-enhancing diet enriched with ω-3 fatty acids, arginine, and RNA or a standard enteral diet, these findings were not substantiated. Although patients greater than 4 years of age were entered into the study, the average age of the patients receiving the immune-enhancing diet was 35 vs. 37 for the standard diet. Total length of stay, length of stay per percent body burn, ventilator days, and hospital charges were very similar. This study, however, compared an immune-enhancing diet with a high-protein enteral diet, which may have blunted differences between the two patient populations.

SUMMARY

Clinical data from burn patients again substantiate that the delivery of nutrients via the gastrointestinal tract appears to provide significant benefit when compared with IV feeding. Enteral feeding must be started early—within 24 hours—to gain the benefit of reduced septic morbidity, a reduction in mortality, and a blunting of the hypermetabolic response. Immune-enhancing diets are effective in pediatric burn patients but have not been shown to provide any additional benefit over a high-protein enteral diet in burned adults.

SEVERE HEAD INJURIES

Data suggesting that enteral feeding improves outcome after closed-head injuries are much less compelling than for blunt or penetrating injuries or burns (Table 3). Rapp et al.[41] at the University of Kentucky examined the effect of route of nutrient administration after severe closed-head injury. Patients were randomized to receive either early IV nutrition or intragastric feeding once gastric atony had resolved, usually 5 to 8 days after injury. Clearly, the enterally fed group was underfed. Of the 18 patients randomized to enteral feeding, all received fewer than 600 calories per day during the first 10 days, and none received more than 1,000 calories per day during the first 14 days. Because no attempt was made to pair-feed, this study essentially compared early IV feeding with fasting for at least the first 4 days. Although there were no significant differences in age, albumin, or GCS score, mortality appeared higher in the group randomized to intragastric feeding, and sepsis complicated the course of approximately 30% of these patients. From the manuscript, it is unclear how many patients randomized to receive TPN became septic.

Because of the reduced morbidity with early IV feeding in this first study, the Kentucky group[42] designed a follow-up study of 51 head-injured patients with an admission GCS score between 4 and 10. The patients were monitored for up to 12 months postinjury and were again randomized to receive either IV TPN within 48 hours of admission or enteral feedings once gastric atony had resolved. There were no significant differences in GCS scores, age, or extracranial injuries between groups, although more enteral patients had respiratory paralysis, exhibited more decorticate or decerebrate activity, and more often had intracranial pressure greater than 20 mm Hg than did the TPN group. Even though none of these differences reached statistical significance, it appeared that the enterally fed patients had worse initial prognostic signs. Despite this, no significant differences between the two groups were found in early or late deaths or septic morbidity such as sepsis, pneumonia, brain abscess, or multiple organ dysfunction. A more favorable CNS outcome was found at 3 months in the group randomized to TPN feeding, although there were no significant differences at 1 year. As in the first study, this investigation compared early IV

TABLE 3.
Nutrition Supplementation in Neurotraumatic Head Injuries

Author	Route/Timing	Patient Characteristics	Findings	Comments
Rapp,[41] 1983	Early TPN vs. late enteral	Intracranial injury only	Mortality significantly higher in enteral group. Nitrogen intake significantly higher in TPN group	Enteral group underfed until bowel function returned. Septic morbidity not clearly defined
Young,[42] 1987	Early TPN vs. late enteral	GCS, 4–10	No significant difference in mortality between groups. No significant difference in septic morbidity between groups. Favorable outcome at 3 mo significantly higher in TPN group. Nitrogen intake significantly higher in TPN group	Enteral group received parenteral supplementation if bowel function had not returned by day 7

(continued)

TABLE 3. (continued)

Author	Route/Timing	Patient Characteristics	Findings	Comments
Grahm,[43] 1989	Early jejunal vs. late gastric	GCS, <10	Total infections significantly lower in early group	Total infections included bronchitis, pneumonia, and ventriculitis Head-injured patients tolerate jejunal feeds Less septic morbidity with early jejunal feeds
Borzotta,[44] 1993	Jejunal vs. TPN	GCS, <8	No significant difference in septic morbidity between groups	Early postpyloric cannulation in enteral group Jejunal feeds associated with improved cognitive recovery

Abbreviations: TPN, total parenteral nutrition; GCS, Glasgow Coma Scale score.

feeding and early starvation with enteral feeding only after gastric atony had resolved. This study demonstrated no significant difference in septic morbidity in patients receiving early IV nutrition and those given delayed enteral feeding.

Two studies have compared early enteral vs. early intravenous and early enteral vs. delayed enteral feeding after severe head injury, but the results of these two studies are conflicting. Grahm et al[43] prospectively randomized 32 patients with head trauma to receive a fluoroscopically placed nasojejunal feeding tube or receive an intragastric feeding after gastric atony had resolved (i.e., initial fasting followed by delayed enteral feeding). Feedings were initiated within 36 hours in the early group. There were no significant differences in age, admission GCS, associated injuries, or nitrogen excretion, but as expected, caloric intake was significantly greater in the early-fed group during the first week. Patients were monitored for the development of bronchitis (positive sputum cultures of pathogenic bacteria with polymorphonucleocytes), pneumonia (bronchitis with infiltrate present on the chest radiograph), and ventriculitis. With these infectious criteria, significantly fewer total infections developed in the early-fed group than in the late-fed group.

The most significant difference between the Grahm study[43] and the Kentucky studies[41, 42] was the use of direct jejunal feeding. Grahm and colleagues bypassed the dysfunctional stomach and provided nutritional support to the small bowel, which maintained normal motility. Although these results would suggest that direct nasojejunal feeding might be beneficial after severe head injury, Borzotta et al.[44] studied 57 patients prospectively randomized to receive TPN or enteral feedings within 72 hours of injury. Although both routes were equally effective in meeting the calculated goals, no difference in infectious complications was detected between groups, which was not consistent with the results of Grahm and associates. Whereas the Kentucky studies demonstrated no difference in infectious complications between delayed enteral feeding and TPN, Grahm's work suggested a reduction in septic complications with direct jejunal feeding when compared with patients who were fasted. This finding, however, was not substantiated in the Borzotta study. As a result of these data, it is has not been the policy at our institution to institute early postpyloric feedings through either endoscopic or fluoroscopic placement of feeding tubes.

SUMMARY OF THE STUDIES

In reviewing all the literature comparing early enteral feeding with early fasting (delayed intragastric feeding) or IV TPN, enteral feeding—usually through direct small-bowel feeding—improves outcome in certain patient populations.[12, 14–16] This is best substantiated in patients sustaining blunt and penetrating trauma, particularly if the patients had a high ATI or high ISS and were at risk of intra-abdominal infections and/or the development of pneumonia.[15] In this situation, early post–ligament of Treitz feeding reduces septic complications. In this most severely injured patient population, the early use of an immune-enhancing diet is even more effective in reducing septic morbidity.[19] In burn patients, a protein-supplemented enteral diet benefits both pediatric[38] and adult burn patients,[40] and results may be further improved in the pediatric population[39] through the use of an immune-enhancing diet. In burned patients, as well as blunt and penetrating trauma patients, a higher complication rate occurs with IV nutrition.[36]

The data are not as clear in patients with severe closed-head injuries. Although one study suggests that direct small-bowel feeding is beneficial,[43] this finding has not been substantiated.[44] The incidence of septic complications after severe head injury is approximately equal in patients fed IV TPN early and patients in whom enteral feeding is delayed until gastric atony resolves.[41, 42]

INDICATIONS FOR DIRECT SMALL-BOWEL CANNULATION

BLUNT AND PENETRATING TRAUMA REQUIRING CELIOTOMY

Patients requiring a celiotomy for trauma with a calculated ATI of 25 or greater or with an ISS greater than 20 should have access obtained beyond the ligament of Treitz.[15] The ATI can be rapidly calculated at the operating table to identify those patients with a high ATI[22] and the gastrointestinal tract cannulated with little additional risk of complications.[45] Isolated injuries to single intra-abdominal organs almost never necessitate cannulation, with several exceptions. Patients with major colon injuries requiring resection with anastomosis or colostomy should have access and institution of feedings with an immune-enhancing diet.[19] Major injuries to the pancreas requiring resection or drainage should also have access so that if pancreatitis or a pancreatic fistula should develop, enteral feedings can be instituted beyond the ligament of Treitz. Feedings at this point stimulate no more pancreatic output than TPN does[46] and are well tolerated with pancreatitis.[47] Major duodenal injuries—usually associated with simultaneous pancreatic injuries—should also have access so that if delayed gastric emptying occurs because of fistula development, delayed gastric emptying, or abscess formation, prolonged TPN can be avoided. We typically obtain access in patients with distal stomach injuries either at or just proximal to the pylorus because of the potential for delayed gastric emptying in patients with these conditions as well.

Access beyond the ligament of Treitz should also be obtained in patients undergoing celiotomy in some circumstances in which minor intra-abdominal injuries are present and the ATI is less than 25. Access should be obtained in patients with severe closed-head injury, spinal cord injury, severe chest injuries likely to need prolonged ventilator support, or multiple lower extremity fractures or major soft tissue injuries necessitating frequent trips to the operating room; in the elderly; and in the debilitated. Many of these patients will have delayed oral intake despite the fact they have insignificant intra-abdominal injuries and will require IV TPN or intragastric feeding if access is not obtained. Intragastric feeding is often unsuccessful, however, because septic complications of these injuries produce gastroparesis. Although transpyloric placement of tubes into the jejunum by fluoroscopy or endoscopic technique is possible, delays of a week or more are not uncommon. Fluoroscopic or endoscopic access techniques create additional costs that are unnecessary if an extra 10 minutes is taken to obtain postpyloric access before closure of the abdomen.

BURN PATIENTS

Early, direct intragastric feeding in burn patients is often well tolerated and appears to minimize the onset of subsequent gastroparesis.[37] After the first 8 to 16 hours of aggressive resuscitation, gastric feedings should be instituted at 25 mL/hr and rapidly progressed as tolerated up to the goal rate. Although gastric atony may develop in a few of these patients, the majority of patients will have continued gastric function and tolerate these feedings, thus eliminating the need for either direct small-bowel cannulation by endoscopic or fluoroscopic technique or the use of IV nutrition.

HEAD INJURIES

Because of the paucity of data suggesting any benefit with early enteral feeding in patients with severe closed-head injury, a nasogastric tube should be initially placed for decompression of the stomach. The majority of patients will resolve their gastroparesis by 4 days,[34] and the nasogastric tube can be replaced at that time with a small-bowel feeding tube with successful advancement of intragastric feedings. If at 4 days nasogastric drainage is still high (>250 mL per shift), the nasogastric tube should be clamped and residuals checked every 4 hours. Many of the patients with relatively high nasogastric output while receiving continuous suction have no gastroparesis and empty their stomach adequately when the nasogastric tube is clamped. The tube can then be removed and replaced with a small-bore tube for feeding. If gastric residuals remain high at 4 to 5 days, gastric motility agents may be successful. If no response is seen by day 6 or 7, either direct small-bowel access can be used or IV nutrition can be instituted with transition to enteral feeding as the gastroparesis resolves.

CHOICE OF TUBE FOR SMALL-BOWEL ACCESS

Although jejunostomies—either needle catheters or large-bore red rubber catheters—are the most popular form of access beyond the ligament of Treitz, transgastric jejunostomy tubes[48] have been developed to provide both gastric decompression and direct small-bowel access. Tubes designed to decompress the stomach but deliver nutrients into the *duodenum* are less desirable because in our experience, excessive gastric and duodenal secretions are produced as a result of hormonal stimulation by duodenal delivery of nutrients. This can produce 3 to 4 L of gastric and duodenal secretions and complicate fluid and electrolyte management. This does not occur when feedings are delivered beyond the ligament of Treitz. In this case, there is essentially no increase in pancreatic or biliary secretions over the resting state. Finally, a tube can be manipulated transnasally through the stomach and into the small intestine. These tubes should probably be bridled because in our experience, they are frequently dislodged into the stomach or entirely from the patient during transport and nursing care.

REFERENCES

1. Amaral JF, Caldwell MD: Metabolic response to starvation, stress, and sepsis, in Miller TA (ed): *Physiologic Basis of Modern Surgical Care.* St Louis, Mosby, 1988, pp 1–35.
2. Bessey PQ: Metabolic response to critical illness, in Wilmore DW, Brennan MF, Harken AH, et al (eds): *Care of the Surgical Patient.* New York, Scientific American, 1989, pp 1–23.
3. Johnson LR, Copeland EM, Dudrick SJ, et al: Structural and hormonal alterations in the gastrointestinal tract of parenteral fed rats. *Gastroenterology* 68:1177–1183, 1975.
4. Li J, Langkamp-Henken B, Suzuki K, et al: Glutamine prevents parenteral nutrition–induced increases in intestinal permeability. *JPEN J Parenter Enteral Nutr* 18:303–307, 1994.
5. Deitch EA, Winterton J, Ma L, et al: The gut as a portal of entry for bacteremia: Role of protein malnutrition. *Ann Surg* 205:681–692, 1987.
6. Alverdy JC, Aoys E, Moss G: Total parenteral nutrition promotes bacterial translocation from the gut. *Surgery* 104:185, 1988.

7. Li J, Kudsk KA, Gocinski B, et al: Effects of parenteral and enteral nutrition on gut-associated lymphoid tissue. *J Trauma* 39:44–52, 1995.

8. Deitch EA: Intestinal permeability is increased in burn patients shortly after injury. *Surgery* 107:411–416, 1990.

9. Janu P, Li J, Minard G, et al: Systemic interleukin-6 (IL-6) correlates with intestinal permeability. *Surg Forum* 47:7–9, 1996.

10. Zeigler TR, Smith RJ, O'Dwyer ST, et al: Increased intestinal permeability associated with infection in burn patients. *Arch Surg* 123:1313–1319, 1988.

11. Ambrose NS, Johnson M, Burdon DW, et al: Incidence of pathogenic bacteria from mesenteric lymph nodes and ileal serosa during Crohn's disease surgery. *Br J Surg* 71:624–625, 1984.

12. Moore EE, Jones TN: Benefits of immediate jejunostomy feeding after major abdominal trauma: A prospective, randomized study. *J Trauma* 26:874–881, 1986.

13. Adams S, Dellinger EP, Wertz MJ, et al: Enteral versus parenteral nutritional support following laparotomy for trauma: A randomized prospective trial. *J Trauma* 26:882–891, 1986.

14. Moore FA, Moore EE, Jones TN, et al: TEN vs. TPN following major abdominal trauma—reduced septic morbidity. *J Trauma* 29:916–923, 1989.

15. Kudsk KA, Croce MA, Fabian TC, et al: Enteral vs. parenteral feeding: Effects on septic morbidity following blunt and penetrating abdominal trauma. *Ann Surg* 215:503–513, 1992.

16. Moore FA, Feliciano DV, Andrassy RJ, et al: Early enteral feeding, compared with parenteral, reduces postoperative septic complications: The results of a meta-analysis. *Ann Surg* 216:172–183, 1992.

17. Eyer SD, Micon LT, Konstantinides FN, et al: Early enteral feeding does not attenuate metabolic response after blunt trauma. *J Trauma* 34:639–644, 1993.

18. Moore FA, Moore EE, Kudsk KA, et al: Clinical benefits of an immune-enhancing diet for early postinjury enteral feeding. *J Trauma* 37:607–615, 1994.

19. Kudsk KA, Minard G, Croce MA, et al: A randomized trial of isonitrogenous enteral diets following severe trauma: An immune-enhancing diet (IED) reduces septic complications. *Ann Surg* 224:531–543, 1996.

20. Kudsk KA, Carpenter G, Petersen SR, et al: Effective enteral and parenteral feeding in malnourished rats with hemoglobin–E. coli adjuvant peritonitis. *J Surg Res* 31:105–110, 1981.

21. Kudsk KA, Stone JM, Carpenter G, et al: Enteral and parenteral feeding influences mortality after hemoglobin–E. coli peritonitis in normal rats. *J Trauma* 23:605–609, 1983.

22. Borlase BC, Moore EE, Moore FA: The Abdominal Trauma Index—a critical reassessment and validation. *J Trauma* 30:1340–1344, 1990.

23. Jones TM, Moore FA, Moore EE, et al: Gastrointestinal symptoms at-

tributed to jejunostomy feeding after major abdominal trauma—a critical analysis. *Crit Care Med* 17:1146–1150, 1989.
24. Fagon JY, Chastre J, Hance AJ, et al: Detection of nosocomial lung infection in ventilated patients. Use of a protected specimen brush and quantitative culture techniques in 147 patients. *Am Rev Respir Dis* 138:110–116, 1988.
25. Heyland DK, Cook DJ, Guyatt GH: Does the formulation of enteral feeding products influence infectious morbidity and mortality rates in the critically ill patient? A critical review of the evidence. *Crit Care Med* 22:1192–1202, 1994.
26. Burke DJ, Alverdy JC, Aoys E, et al: Glutamine-supplemental total parenteral nutrition improves gut immune function. *Arch Surg* 124:1396–1399, 1989.
27. Gurr MI: The role of lipids in the regulation of the immune system. *Prog Lipid Res* 22:257–287, 1983.
28. Alverdy JD, Aoys E, Weiss-Carrington P, et al: The effect of glutamine-enriched TPN on gut immune cellularity. *J Surg Res* 52:34, 1992.
29. Kinsella JE, Lokesh B, Broughton S, et al: Dietary polyunsaturated fatty acids and eicosanoids: Potential effects on the modulation of inflammatory and immune cells: An overview. *Nutrition* 6:24–44, 1990.
30. Daly JM, Lieberman MD, Goldfine J, et al: Enteral nutrition with supplemental arginine, RNA, and omega-3 fatty acids in patients after operation: Immunologic, metabolic, and clinical outcome. *Surgery* 112:56–67, 1992.
31. Bower RH, Cerra FB, Bershadsky B, et al: Early enteral administration of a formula supplemented with arginine, nucleotides, and fish oil in intensive care unit patients: Results of a multicenter prospective, randomized, clinical trial. *Crit Care Med* 23:436–449, 1995.
32. Cerra FB, Lehmann S, Konstantinides N, et al: Improvement in immune function in ICU patients by enteral nutrition supplemented with arginine, RNA and Menhaden oil is independent of nitrogen balance. *Nutrition* 7:193–199, 1991.
33. Korretz RL: Nutritional supplementation in the ICU: How critical is nutrition for the critically ill? *Am J Respir Crit Care Med* 151:570–573, 1995.
34. Kirby DF, Clifton GL, Turner H, et al: Early enteral nutrition after brain injury by percutaneous endoscopic gastrojejunostomy. *JPEN J Parenter Enteral Nutr* 15:298–302, 1991.
35. Herndon DN, Stein MD, Rutan TC, et al: Failure of TPN supplementation to improve liver function, immunity, and mortality in thermally injured patients. *J Trauma* 27:195–204, 1987.
36. Herndon DN, Barrow RE, Stein M, et al: Increased mortality with intravenous supplemental feeding in severely burned patients. *J Burn Care Rehabil* 10:309–313, 1989.
37. Chiarelli A, Giuliano E, Casadei A, et al: Very early nutrition supplementation in burned patients. *Am J Clin Nutr* 51:1035–1039, 1990.

38. Alexander JW, MacMillan BG, Stinnet JD, et al: Beneficial effects of aggressive protein feeding in severely burned children. *Ann Surg* 192:505–517, 1980.
39. Gottschlich MM, Jenkins M, Warden GD, et al. Differential effects of 3 enteral dietary regimens on selected outcome variables in burn patients. *JPEN J Parenter Enteral Nutr* 14:225–236, 1990.
40. Saffle JR, Wiebke G, Jennings K, et al: A randomized trial of immune-enhancing enteral nutrition in burn patients (abstract). Presented at the American Association for the Surgery of Trauma 1996 Annual Meeting, Houston, Sep 20, 1996.
41. Rapp RP, Young B, Twyman D, et al: The favorable effect of early parenteral feeding on survival in head-injured patients. *J Neurosurg* 58:906–912, 1983.
42. Young B, Ott L, Twyman D, et al: The effect of nutritional support on outcome from severe head injury. *J Neurosurg* 67:668–676, 1987.
43. Grahm TW, Zadrozny DB, Harrington T: The benefits of early jejunal hyperalimentation in the head-injured patient. *Neurosurgery* 25:729–735, 1989.
44. Borzotta AP, Osborne A, Bledsoe F, et al: Enteral nutritional support enhances cognitive recovery after severe closed head injury. *Surg Forum* 42:29, 1993.
45. Dent D, Kudsk K, Minard G, et al: Risk of abdominal septic complications following feeding jejunostomy placement in patients undergoing splenectomy for trauma. *Am J Surg* 166:686–689, 1993.
46. Bodoky G, Harsanyi L, Pap A, et al: Effect of enteral nutrition on exocrine pancreatic function. *Am J Surg* 161:144–148, 1991.
47. Kudsk KA, Campbell SM, O'Brien T, et al: Postoperative jejunal feedings following complicated pancreatitis. *Nutr Clin Pract* 5:14–17, 1990.
48. Winkler MJ, Koruda MJ, Garmhausen L, et al: Jejunal cannulation via Stamm gastrostomy: An improved technique for feeding jejunostomy at laparotomy. *Surg Rounds* 18(11):469–474, 1995.

CHAPTER 4

The Role of Sentinel Lymph Node Mapping for Melanoma

Kenneth K. Tanabe, M.D.

Surgical Director, Pigmented Lesion Clinic and Melanoma Center, Massachusetts General Hospital, Boston, Massachusetts; Assistant Professor of Surgery, Harvard Medical School, Boston, Massachusetts

Douglas Reintgen, M.D.

Program Leader, Cutaneous Oncology, Moffit Cancer Center, Tampa, Florida; Professor of Surgery, University of South Florida, Tampa, Florida

I t is well recognized that tumor cells may spread via lymphatic channels or through the bloodstream and thereby give rise to regional lymph node and distant metastases. Melanoma provides no exception to this pattern of tumor progression. Once a diagnosis of melanoma is made, the most urgent question is whether it has spread to other sites. Although some patients may have clinical signs and symptoms of melanoma metastases, most will have a primary melanoma and no clinical evidence of regional or distant metastases.[1] Appropriate management of the regional lymph nodes in these patients has long been debated, with advocates and opponents of elective lymph node dissection.[2, 3] The introduction of intraoperative sentinel lymph node mapping may help define the optimal management of these patients with early-stage melanoma.

In this chapter we present an analysis of the biological significance of metastatic melanoma in regional lymph nodes, technical details of intraoperative sentinel lymph node mapping, methods for detection of occult melanoma in sentinel lymph nodes, results of clinical trials using intraoperative sentinel lymph node mapping, and its role in the management of patients with melanoma.

Advances in Surgery®, vol. 31
© 1998, Mosby–Year Book, Inc.

BIOLOGICAL SIGNIFICANCE OF MELANOMA LYMPH NODE METASTASES

The single most powerful predictor of survival in patients with melanoma is the presence or absence of regional lymph node metastases.[4] The presence of lymph node metastases decreases the 5-year survival rate of patients approximately 40% when compared with those who have no evidence of lymph node metastases.[5] Although the current system for staging of melanoma as adopted by the American Joint Commission on Cancer stratifies stage and overall survival by the size of lymph node metastases,[5] careful retrospective analysis indicates that the number rather than the size of lymph node metastases is the single most important prognostic variable to predict survival.[6] Ten-year survival rates for patients with metastatic melanoma in one node, two to four nodes, and five or more nodes are approximately 40%, 26%, and 15%, respectively.[4] Once patients have metastatic melanoma in their regional lymph nodes, prognostic factors derived from an analysis of their primary tumor add very little prognostic information in comparison to the number of lymph nodes that contain metastatic melanoma. After accounting for the number of nodes with metastatic melanoma, factors such as tumor thickness, gender, Clarke's level, histologic type, and lymphocytic invasion add little to a prognostic model for survival.[4]

The strong correlation between the presence of lymph node metastases and subsequent death from metastatic disease in patients with melanoma led some investigators to forward a model of tumor progression in which metastatic melanoma cells spread to regional lymph nodes before their spread to distant metastatic sites. In this scenario, patients in whom regional lymph node metastases had developed but in whom distant metastases had not yet developed could potentially be cured by surgical removal of all the lymph nodes containing metastatic melanoma. Accordingly, removal of regional lymph nodes before the development of palpable metastatic disease in them, referred to as *elective lymph node dissection,* was championed by surgeons who subscribed to this theory of tumor progression.[3, 7, 8]

The results of prospective randomized trials designed to evaluate the benefit of elective lymph node dissection in patients with melanoma have been difficult to interpret because of significant problems with trial design.[3, 9, 10] In the most recently reported prospective randomized trial designed to evaluate the benefit of elective lymph node dissection, overall survival was not significantly different between patients randomized to wide local excision of their primary melanoma combined with elective lymph node dissection and those randomized to wide local excision alone.[11] However, two defined subsets of patients demonstrated a significant increase in overall survival after elective lymph node dissection. Patients with melanomas between 1.1 and 2.0 mm in thickness and patients younger than age 60 randomized to receive elective lymph node dissection experienced a survival benefit when compared with similar groups of patients who were randomized to receive just wide local excision of their primary sites without elective lymph node dissection. Even though patients were stratified at time of randomization according to melanoma thickness, analysis of subgroups complicates interpretation of the trial results. Presumably, a subset of patients with metastatic melanoma in their regional lymph nodes exist that have either no systemic melanoma spread or limited systemic tumor burden that can be controlled by their own immune system. Although this subset of patients would stand to benefit from elective lymph node dissection, it is still not possible to accurately identify this subgroup of patients *a priori.* The absence of a clear survival benefit from elective lymph node dissection for patients with melanoma suggests that occult distant metastases have already developed in a significant proportion of patients with regional lymph node metastases.

Although removal of regional lymph nodes may not alter survival, identification of patients with metastatic melanoma in their lymph nodes defines a group of patients who have a very high risk of harboring occult distant metastases and who may benefit from adjuvant therapy. Careful staging for the presence or absence of metastatic melanoma in lymph nodes can improve survival by identification of patients who should receive adjuvant therapy. The well-received recent report of a multicenter, prospective, randomized trial that demonstrated a survival advantage for patients with melanoma lymph node metastases who are treated with interferon alfa-2b underscores the potential importance of accurate identification of patients with regional lymph node metastases.[12] In other words, removal of regional lymph nodes that contain occult metastatic melanoma may not improve survival per se; however, these lymph nodes contain extraodinarily important prognostic information that may be used to improve survival with the use of an effective adjuvant therapy such as interferon alfa-2b. In essence, sentinel lymph node mapping serves as a valuable staging procedure.

DEVELOPMENT OF INTRAOPERATIVE SENTINEL LYMPH NODE MAPPING

In an attempt to identify patients with melanoma metastases in their regional lymph nodes without subjecting them to the morbidity of elective lymph node dissection, researchers at the UCLA Medical Center examined two hypotheses: (1) defined patterns of lymphatic drainage allow identification of the first (sentinel) lymph node in a regional lymph node basin from any cutaneous site, and (2) the absence of metastatic melanoma in the sentinel lymph node accurately predicts the absence of melanoma in the remaining nodes in the basin. These investigators developed a feline model to examine their hypothesis[13] because unlike most laboratory rodents that have only a single inguinal lymph node, cats have three inguinal lymph nodes on each side. Intradermal injections of isosulfan blue into specific cutaneous sites always resulted in accumulation of the blue dye in a single lymph node. Intradermal injection into the medial aspect of the thigh resulted in coloration of a central node, whereas intradermal injection into the abdominal wall and lateral aspect of the thigh stained the lateral node. Intradermal injections into the skin of the perineum resulted in coloration of only the most medial lymph node. In this model, as in humans, the sentinel lymph node was not necessarily the closest node to the primary site. Dr. David Krag and his colleagues at the University of Vermont used a feline model to demonstrate that radiocolloid intradermal injections also localize in the sentinel lymph node and that a handheld gamma radiation detector simplifies identification and excision of the radioactive sentinel lymph node.[14]

Dr. Donald Morton and his colleagues at the UCLA Medical Center then tested their second hypothesis by performing sentinel lymph node mapping with isosulfan blue in 223 patients.[15] In addition to excision of the sentinel lymph node, all patients underwent a complete regional lymphadenectomy to allow comparison of the histology of the sentinel lymph node with that of the remaining lymph nodes. They successfully identified sentinel node(s) in 194 of 237 (82%) lymphatic basins. Metastases were present in 47 of 259 (18%) sentinel lymph nodes, whereas nonsentinel lymph nodes were the sole site of metastasis in only 2 of 3,079 (0.006%) lymph nodes. Only 2 patients whose sentinel lymph nodes had no evidence of melanoma had melanoma in nonsentinel regional lymph nodes. These data strongly supported the concepts that defined patterns of lymphatic drainage allow identification of the sentinel lymph node and that absence of melanoma in the sentinel lymph node accurately predicts the absence of melanoma in surrounding regional lymph nodes.

Dr. Krag and his colleagues then performed a pilot trial using radiocolloid and a handheld gamma probe for sentinel lymph node mapping in ten patients with melanoma. They successfully identified a sentinel lymph node in all ten patients (100%), thus suggesting that the use of radiocolloid for lymphatic mapping is associated with a higher technical success rate.[14] In larger trials, the highest success rates for identification of the sentinel lymph node have been reported with the use of a combination of vital blue dye and radiocolloid.[16]

TECHNIQUE OF SENTINEL LYMPH NODE MAPPING

There is great variation from hospital to hospital in the technique of intraoperative sentinel lymph node mapping. The following is a description of the technique as performed at the Massachusetts General Hospital and the Moffitt Cancer Center. Many details are subtle, yet critical for successful mapping.

Except in rare circumstances, we routinely plan to limit the first operative procedure to intraoperative sentinel lymph node mapping with lymph node biopsy and then wide excision of the primary melanoma. These procedures can nearly always be performed on an outpatient basis under local anesthesia with or without IV sedation. Only 12% to 15% of patients who undergo sentinel lymph node mapping will have metastatic melanoma identified in their sentinel lymph nodes.[16, 17] We do not plan to simultaneously perform a completion lymphadenectomy for patients whose sentinel lymph nodes are found to contain metastatic melanoma on frozen section evaluation. Instead, we plan to bring these patients back to the operating room at a subsequent date to perform a completion lymphadenectomy under general anesthesia. This strategy has several advantages. It allows for a more accurate match between the extent of surgery and the required type of anesthesia, nursing staff, operating room resources, and postoperative care resources. Operations are not extended after the results of frozen section analysis of the sentinel nodes are determined, and therefore this strategy allows more accurate estimates of operative times. This approach also allows pathologists time to carefully review paraffin sections before rendering a diagnosis. Frozen section analysis of lymph nodes misses metastatic melanoma cells that are subsequently detected on examination of paraffin sections in approximately 5% of cases.[18]

Patients arrive in the nuclear radiology area approximately 3 hours before their scheduled operation and receive an injection of 450 μCi of filtered ^{99m}Tc–labeled sulfur colloid into the dermis around the site of their primary melanoma. Typically, four injections are made circumferentially around the primary melanoma or around the scar from the previous biopsy. On occasion, the total dose of radiocolloid is split into more than four injections to prevent injections from being separated by more than 2 cm. It is critically important for the radiocolloid to be injected into the dermis and not into the subcutaneous tissue in order to map the dermal lymphatics, which are the channels by which melanoma cells metastasize. Inadvertant injection into the subcutaneous tissue may lead to identification of an incorrect sentinel lymph node or technical failure because of inadequate lymphatic migration of the radiocolloid. Dynamic scans of all lymphatic basins at risk for metastatic disease are performed 5 to 10 minutes after the injection (Fig 1). The location of each sentinel lymph node may be marked with an intradermal tattoo if desired.

The patient is then moved to the operating room and 1 mL of 1% isosulfan blue (Lymphazurin, Zenith Parenterals, Rosemont, Ill) is injected into the dermis in the exact same locations as the radiocolloid injections. We do not mix the isosulfan blue with the radiocolloid to allow a single injection session because the isosulfan blue begins to wash through the sentinel lymph node within 45 minutes whereas the radiocolloid is concentrated in the sentinel lymph node over a period of 2 to 4 hours.[16, 19] Instead, we inject the isosulfan blue in the operating suite just before the operation. A few minutes of exercise of the area of injection enhances movement of the isosulfan blue to the sentinel lymph node. Isosulfan blue does not interfere with pulse oximeter measurements of oxygen saturation. Patients should be counseled that their urine will turn blue for up to 24 hours after the procedure.

FIGURE 1.

A, preoperative lymphoscintigraphy in a patient with a melanoma of "intermediate" thickness on the left scapula. Filtered technetium sulfur colloid, 450 μCi, was injected in the dermis around the primary melanoma site. A scan obtained 10 minutes later shows two well-defined afferent lymphatics coalescing into single left axillary sentinel lymph node *(arrow)*. **B,** preoperative lymphoscintigraphy in a patient with a melanoma measuring 2.0 mm in thickness on the top of the left shoulder. A scan at 10 minutes shows bidirectional lymphatic flow *(arrows)* to the left posterior cervical triangle and to the left axilla. One sentinel lymph node is located in each basin, and both are at risk for metastatic disease.

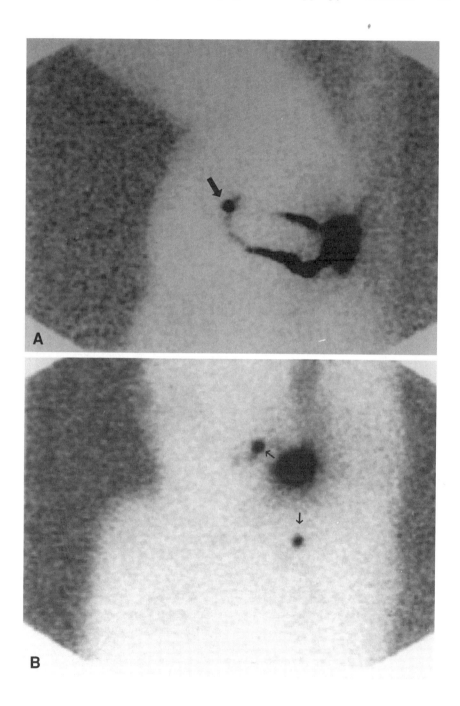

A handheld gamma probe (C-Trak, Care Wise Medical Products, Morgan Hill, Calif, or Neoprobe Corporation, Dublin, Ohio) is used to identify the exact location of the "hot spot" representing the location of the underlying sentinel lymph node in each regional lymph node basin. More than a single hot spot may be identified in any given regional lymph node basin. Gamma rays emitted from ^{99m}Tc easily penetrate tissue, and accordingly, when scanning for hot spots, the probe should be angled so that it is not pointing toward the primary injection site, thereby avoiding "shine-through" from the primary tumor radiocolloid injection. Inadvertent detection of shine-through may lead to unnecessary surgical exploration of sites that are mistakenly thought to contain radioactive lymph nodes. If this problem is unavoidable because of close proximity between the primary melanoma and the regional lymph node basin, it may be necessary to first perform a wide local excision of the primary tumor before searching for sentinel lymph nodes. However, in most instances we dissect out the sentinel lymph node before performing a wide excision of the primary melanoma.

Typically, we will wait at least 10 minutes after the isosulfan blue injection before making an incision over the regional lymph node basin to allow sufficient time for the blue dye to travel to the sentinel lymph node. A small incision is made directly over the hot spot, and use of the gamma probe allows dissection straight down to the radioactive lymph node; it should not be necessary to create significant flaps to identify the sentinel lymph node. Surgical dissection is aided both by visualization of the stained afferent lymphatics down to the blue-stained node and by use of the handheld gamma probe. The gamma probe will define whether a blue-stained lymphatic channel represents an afferent channel leading toward the sentinel node or an efferent channel leading away from the sentinel node. The sentinel node is identified and removed (Fig 2); afferent and efferent lymphatic channels are securely tied or clipped to minimize the risk of subsequent seroma formation.

The level of radioactivity in the excised lymph node is measured and recorded, as well as the level of radioactivity in the basin. If radioactivity has not decreased to background levels in the basin, the gamma probe is used to direct additional dissection to locate and excise additional sentinel lymph nodes. After completion of the lymph node excisions, the basin is again scanned with the gamma probe to ensure that all sentinel lymph nodes have been removed and that radioactivity in the basin has returned to background levels. Sulfur colloid has a retention time in the sentinel lymph nodes of at least 4 hours, whereas isosulfan blue has a re-

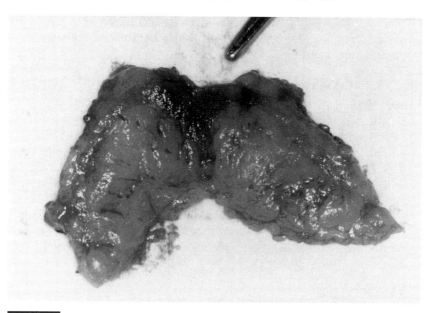

FIGURE 2.

Sentinel lymph node harvested from the patient whose lymphoscintigraphy is shown in Figure 1, A. Radiocolloid and a vital blue dye were used to intraoperatively identify the location of the sentinel lymph node. The harvested sentinel lymph node has been bisected, and the blue dye was identified in the subcortical sinus and cortex of the lymph node. This is the same location in which metastatic melanoma cells were identified.

tention time of only 45 minutes. A repeat injection of isosulfan blue around the primary melanoma may be helpful if difficulty in sentinel lymph node identification results in a prolonged dissection.

After removal of all the sentinel lymph nodes and confirmation with use of the gamma probe that no sentinel lymph nodes have been left behind, the biopsy incision is closed and attention is directed to excision of the primary melanoma with appropriate margins. We have not routinely performed sentinel lymph node mapping if a wide local excision of the primary melanoma has already been performed. In this situation, the lymphatic pathways that lead from the primary melanoma to the sentinel lymph node may have been disrupted, thereby resulting in inaccurate lymph node mapping. Residual isosulfan blue may be left behind after removal of the primary melanoma, and this occurs more frequently after 1-cm margin excisions than after 2-cm margin excisions. Accordingly, patients should be counseled in advance that they may have a fading blue area around their primary melanoma excision scar for up to 6 months postoperatively. Residual dye in head and neck cutaneous sites fades more rapidly because of the rich lymphatics of this region.

TECHNICAL FACTORS
BLUE DYE
Dr. Morton and his colleagues examined a variety of dyes in their initial mapping experiments in animals.[13] These included methylene blue, isosulfan blue, patent blue-V, Cyalume, and fluorescein dye. Patent blue-V and isosulfan blue produced the best results, with significant entry into the lymphatics, minimal diffusion into surrounding tissue, and easily detectable accumulation in the sentinel lymph node. Fluorescein and Cyalume were readily visualized, but only in a dark room. Methylene blue diffused out of the lymphatic channels and accumulated poorly in the sentinel lymph node.

RADIOCOLLOID
The ideal radiocolloid for intraoperative sentinel lymph node mapping should consist of particles of appropriate size that are readily taken up by dermal lymphatics, transported to the node basin, and trapped in the sentinel lymph node. Uniform particle size would theoretically result in a constant and predictable rate of uptake and transport to the lymph node. Furthermore, the ideal radiocolloid would have a short radioactive half-life to simplify handling of excised radioactive specimens, soiled drapes, sponges, and waste from the operating room. The liver scanning agent ^{99m}Tc-labeled sulfur colloid satisfies many of these requirements because it emits γ-particles and possesses a relatively short half-life. This compound is rapidly transported to regional lymph nodes after interstitial injection.[20] An investigational agent, antimony sulfide, became available in 1979. It has a smaller and more uniform particle size (3 to 12 μm). When labeled with ^{99m}Tc, antimony sulfide serves as an excellent agent for lymphoscintigraphic imaging. The surgeons and radiologists in the Sydney Melanoma Unit prefer ^{99m}Tc-labeled antimony sulfide for lymphoscintigraphy, as well as for intraoperative sentinel lymph mapping.[21] The major disadvantage of this compound is that it is investigational and not readily available; it is presently not available for use in the United States.

Sulfur colloid has a relatively broad spectrum of particle sizes (100 to 1,000 nm). It migrates rapidly and is well trapped by the sentinel lymph node. Sulfur colloid is the preferred radiocolloid for intraoperative lymphatic mapping for many investigators.[17]

However, lymphoscintigraphic images (see later) generated by this compound are generally poor. In comparison, 100-μm–filtered ^{99m}Tc-labeled sulfur colloid has a much more uniform particle size and appears to produce superior lymphoscintigram images when compared with unfiltered ^{99m}Tc-labeled sulfur colloid. Accordingly, filtered ^{99m}Tc-labeled sulfur colloid is the agent of choice for surgeons and radiologists in the Moffitt Cancer Center.[16]

HANDHELD GAMMA PROBE

The gamma probe is a sodium iodide crystal coupled to a photomultiplier tube and is approximately the size of a marking pen. The detector element is well columnated to minimize background noise and allow precise directional detection of emitted radioactive particles. This detector element is connected to a preamplifier and a signal processor with a digital readout of radioactivity and an audible sound that varies in pitch according to the level of detected radioactivity. Two handheld gamma probes suitable for use in the operating room are now available, the C-Trak and the Neoprobe. The C-trak's audible pitch can vary over a significantly greater range of radioactivity level than that of the Neoprobe. However, the two probes appear to provide equally successful sentinel lymph node identification rates in patients with melanoma.[16, 17]

RADIOCOLLOID VS. ISOSULFAN BLUE

Although intraoperative sentinel lymph node mapping was first performed with only vital dye, the use of radiocolloid as an adjunct proved to be extremely valuable. The location of the sentinel lymph node within a regional node basin cannot be predicted from the anatomical location of the primary melanoma. Accordingly, intraoperative lymphatic mapping with the use of only vital blue dye requires larger incisions and more extensive dissection to identify the sentinel lymph node than does the use of radiocolloid. In addition, the mere identification of one blue sentinel lymph node does not preclude the presence of others, and consequently, further dissection is necessary to identify or exclude the presence of additional sentinel lymph nodes. The technical difficulties associated with sentinel lymph node mapping using only vital dye led Dr. Morton and his colleagues to suggest that a surgeon would become proficient with the technique after practicing on 60 patients, a number of melanoma patients that is more than many surgeons see in their entire career.[15]

In contrast, gamma probe–guided resection of radiolabeled lymph nodes is more readily mastered and provides higher successful sentinel node localization rates.[16, 17] The addition of radio-colloid reduces the size of the incision and dissection necessary for sentinel node identification when compared with the use of iso-sulfan blue alone. The presence of high levels of radioactivity in the excised lymph node easily identifies it as the sentinel lymph node. Furthermore, the presence of additional radioactivity in the basin detected by the gamma probe serves as a sensitive indicator of additional sentinel lymph nodes that should be excised. A sig-nificant proportion of patients will have more than one sentinel lymph node in any basin because of parallel lymphatic channels from the primary tumor. We prefer to use both isosulfan blue and radiocolloid because the vital blue dye allows rapid visualization of the sentinel node once gamma-probe–directed dissection is be-gun. However, if a wide excision of the primary melanoma is not planned after injection of the isosulfan blue, the intense blue stain may require 3 to 6 months to fade, and in some cases it leaves a small but permanent tattoo. Accordingly, in select cases we per-form intraoperative sentinel lymph node mapping using only ra-diocolloid.

PREOPERATIVE LYMPHOSCINTIGRAPHY

It is well accepted that lymph node drainage patterns can be ex-ceedingly difficult to accurately predict based solely on location of the primary melanoma.[22, 23] Lymphoscintigraphy has been demon-strated to accurately predict lymphatic basins at risk for the devel-opment of metastases from cutaneous melanoma. Drainage patterns identified by lymphoscintigraphy as compared with those pre-dicted by historical anatomical guidelines are discordant in 26% to 32% of cases and discordant in 63% of the patients with primary melanomas on the head and neck.[23, 24] In a series of over 600 pa-tients with clinical stage I and II melanoma studied by lymphoscin-tigraphy at the Moffitt Cancer Center with a mean follow-up of 5 years, there has not been a single recurrence in any lymph node ba-sin that was not predicted by lymphoscintigraphy.[25]

Preoperative lymphoscintigraphic images may be helpful in successful intraoperative sentinel lymph node mapping. The im-ages identify all lymph node basins at risk as well as any *in transit* lymph nodes or lymph nodes in aberrant locations. The images may also help estimate the number of sentinel lymph nodes in the regional basin that should be harvested. The absolute requirement for preoperative lymphoscintigraphy has been somewhat dimin-ished with use of the handheld gamma probe. Careful scanning of all areas lying between the primary melanoma and all potential regional lymph node basins with the gamma probe can accurately localize sentinel lymph nodes. Furthermore, after excision of radioactive sentinel lymph nodes, careful examination of the remainder of the basin with the gamma probe will ensure that all sentinel lymph nodes are excised. Nonetheless, preoperative lymphoscintigraphy can be of significant help to surgeons first learning the technique of sentinel lymph node mapping by providing a road map of all the basins at risk for metastatic disease.

INFLUENCE OF PRIOR WIDE LOCAL EXCISION OF THE PRIMARY MELANOMA

Optimal accuracy of sentinel lymph node mapping is achieved when the technique is applied to patients who have had minimal surgical disruption of their primary tumor site. Virtually all the reported results of sentinel lymph node mapping involved patients who had undergone only a biopsy or simple excision of their primary melanoma before the lymphatic mapping procedure. Wide local excision of the primary melanoma, especially with a rotation flap closure, distorts the true lymphatic pathways of the lesion and may lead to excision of incorrect sentinel lymph nodes. Accordingly, the accuracy of sentinel lymph node mapping after wide local excision of a primary melanoma has not been established.

In patients who have already had a wide local excision of their primary melanoma, circumferential injection of radiocolloid and vital blue dye around the resulting scar or skin graft should theoretically allow uptake into lymphatics that drain to the "correct" sentinel node. However, other nonrelevant lymphatic channels would also presumably take up the injected tracer, thereby possibly *overestimating* the potential routes of lymphatic drainage and increasing the number of radioactive lymph nodes that are excised or basins dissected. This approach may be most applicable to patients with extremity melanomas, in which case the lymphatic drainage is unidirectional to a single basin. Further studies are necessary to determine whether sentinel lymph node mapping is accurate in patients who have already undergone wide local excision of their primary melanoma.

DETECTION OF TUMOR IN LYMPH NODES

Routine histologic analysis of lymph nodes by hematoxylin and eosin (H&E) staining of slides prepared from bisected lymph nodes examines less than 1% of the submitted material. Nonetheless, prognoses are assigned and treatment decisions are based on this relatively cursory examination. Metastatic melanoma cells initially travel to lymph nodes as either individual cells or clumps of cells that are easily missed if a lymph node is simply bisected for analysis. The sensitivity of routine histologic examination allows the detection of 1 abnormal melanoma cell in a background of approximately 10,000 normal lymphocytes.[25] Analysis of multiple levels of the lymph node enhances sensitivity of the examination. Immunohistochemical staining for S100, NK1/C3, and HMB45 proteins has enhanced detection of metastatic melanoma in lymph nodes in the hands of some investigators[15, 18]; however, the added benefit of this costly technique above that of H&E staining of multiple levels remains to be clearly demonstrated.

Nonetheless, it is well accepted that some patients have microscopic metastases in their regional lymph nodes that are missed by routine examination. For example, the incidence of detected microscopic metastases in patients in a prospective, randomized trial who underwent elective lymphadenectomy was 21%. However, in 56% of the patients randomized to observation of the lymph node basin in this trial, palpable lymph node metastases ultimately developed and required therapeutic lymph node dissection.[9, 26] Some of the difference between these two figures (21% and 56%) may represent microscopic metastases missed by routine histologic examination.

In an attempt to develop a more sensitive assay, investigators at the Moffitt Cancer Center proposed a cell culture technique in which the regional nodes are bisected, with half the node evaluated by routine histologic examination and the other half placed into tissue culture.[27] Several patients with histologically negative nodes had melanoma cells grow in their regional node culture, and detailed immunohistochemical and electron microscopic evaluation of these tissue culture cells confirmed that they were melanoma cells. Thirty-one percent of the patients who were histologically node-negative were found to have metastatic melanoma cells in their lymph node cultures. Although the clinical correlation between lymph node culture and disease-free survival was very good, this technique was extraordinarily labor-intensive and believed to be too complex to be widely applicable.

Investigators at the Moffitt Cancer Center have subsequently developed an alternative assay to detect micrometastases in lymph nodes that is more economical and efficient to perform and relies on polymerase chain reaction (PCR) amplification detection of tyrosinase messenger RNA (mRNA). The hypothesis was that the presence of tyrosinase mRNA preparations from lymph nodes would indicate the presence of melanoma cells. Polymerase chain reaction amplification of reverse-transcribed complementary DNA from lymph node mRNA preparations could theoretically be an extremely sensitive method of melanoma cell detection. In cell-mixing experiments, 1 melanoma cell in 1 million normal lymphocytes could be detected by two rounds of PCR amplification, thus suggesting that this technique is two orders of magnitude more sensitive than routine H&E examination of lymph nodes.

The clinical outcome of 124 patients with a median follow-up of 18 months has been correlated with an examination of their sentinel lymph nodes by both PCR and routine histologic evaluation (Table 1). Patients whose sentinel lymph nodes were negative for metastatic melanoma cells by both routine histologic evaluation and PCR analysis had a recurrence rate of 2.0%. In contrast, patients whose sentinel lymph nodes were positive by both assays had a recurrence rate of 64%. Interestingly, patients whose sentinel lymph nodes were histologically negative but PCR-positive for metastatic melanoma cells had an intermediate prognosis, with a recurrence rate of 10%. Within the group of patients whose sentinel lymph nodes were negative for melanoma based on routine histologic evaluation, PCR analysis changed the stage in 47% of these patients and correlated with disease-free survival. This difference in disease-free survival between these two groups of patients borders on statistical significance, with a *P* value of 0.07. Furthermore, PCR analysis correlated with the most dominant primary tumor–based prognostic factor, namely, melanoma thickness. Thirty-three percent of the patients with primary melanomas between 0.76 and

TABLE 1.

Correlation Between Clinical Outcome and Sentinel Lymph Node Analysis

Sentinel Lymph Node Status	Number of Patients	Total Recurrences	Local-Regional Recurrences
Histology-positive, RT-PCR–positive	22	14 (64%)	8 (36%)
Histology-negative, RT-PCR–positive	59	6 (10%)	2 (3%)
Histology-negative, RT-PCR–negative	43	1 (2%)	1 (2%)

Abbreviation: RT-PCR, reverse transcriptase polymerase chain reaction.

1.50 mm in thickness have PCR-detectable tyrosinase mRNA in their sentinel lymph nodes, whereas 70% of the patients with melanomas thicker than 4.0 mm have PCR-detectable tyrosinase mRNA in their sentinel lymph nodes, and it has been well established that overall survival correlates closely with tumor thickness.

The occasional but normal presence of nevoid rests in some lymph nodes presents a theoretical concern that PCR detection of tyrosinase mRNA may not be specific for melanoma cell metastases in lymph nodes and may occasionally detect tyrosinase mRNA in nevoid rests. To address this concern, several normal lymph nodes removed from patients who did not have melanoma have served as controls, and tyrosinase mRNA has not been detected in any of these nodes. However, the possible lack of specificity of the PCR assay remains of concern, and this concern is underscored by data that demonstrate a 33% incidence of PCR-detectable tyrosinase mRNA in patients whose primary melanomas were between 0.76 and 1.5 mm in thickness.[25] This incidence of PCR-detectable tyrosinase appears to be much higher than historical recurrence rates in this group of patients. More definitive conclusions about the utility of PCR analysis of sentinel lymph nodes will necessarily await additional clinical trials. Nonetheless, the increased sensitivity of the assay when compared with routine histologic evaluation holds significant promise of providing more accurate staging information for patients with melanoma.

RESULTS OF SENTINEL LYMPH NODE MAPPING

In the first reported clinical trial of intraoperative sentinel lymph node mapping for melanoma, Dr. Donald Morton and colleagues used isosulfan blue dye and attempted sentinel lymph node biopsy on 223 patients with melanoma, followed by complete regional lymphadenectomy.[15] Overall, metastatic melanoma was detected in 21% of the dissected regional lymph node basins either by routine H&E staining (12%) or by immunohistochemical staining (9%). Of the 40 patients with histologically positive nodes, 38 were found to have metastatic melanoma in their sentinel lymph node (5% false negative rate). The participating surgeons successfully identified the sentinel node in 72% to 96% of the patients, depending on where the surgeon was on the "learning curve." Groin mappings accounted for the highest technical success rate (89%). This landmark study demonstrated the feasibility of this new technique to accurately identify patients with occult regional lymph node metastases.

Based on these results, a second study was performed by surgical investigators at the Moffitt Cancer Center, M.D. Anderson

Cancer Center, and Duke University Medical Center. Intraoperative sentinel lymph node mapping with biopsy of the sentinel lymph node was performed in 42 patients with intermediate-thickness melanoma, and completion lymphadenectomy was performed in all patients.[28] With only isosulfan blue used intraoperatively, the sentinel lymph node was successfully identified in 90% of the patients. Thirty-four patients had histologically negative sentinel lymph nodes, and the remaining lymph nodes in those basin were also negative. In all 8 patients with histologically positive nodes, the sentinel lymph node was histologically positive. Thus no patients in this study had skip metastases. These results confirmed the hypothesis that melanoma metastases to regional lymph nodes can be identified with minimal morbidity by the use of intraoperative sentinel lymph node mapping.

However, the use of only isosulfan blue was associated with a technical failure rate of 10% to 28%, and Dr. Morton's experience suggested that a learning experience of at least 60 patients was necessary to obtain adequate expertise.[15] Dr. David Krag first introduced the concept of using a radiocolloid together with a handheld gamma probe for intraoperative sentinel lymph node mapping to allow easier identification and excision of the sentinel lymph node. [29] He first demonstrated that ^{99m}Tc-labeled sulfur colloid injected into the dermis of a cat is rapidly transported to the regional lymph node basin by lymphatics and accumulates in the primary lymph node. Identification of the precise location of this radioactive lymph node was greatly simplified by using a handheld gamma probe. After first demonstrating the technical ease of this procedure in a pilot trial, Dr. Krag then directed a multi-institutional study of 121 melanoma patients who underwent sentinel lymph node mapping using ^{99m}Tc sulfur colloid.[17] Some patients also received intradermal injections of isosulfan blue to aid in the mapping procedure. Only patients with metastatic melanoma in their sentinel lymph nodes underwent completion lymphadenectomy, and the remaining patients were observed. The overall technical success rate was 98% in this trial, in which several surgeons practicing in a variety of settings, including community practice, participated. This successful localization rate was markedly better than that reported with the use of isosulfan blue alone, and it was believed that surgeons mastered the technique after significantly fewer cases than with isosulfan blue alone.

The improved accuracy of sentinel lymph node mapping with the use of radiocolloid and a handheld gamma probe was confirmed in a trial performed at the Moffitt Cancer Center in which 106 consecutive patients underwent sentinel lymph node mapping after injection of a mixture of ^{99m}Tc-labeled sulfur colloid and iso-sulfan blue.[25] A sentinel lymph node was successfully identified in 96% of the lymph node basins that were sampled. Seventy percent of the sentinel lymph nodes were stained with isosulfan blue, whereas 84% of the sentinel lymph nodes were radioactive. Micrometastases were identified in 2 patients' sentinel lymph nodes that were radioactive but not stained blue. After excision of one sentinel lymph node, the presence of an additional sentinel lymph node was suggested only by use of the handheld gamma probe in several patients. These results confirm the importance of radiocolloid and a handheld gamma probe in sentinel lymph node mapping not only to improve the ease with which the sentinel lymph node can be identified but also to signal the presence of additional sentinel lymph nodes not easily identified with the dye technique alone. Several other centers have confirmed these findings.

The initial trials that examined the accuracy of sentinel lymph node mapping compared the results of histologic analysis of the sentinel lymph node with the results of histologic analysis of the remainder of the lymph nodes in the regional node basin. However, in more recent trials, patients who undergo sentinel lymph node mapping have the remainder of the lymph nodes in the basin excised only if their sentinel lymph nodes contain metastatic melanoma. Accordingly, the false negative rate can only be determined with prolonged and careful follow-up of the patients whose sentinel lymph nodes contain no evidence of metastatic melanoma. The most mature data that address this issue come from the M.D. Anderson Cancer Center and the Moffitt Cancer Center in a study of patients with cutaneous melanomas at least 1.0 mm in thickness or Clark level IV who underwent sentinel lymph node mapping and biopsy. Some patients had their intraoperative lymph node mapping performed with vital blue dye injection alone; however, all patients underwent preoperative lymphoscintigraphy. Only patients with metastatic melanoma in their sentinel lymph node underwent subsequent completion lymphadenectomy. Patients whose sentinel lymph nodes contained no evidence of metastatic melanoma were observed. Six hundred eighteen patients underwent mapping with successful identification of at least one sentinel lymph node. Five hundred eighteen (84%) of these patients had no evidence of melanoma in their sentinel lymph node. With a median follow-up of 18 months, 9 of the 518 patients (1.7%) had their first recurrence in a previously mapped lymph node basin that had a histologically negative sentinel lymph node.[25] These results strongly suggest that sentinel lymph node mapping is an accurate technique to stage regional lymph node basins and that the absence of metastatic melanoma in a sentinel lymph node is associated with a very low incidence of subsequent melanoma recurrence in that node basin. Recurrence in the lymph node basin can theoretically be attributed to either excision of the incorrect sentinel lymph node, missed identification of metastatic melanoma cells in the sentinel lymph node by the pathologist, or *in transit* tumor cells that arrived in the lymph node basin after sentinel lymph node biopsy.

A prospective trial sponsored by the National Cancer Institute is now being performed at several centers in which patients are randomized to receive wide local excision of their primary melanoma with sentinel lymph node biopsy or receive only wide local excision of their primary melanoma. Only patients with metastatic melanoma in their sentinel lymph nodes undergo completion lymphadenectomy. The principal goal of this trial is to determine whether staging of the regional lymph node basins with sentinel lymph node mapping alters overall survival. Mature data that address this end point are not expected to be available until after 2000.

PATIENT SELECTION

The rationale for removal of regional lymph nodes in patients with melanoma is similar to the rationale in many other types of cancer: (1) enhance local control, (2) provide more accurate staging information, and (3) improve survival. Sentinel lymph node mapping and selective lymphadenectomy probably provide only minimal advantage for obtaining local control in regional lymph node basins when compared with careful observation and therapeutic lymphadenectomy for patients with palpable metastatic disease in the basin. However, sentinel lymph node mapping and selective lymphadenectomy may improve survival, and the technique definitely provides accurate staging information.

Trials designed to evaluate the effect of elective lymphadenectomy on survival in patients with melanoma have failed to conclusively demonstrate a survival advantage in patients randomized to undergo elective lymphadenectomy.[9, 10, 26] Results from the latest trial to address this question were recently published, and as discussed earlier, they do not conclusively demonstrate a survival advantage for those patients who undergo elective lymphadenectomy.[11] Nonetheless, the large subgroups of patients with melanomas between 1.1 and 2.0 mm in thickness or who were younger than 60 year of age experienced enhanced survival if they were randomized to undergo elective lymph node dissection. Analysis of subgroups reduces the statistical significance of these results, and therefore the survival benefit of elective lymphadenectomy remains unclear. Results from a current trial comparing survival in patients randomized to either wide local excision alone or wide local excision and sentinel lymph node mapping with selective lymphadenectomy are not expected to shed any new light on this issue until after 2000. Accordingly, it remains unproved whether removal of regional lymph nodes containing metastatic melanoma enhances survival. Nonetheless, in comparison to trials in which a large proportion of the patients underwent elective lymphadenectomy and had no melanoma detected in any of their lymph nodes, the use of intraoperative sentinel lymph node mapping and selective lymphadenectomy ensures that only patients who truly have regional metastatic disease are subjected to the morbidity of a complete lymphadenectomy.

Enhanced staging of patients with melanoma is most advantageous in the setting in which effective therapies can be accurately applied to patients who are most likely to benefit from accurate staging information. As discussed earlier, the presence or absence of lymph node metastases is the single most important prognostic factor for overall survival in patients with melanoma. Furthermore, results from a recent trial indicate that high-dose interferon alfa-2b administered as an adjuvant to patients with melanoma lymph node metastases enhances overall survival. Patients in the Eastern Cooperative Oncology Group (ECOG) trial EST 1684 with melanoma metastatic to lymph nodes who were randomized to receive interferon alfa-2b enjoyed enhanced overall survival when compared with patients randomized to observation.[12] These data suggest that it is beneficial to identify patients with melanoma who have lymph node metastases so that they can receive adjuvant therapy with interferon alfa-2b. It should be noted that a majority of the patients enrolled in this trial had palpable lymph node metastases and had undergone therapeutic lymphadenectomy. Patients with occult regional lymph node metastases only accounted for 12% of the patients enrolled into ECOG EST 1684. Consequently, additional trials are required to determine whether patients whose metastatic melanoma is detected only by sentinel lymph node mapping definitely benefit from adjuvant therapy with interferon alfa-2b.

Outside the setting of a clinical trial, we offer sentinel lymph node mapping to patients who have at least a 5% risk of regional

TABLE 2.
Risk of Occult Regional and Distant Metastases

Location of the Primary Melanoma	Risk of Occult Regional Metastases Only,* %	Risk of Occult Distant Metastases,* % (With or Without Regional Metastases)
Female extremity		
<0.76 mm	2	1
0.76–1.49 mm	5–7	7–10
1.50–3.99 mm	7–19	10–24
≥4.00 mm	0	48
Male extremity		
<0.76 mm	2	2
0.76–1.49 mm	22–24	22–24
1.50–3.99 mm	24–29	24–34
≥4.00 mm	0	70
Female axial		
<0.76 mm	8	10
0.76–1.49 mm	14–17	21–29
1.50–3.99 mm	17–21	29–41
≥4.00 mm	0	60
Male axial		
<0.76 mm	9	14
0.76–1.49 mm	27–28	29–32
1.50–3.99 mm	28–30	32–45
≥4.00 mm	0	79

*Estimated risk for microscopic metastases at the time of initial diagnosis in patients with clinically localized cutaneous melanoma based on a mathematical model that included ulceration as a factor. (Courtesy of Balch CM, Houghton A, Milton GW, et al (eds): *Cutaneous Melanoma,* ed 2. Philadelphia, JP Lippincott, 1993, p 350.)

metastatic disease based on an analysis of prognostic variables (Table 2) and who would be candidates for high-dose interferon alfa-2b adjuvant therapy. Patients whose melanoma is less than 0.76 mm in thickness and located on an extremity have less than a 2% chance of regional lymph node or distant metastatic disease, and there is little justification in offering sentinel lymph node mapping to these patients. However, patients whose melanoma is less than 0.76 mm in thickness but located on the trunk, head, or neck have a 8% to 9% risk of occult regional lymph node metastases, and it is reasonable to offer sentinel lymph node mapping to these patients. Females with extremity melanomas between 0.76 mm and 1.49 mm in thickness have a 5% to 7% risk of occult lymph node metastases, and this risk is 22% to 24% in males with similar-thickness extremity melanomas. Prognostic factors have been analyzed for patients with "thin" melanomas who may be at greater risk for metastatic disease. This analysis demonstrates that patients with "thin" melanomas that are Clark level III or greater, regressed, ulcerated, or axial in location have approximately a 10% risk of recurrence.[30] These data underscore the importance of accounting for prognostic variables other than just tumor thickness to estimate the risk of regional lymph node metastases.

We also offer sentinel lymph node mapping to patients with thick primary melanomas who would be candidates for adjuvant therapy with high-dose interferon alfa-2b. These patients have a high rate of occult distant metastases, and elective lymph node dissection has not been previously recommended. However, the discovery of an effective adjuvant therapy changes this strategy. Patients with thick primary melanomas who have no documented metastatic disease should undergo sentinel lymph node mapping for staging to allow those with metastatic melanoma in their lymph nodes to receive adjuvant therapy, a therapy that has been demonstrated to be effective in patients with metastatic melanoma in their lymph nodes.

CONCLUSION

Regional lymph nodes are a common site of melanoma metastases, and the presence or absence of melanoma in regional lymph nodes is the single most important prognostic factor for predicting survival. Furthermore, identification of metastatic melanoma in lymph nodes and excision of these nodes may enhance survival in a subgroup of patients whose melanoma has metastasized only to their regional lymph nodes and not to distant sites. Sentinel lymph node mapping allows identification of patients with metastatic melanoma in their regional lymph nodes with minimal morbidity. The presence or absence of metastatic melanoma in the sentinel lymph node accurately predicts the presence or absence of metastatic melanoma in that lymph node basin. The use of radiocolloid and a handheld gamma probe during sentinel lymph node mapping greatly facilitates the procedure and enhances its accuracy.

The procedure can nearly always be performed with local anesthesia and is associated with very little morbidity. The results of reported trials indicate that the absence of metastatic melanoma in the sentinel lymph node is associated with less than a 2% rate of subsequent recurrence in that lymph node basin. Standard pathologic evaluation of bisected lymph nodes may miss metastatic melanoma cells. More sensitive techniques to examine regional lymph nodes have been developed, such as serial sectioning and PCR amplification of tyrosinase mRNA. Sentinel lymph node mapping produces a very limited number of lymph nodes to evaluate, thereby allowing application of these more sensitive techniques. The recently reported results of a prospective randomized trial demonstrate that adjuvant therapy with interferon alfa-2b administered in high doses enhances survival in patients whose melanoma has spread to their regional lymph nodes. Identification of patients with melanoma in their regional lymph nodes and removal of these lymph nodes provide important prognostic information and may enhance their survival. Accordingly, sentinel lymph node mapping should be offered to virtually all patients who are at risk for harboring occult melanoma metastases in their regional lymph nodes.

REFERENCES

1. Balch CM, Soong S-J, Shaw HM, et al: Changing trends in the clinical and pathologic features of melanoma, in Balch CM, Houghton AN, Milton GW, et al (eds): *Cutaneous Melanoma,* ed 2. Philadelphia, JB Lippincott, 1992, pp 40–45.
2. Crowley NJ: The case against elective lymphadenectomy. *Surg Oncol Clin North Am* 1:223–246, 1992.
3. Ross MI: The case for elective lymphadenectomy. *Surg Oncol Clin North Am* 1:205–222, 1992.
4. Balch CM, Soong S-J, Shaw HM, et al: An analysis of prognostic factors in 8500 patients with cutaneous melanoma, in Balch CM, Houghton AN, Milton GW, et al (eds): *Cutaneous Melanoma,* ed 2. Philadelphia, JB Lippincott, 1992, pp 165–187.
5. Beahrs OH, Henson DE, Hutter RVP, et al (eds): *Manual for Staging of Cancer,* ed 4. Philadelphia, JB Lippincott, 1992, pp 143–150.
6. Buzaid AC, Tinoco LA, Jendiroba D, et al: Prognostic value of size of lymph nodes metastases in patients with cutaneous melanoma. *J Clin Oncol* 13:2361–2368, 1995.
7. Balch CM, Milton GW, Cascinelli N, et al: Elective lymph node dissection: Pros and cons, in Balch CM, Houghton AN, Milton GW, et al (eds): *Cutaneous Melanoma,* ed 2. Philadelphia, JB Lippincott, 1992, pp 345–366.

8. Balch CM, Soong S-J, Milton GW, et al: A comparison of prognostic factors and surgical results in 1,786 patients with localized (stage I) melanoma treated in Alabama, USA, and New South Wales, Australia. *Ann Surg* 196:677–684, 1982.

9. Veronesi U, Adamus J, Bandiera DC, et al: Inefficacy of immediate node dissection in stage I melanoma of the limbs. *N Engl J Med* 297:627–630, 1977.

10. Sim FH, Taylor WR, Pritchard DJ, et al: Lymphadenectomy in the management of stage I malignant melanoma: A prospective randomized study. *Mayo Clin Proc* 61:697–705, 1986.

11. Balch CM, Soong S-J, Bartolucci AA, et al: Efficacy of an elective regional lymph node dissection of 1 to 4 mm thick melanomas for patients 60 years of age and younger. *Ann Surg* 224:255–266, 1996.

12. Kirkwood JM, Strawderman MH, Ernstoff MS, et al: Interferon alfa-2b adjuvant therapy of high-risk resected cutaneous melanoma: The Eastern Cooperative Oncology Groups trial EST 1684. *J Clin Oncol* 14:7–17, 1996.

13. Wong JH, Cagle LA, Morton D: Lymphatic drainage of skin to a sentinel lymph node in a feline model. *Ann Surg* 214:637–641, 1991.

14. Alex JC, Weaver DL, Fairbank JT, et al: Gamma-probe–guided lymph node localization in malignant melanoma. *Surg Oncol* 2:303–308, 1993.

15. Morton DL, Wen D-R, Wong JH, et al: Technical details of intraoperative lymphatic mapping for early stage melanoma. *Arch Surg* 127:392–399, 1992.

16. Albertini JJ, Cruse CW, Rapaport D, et al: Intraoperative radiolymphoscintigraphy improves sentinel lymph node identification for patients with melanoma. *Ann Surg* 223:217–224, 1996.

17. Krag DN, Meijer SJ, Weaver DL, et al: Minimal-access surgery for staging of malignant melanoma. *Arch Surg* 130:654–658, 1995.

18. Morton DL, Wen D-R, Cochran AJ: Management of early-stage melanoma by intraoperative lymphatic mapping and selective lymphadenectomy. *Surg Oncol Clin North Am* 1:247–259, 1992.

19. Nathanson DS, Anaya P, Karvelis KC, et al: Sentinel lymph node uptake of two different technetium-labelled radiocolloids. *Ann Surg Oncol,* in press.

20. Hauser W, Atking HL, Richards P: Lymph node scanning with 99mTc-sulfur colloid. *Radiology* 92:1369, 1969.

21. Uren RF, Howman-Giles R, Thompson JF, et al: Lymphoscintigraphy to identify sentinel lymph nodes in patients with melanoma. *Melanoma Res* 4:395–399, 1994.

22. Meyer CM, Lecklitner ML, Logic JR, et al: Technetium-99m sulfur-colloid cutaneous lymphoscintigraphy in the management of truncal melanoma. *Radiology* 131:205–209, 1979.

23. Norman J, Cruse CW, Wells K, et al: A redefinition of skin lymphatic drainage by lymphoscintigraphy for malignant melanoma. *Am J Surg* 162:432–437, 1991.

24. Lamki LM, Logic JR: Defining lymphatic drainage patterns with cutaneous lymphoscintigraphy, in Balch CM, Houghton AN, Milton GW, et al (eds): *Cutaneous Melanoma,* ed 2. Philadelphia, JB Lippincott, 1992.

25. Reintgen D, Rapaport D, Tanabe KK, et al: Lymphatic mapping and accurate assessment of lymph node staging, in Balch CM, Houghton AM, Sober AJ, et al (eds): *Cutaneous Melanoma,* ed 3. St Louis, Quality Medical Publishing, in press.

26. Veronesi U, Adamus J, Bandiera DC, et al: Delayed regional lymph node dissection in stage I melanoma of the skin of the lower extremities. *Cancer* 49:2420–2430, 1982.

27. Heller R, Becker J, Wassalle J, et al: Detection of submicroscopic lymph node metastases in patients with malignant melanoma. *Arch Surg* 126:1455–1460, 1991.

28. Reintgen D, Cruse CW, Wells K, et al: The orderly progression of melanoma nodal metastases. *Ann Surg* 220:759–767, 1994.

29. Alex JC, Krag DN: Gamma-probe–guided localization of lymph nodes. *Surg Oncol* 2:137–144, 1993.

30. Reintgen DS, Cox EB, McCarthy KS, et al: Efficacy of elective lymph node dissection in patients with intermediate thickness primary melanoma. *Ann Surg* 198:379–385, 1983.

CHAPTER 5

Small-Diameter Portocaval Shunt vs. Transjugular Intrahepatic Portosystemic Shunt for Portal Hypertension

Emmanuel E. Zervos, M.D.

Fellow, Digestive Disorders Center, Department of Surgery, University of South Florida, Tampa, Florida

Alexander S. Rosemurgy, M.D.

Professor and Chief, Division of General Surgery, University of South Florida, Tampa, Florida

D ebate surrounding the surgical management of portal hypertension began soon after reports of the first successful portosystemic shunt. Opinions regarding the advantages of selective vs. nonselective shunts, total vs. partial shunts, and liver transplantation vs. shunts were not close to consensus when in the early 1990s yet another option was introduced. The transjugular intrahepatic portosystemic shunt (TIPS) surfaced in 1991 amidst unresolved disputes regarding the best means of managing the complications of medically refractory portal hypertension. Inspired by growing concern over the physiologic impact of shunt surgery in a fragile population of patients and promising early results, TIPS has achieved considerable regard within the medical community, especially among invasive radiologists and gastroenterologists. Initially, the prospect of portal decompression through nonsurgical means was met with great enthusiasm because it not only provided another option for a difficult disease but also lightened the yoke borne by the surgeon in managing those patients refractory to medical therapy.

Advances in Surgery®, vol. 31
© 1998, Mosby–Year Book, Inc.

As early problems in the evolution of TIPS resolved with experience and improved technical facility, investigators began to focus on the longer-term implications and outcomes of transhepatic portal decompression. When considered alone, early and intermediate-term results of TIPS compare favorably with the established long-term outcomes and complications associated with surgical shunting in the opinion of many. Because of their minimal expectations regarding the treatment of portal hypertension and variceal hemorrhage, advocates were encouraged that TIPS through partial portal decompression, alleviated the variceal bleeding of portal hypertension with acceptable 1- to 3-year outcomes. Until recently, however, no investigator has defined the true role of TIPS by comparing it in a prospective and randomized fashion with an established and accepted means of surgical shunting. This monograph summarizes the current status of partial portal decompression as attained by TIPS and small-diameter prosthetic H-graft portacaval shunting (HGPCS), as well as updated results of an ongoing prospective randomized trial comparing small-diameter portacaval shunts with TIPS at our institution.

SURGICAL MANAGEMENT OF BLEEDING ESOPHAGEAL VARICES
HISTORY

Throughout this century, all surgeons faced with the complications of portal hypertension have been challenged not only by the complexity of this disease but also by the skill required to treat it surgically. More than 25 years after Eck successfully placed a portacaval anastomosis in a dog in 1877,[1] the first successful portacaval anastomosis in humans was achieved by Vidal.[2] The medical community was slow to appreciate the potential impact of Vidal's achievement, however, inasmuch as the next 40 years were characterized by procedures such as devascularization that were either ineffective or carried unacceptably high morbidity.[3, 4] The modern era of surgical shunting was heralded by Whipple's seminal report of ten successful portacaval and splenorenal shunts in 1945,[5] a report that launched an area of basic science and clinical research into the pathophysiology and treatment of medically refractory portal hypertension that continues to this day.

Eck's fistula completely diverted portal hepatic inflow and, as predicted by the physiologist Pavlov, resulted in high rates of encephalopathy and liver failure when applied in humans. This morbidity led several pioneers of modern shunt surgery to advocate the distal splenorenal shunt because of its efficacy and low rate of encephalopathy.[6] The distal splenorenal shunt would further minimize encephalopathy while theoretically maintaining portal perfusion by "selectively" decompressing bleeding varices and veins of the esophagus and stomach into the renal vein.[7] Although selective shunts have generally maintained a low incidence of rebleeding and encephalopathy, controlled studies demonstrating poor long-term maintenance of portal perfusion and recollateralization of varices, in addition to the inherent difficulties posed by the procedure, have precluded their widespread acceptance.[8, 9] Interestingly, optimal outcomes after distal splenorenal shunting occur in patients whose portal pressures decrease with shunting, although not to pressures equivalent to those of the inferior vena cava. Stated differently, patients do best after distal splenorenal shunting if they achieve partial portal decompression.

The technical difficulty associated with the distal splenorenal shunt inspired other investigators to seek alternative means of decompression while maintaining portal blood flow. Drapanas believed that the superior mesenteric vein was of sufficiently small diameter that mesocaval shunting would decrease but not eliminate portal flow.[10] Early data supporting his contention were later found to be erroneous, however, because of a radiologic misinterpretation.[11, 12] Shunt patency also proved to be a problem in early mesocaval shunts.[13] Drapanas' work was not lost, however, inasmuch as Cameron and others[14, 15] refined the mesocaval shunt to achieve those characteristics that inspired its design and ultimately seat it firmly into the armamentarium of surgical options for portal decompression. The common characteristic of these and most other shunts being used today is a recognition that total diversion of portal flow and/or equilibration of portal and inferior vena cava pressures is clearly detrimental in the long term.

PARTIAL SHUNTS

Partial portacaval shunts were inspired by the unacceptably high rates of liver failure and hepatic encephalopathy after totally diverting shunts.[16, 17] Bismuth et al. believed that there existed a critical portal pressure threshold below which variceal bleeding could not occur but at which portal perfusion could still occur. They were unable to achieve that pressure with 15-mm shunts because they could not maintain prograde flow.[18] Marion and colleagues, who also believed in a critical threshold, were the first to systematically reduce the aperture of a shunt side to side to achieve a desired pressure gradient while maintaining prograde flow.[19] Sarfeh et al. built on Marion's work by standardizing the constriction of the shunt by using sequentially smaller-diameter prosthetic interposition grafts.[20] Their group noted in the laboratory and clinically that hepatopedal flow could be maintained in nearly half the subjects undergoing 10-mm prosthetic HGPCS and in more than 80% of those receiving 8-mm shunts.[21, 22] These findings supported the theory that partial portal decompression could be achieved at a theoretical threshold below which variceal bleeding would not recur and at which nutrient hepatic flow would be maintained. Subsequent clinical trials by Sarfeh and Rypins that compared small-diameter with large-diameter total H-graft shunts documented comparably low rates of rebleeding and mortality with significantly longer encephalopathy-free survival when smaller shunts were used.[23] These findings led other centers to investigate Sarfeh and colleagues' encouraging results, and by and large, they were confirmed.[24–26] With similar intent, Johansen constructed "native" side-to-side portacaval shunts in an attempt to achieve a portal vein–inferior vena cava gradient similar to Sarfeh's. In contradistinction to Sarfeh, his studies showed that partial portal decompression can produce exceptional clinical outcomes even when hepatopedal flow is lost.[27]

In all, partial portal decompression as attained in varying ways by numerous authors has produced satisfying results, although the underlying mechanism explaining these results has not been defined. It is probably too simplistic to assume that preservation of portal blood flow alone is responsible for these outcomes. Although a comparison of the different types of surgical shunts is beyond the scope of this monograph, based on current data it is not unreasonable to assume that in capable hands and in the absence of confounding variables such as portal vein thrombosis, small-diameter shunts are comparable to other superior forms of surgical shunting in terms of mortality, rehemorrhage, thrombosis, and postprocedure encephalopathy. Acceptance of parity among currently used surgical shunts is important if the results of a comparative trial involving TIPS and surgical shunting techniques are extrapolated to represent a trial comparing nonoperative TIPS with surgical shunting in general.

EVOLUTION OF TRANSJUGULAR INTRAHEPATIC PORTOSYSTEMIC SHUNTING IN THE MANAGEMENT OF BLEEDING VARICES

The first TIPS procedure was accomplished by Rosch et al. in 1969 in a dog.[28] Rosch's work in animals led to the first successful report of TIPS in humans by Colapinto and associates in 1983.[29] Colapinto's procedure involved the construction of an intrahepatic tract between a branch of the hepatic and portal veins and subsequent balloon dilation of the tract for 12 hours. These investigators went on to undertake this procedure in 20 patients, all of whom did poorly because without a stent, the parenchymal channel quickly collapsed under the intrinsic elasticity of the liver.[30]

A major advance prompted by Colapinto's series was the development of an implantable metal stent designed to maintain patency of the intrahepatic tract. Palmaz was the first to design such a stent, but it was cumbersome and required both transjugular and transhepatic portal venous access to insert.[31] Ring and colleagues simplified and made the technique safer by using the flexible Wallstent.[32, 33] Not only did application of the flexible and self-expanding Wallstent simplify the procedure, it also considerably shortened the length of time necessary to complete it. Refinements in each of these stents led to promising results in subsequent small series of patients undergoing TIPS placement.[30, 34–36] As experience with the use of improved stents for the TIPS procedure increased, encouraging results from several centers have now been reported.[37–40] Despite promising reports, the surgical community remained skeptical toward this new therapy, which had still not been completely tested. Transjugular intrahepatic portosystemic shunting swayed many of its detractors through a turn of events that was neither planned nor expected. As more institutions began performing liver transplants in the late 1980s, waiting lists began to swell and so too did concern over the best means in which to manage bleeding varices in potential transplant recipients. In 13 patients undergoing TIPS while awaiting liver transplantation at the University of California at San Francisco, 7 went on to successful transplants and 2 improved and no longer required one.[34, 41] These encouraging data would help define the major indication for TIPS placement in the mid 1990s as a "bridge to transplantation" while surgeons and internists eagerly awaited long-term follow-up data on early TIPS recipients. As these data now begin to disseminate, TIPS status is once again in flux. Longer-term follow-up suggests that TIPS is prone to stenosis and occlusion, but with closer monitoring and "assisted patency," TIPS can maintain effective portal decompression such that its application has extended beyond that of being just a temporizing measure before transplantation.

PROSPECTIVE COMPARISON BETWEEN TRANSJUGULAR INTRAHEPATIC PORTOSYSTEMIC SHUNTS AND SMALL-DIAMETER H-GRAFT PORTACAVAL SHUNTS

In the years before 1986, the distal splenorenal shunt was the preferred operative procedure in treating bleeding varices secondary to portal hypertension in our institution. Because many of our patients had an advanced Child's class status, a relatively large number had hepatofugal flow, and operative outcomes were complicated by ascites and early deaths, we sought an alternative therapy. In 1986, we began to exclusively use small-diameter prosthetic HGPCS in patients with bleeding varices not amenable to medical management. Our early results are comparable to those of Sarfeh.[42, 43] In 1991, TIPS also became available in our hospital and was becoming an accepted substitute for portal decompression nationally. Realizing the need for a carefully executed, prospective randomized trial comparing this new therapy with a recognized standard of care, in 1993 we began to randomize all patients requiring portal decompression to receive TIPS or HGPCS. In this ongoing prospective trial, all patients fail sclerotherapy or are not candidates for variceal obliteration because of gastric varices or hypertensive gastropathy. For the purposes of this investigation, shunting is offered as definitive therapy only—never as a bridge to transplantation. Portal venous anatomy, including vein patency, is determined in all patients through color-flow Doppler US or visceral angiography before treatment. Once patients are deemed candidates for partial portal decompression, they are randomized to receive either TIPS or HGPCS. Patients with portal vein thrombosis or profound ill health are not randomized. Nonetheless, very few patients are denied portal decompression because of ill health. To date, only 3 patients have been cared for outside of the protocol, 1 because he had previously passed a liver transplant evaluation and 2 because ill health (acute renal failure and hepatic failure) seemed to predict a nearly certain fatal outcome after shunting that would only serve to bias the results. As of this writing, a total of 80 patients have been randomized in pairs to receive either TIPS or HGPCS.

TECHNICAL CONSIDERATIONS

Transjugular Intrahepatic Portosystemic Shunting

In our institution, all TIPS procedures are carried out with the patient under general anesthesia. The procedure is generally accomplished by means of a percutaneous puncture of the right internal jugular vein (one patient has required access via the left internal jugular vein). Modifications of the Seldinger technique and fluoroscopy are used to pass a guide wire and catheter through the right atrium into an intrahepatic branch of a hepatic vein, preferably on the right side. A needle is advanced over the wire and through the substance of the liver in the direction of the portal vein while maintaining negative pressure in the needle. When blood is noted in the catheter, the position within the portal vein is confirmed fluoroscopically. Once that position is confirmed, the needle is exchanged over the guidewire for an 8-mm ultrathin angioplasty balloon (Meditech, Boston Scientific, Watertown, Mass) and the tract dilated. Our institution uses the Schneider Wallstent (Pfizer, New York) to create a permanent tract between the systemic and portal circulation. The stents are dilated to 8 or 10 mm, depending on the portal vein/inferior vena cava pressure gradients observed at the time of TIPS placement.

H-Graft Portacaval Shunt

Our technique of small-diameter prosthetic HGPCS placement has been previously described in detail.[44] Briefly, 8-mm externally reinforced polytetrafluoroethylene (W. L. Gore, Flagstaff, Ariz) is used. The graft measures 3 cm from toe to toe and 1.5 cm from heel to heel, with bevels at each end oriented 90 degrees to one another. A portion of the caudate lobe is usually excised to facilitate shunt placement as close to the portal vein bifurcation as possible. Portal vein and inferior vena cava pressures are transduced intraoperatively before and after shunting. Intraoperative assessment of portal and cava flow is undertaken before and after shunting by using color-flow Doppler US. Extensive efforts are not generally undertaken to ligate collaterals at the time of surgery.

Follow-Up

All patients undergoing TIPS have their shunt studied 2 to 4 days after placement by color-flow Doppler US and transshunt venography. Figure 1 demonstrates a postoperative color-flow Doppler sonogram after successful TIPS insertion. Initially, TIPS patients were monitored with color-flow Doppler every 6 months to assess shunt patency. After it was realized that these patients need to be monitored more closely, especially in the early postoperative period, the latter half of the TIPS recipients were studied with color-flow Doppler US at 6 weeks and then every 3 months for the first year. If any patient (TIPS or HGPCS) is seen sooner with worsening ascites, encephalopathy, or variceal hemorrhage, the shunt is immediately assessed with color-flow Doppler and possibly venographically and revised as indicated. Color-flow Doppler US is undertaken to document TIPS patency and midstent flow velocity, with velocities less than 100 cm/sec generally leading to shunt venography and anticipation of shunt revision.

Surgical shunt patency is assessed venographically on or about the fifth postoperative day via transfemoral cannulation of the shunt. Figure 2 depicts a normally functioning H-graft as assessed venographically on postoperative day 5. At this time, large collaterals, if present and easily accessible, are embolized. All patients

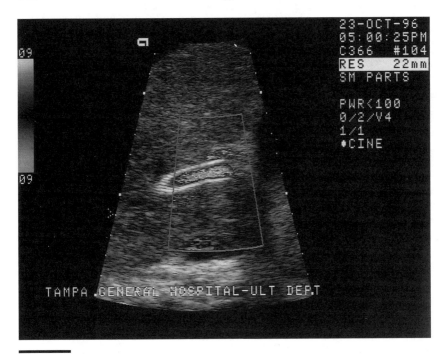

FIGURE 1.
Postoperative color-flow Doppler sonogram demonstrating normal flow through a transjugular intrahepatic portosystemic shunt.

after HGPCS are monitored, at a minimum, with semiannual clinic visits. At 1 year after placement, all shunts are studied by transvenous cannulation, venography, and pressure measurement.

All data reflect complete 1-year follow-up on all patients up to the time of this writing.

RESULTS

Patients

Eighty patients to date have been randomized in pairs to undergo either TIPS or HGPCS. For those undergoing TIPS vs. HGPCS, there was no difference in age, gender, Child's class, incidence of ascites, or incidence of encephalopathy, which was at most mild (Table 1). In patients undergoing TIPS, cirrhosis was caused by alcohol abuse (80%), viral hepatitis (10%), α_1-antitrypsin deficiency (5%), or idiopathic causes (5%). For patients undergoing HGPCS, cirrhosis was caused by alcohol abuse (77%), viral hepatitis (10%), methotrexate toxicity (2.5%), autoimmune hepatitis (2.5%), or unknown causes (8%). No differences between the urgency of shunting existed in either group, and a significant number of emergency procedures were undertaken in both groups. (Table 2)

Efficacy of Portal Decompression

Both TIPS and HGPCS significantly reduce portal pressures and portal vein–inferior vena cava pressure gradients. The magnitude of change in both absolute portal pressures and portal vein–inferior vena cava gradients after HGPCS is significantly greater than that after TIPS, thus documenting that HGPCS more effectively reduces portal pressure (Table 3).

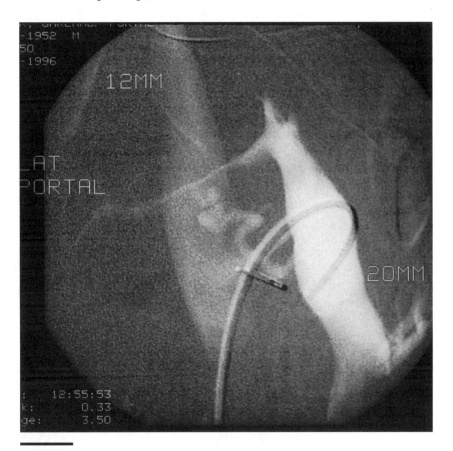

FIGURE 2.

Normal postoperative venogram after successful H-graft placement. Note the catheter traversing the shunt into the portal vein and hemoclips demarcating the H-graft inferior vena cava confluence. In the distance, a variceal collateral from the portal vein is apparent. Flow from the portal vein through the shunt opacifies the cephalad segment of the inferior vena cava.

TABLE 1.
Demographic Data of Patients Undergoing
Transjugular Intrahepatic Portosystemic
Shunting or H-Graft Portacaval Shunting

Patient Characteristics	TIPS	HGPCS
Number	40	40
Age, yr	53 ± 12.5 (SD)	53 ± 13.3
Gender	11F, 29M	17F, 23M
Ascites	70%	75%
Encephalopathy	28%	15%
Child's class	8A, 18B, 14C	8A, 22B, 10C

TABLE 2.
Timing of Shunting

Timing	TIPS	HGPCS
Elective	65%	80%
Urgent	27.5%	7.5%
Emergency	7.5%	12.5%

Abbreviations: TIPS, transjugular intrahepatic portosystemic shunt; *HGPCS,* H-graft portacaval shunt.

TABLE 3.
Efficacy of Portal Decompression

	TIPS		HGPCS	
	Preshunt	Posstshunt	Preshunt	Postshunt
Portal pressure, mm Hg	31 ± 7.3	25 ± 7.1*	30 ± 5.4	20 ± 5.3*†
Gradient, mm Hg	18 ± 5.9	9 ± 3.3*	17 ± 3.9	5 ± 2.8*‡

*Less than preshunt pressure/gradient, $P < 0.01$, paired Student's *t* test.
†Less than portal pressure after TIPS, $P < 0.01$, Student's *t* test.
‡Less than pressure gradient after TIPS, $P < 0.01$, Student's *t* test.
Abbreviations: TIPS, transjugular intrahepatic portosystemic shunt; *HGPCS,* H-graft portacaval shunt.

Shunt Failure

Failure of shunting was defined as an inability to accomplish shunting despite repeated attempts and appropriate anatomy), irreversible shunt occlusion, major variceal rehemorrhage, unexpected liver failure leading to transplantation, or death. Shunt failures are added for each treatment and compared by using the chi-square test. Transjugular intrahepatic portosystemic shunts could not be placed in 2 patients despite repeated attempts and acceptable anatomy. In each case, the liver was too hard to be penetrated to gain access to the portal vein. Twenty-one occlusions (6 early, 15 late) occurred in 13 TIPS patients, 18 of which could be corrected by endovascular methods and 3 of which were irreversible. Figure 3,A demonstrates the appearance of a stenotic TIPS by venography after US revealed a significant decrease in shunt velocity. Figure 3,B and C demonstrates the subsequent balloon dilation and restoration of normal flow in the same patient. One patient continues to do well despite an occluded shunt, 1 has been converted to a surgical shunt, and 1 patient died before definitive therapy could be undertaken. Early occlusion of H-graft shunts occurred in 3 patients, 2 of whom underwent uneventful surgical revisions and 1 was converted to a mesocaval shunt. Late HGPCS occlusion occurred in 1 patient. It was detected at surveillance follow-up and was corrected nonoperatively (Table 4).

Major variceal rehemorrhage occurred in 12 (30%) patients after TIPS, with a fatal outcome in 3 patients. Of these 3 patients, 2 bled more than 30 days after TIPS placement, and in both instances the TIPS was found to be stenotic at revision. No patients rebled after HGPCS. Early deaths (<30 days) occurred in 6 patients each after TIPS and HGPCS. Nine late deaths after TIPS and 3 after HGPCS were not statistically different. In total, 33 incidences of shunt failure occurred in 27 TIPS patients and 10 failures occurred in 10 HGPCS patients. The 6 additional TIPS failures arose in patients who died as a result of recurrent variceal bleeding despite patent TIPS in 5 or irreversible occlusion before death in 1. In all 6 patients, both the predefined shunt failure and the death were counted. In the 5 patients who rebled, mild stenoses were noted in their shunts and the stent was dilated. Failures after TIPS were significantly more frequent than after HGPCS (Table 4).

Encephalopathy and Ascites

Ascites was present preoperatively in 70% of those patients undergoing TIPS and 75% of those undergoing HGPCS. Within 30 days of shunting, ascites was still present in 60% of the patients undergoing each procedure. Except for those patients who suffered periprocedural deaths or were lost to follow-up, 40% of the TIPS patients had incomplete resolution of ascites and 27% of those undergoing HGPCS remained refractory. Interestingly, all the patients suffering periprocedural deaths in both groups had ascites. Patients

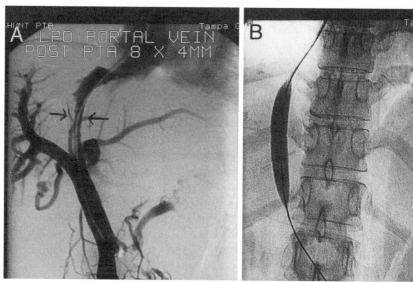

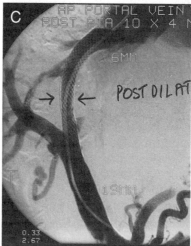

FIGURE 3.

Venogram of a stenotic TIPS as detected by color-flow Doppler US **A,** with balloon dilation **B,** and with subsequent restoration of normal flow **C.**

TABLE 4.

Causes of Shunt Failure After Transjugular Intrahepatic Portosystemic Shunting and Small-Diameter H-Graft Portacaval Shunting

Cause	TIPS	HGPCS
Unable to place shunt	2	0
Irreversible occlusion	3	1
Variceal rehemorrhage	12	0
Liver transplantation	1	0
Early mortality (30 days)	6	6
Late mortality	9	3
Total failures	27*†	10

*Greater than after HGPCS, $P < 0.02$, chi-square test.
†There were 33 occurrences of shunt failure in 27 patients.

suffering periprocedural deaths represented 20% of all patients who had ascites at the time of shunting.

Encephalopathy was present in 11 patients undergoing TIPS and resolved completely in 5. One new case of encephalopathy arose after TIPS. Six TIPS patients died within 30 days of TIPS insertion, never recovering from their procedure. It is difficult to comment on the presence or absence of encephalopathy in these patients because confounding issues surrounding their downward hospital course cloud the issue. Similarly, 6 HGPCS patients were encephalopathic preoperatively and went on to die in the perioperative period. Two new cases of encephalopathy arose in patients undergoing HGPCS, but each was well controlled with lactulose.

Mortality

Early mortality (<30 days) after each procedure was the same. Early deaths secondary to liver failure occurred in five patients after TIPS and HGPCS, the remaining death in each group being due to variceal rehemorrhage and adult respiratory distress syndrome, respectively. With follow-up in all patients at 1 year, late mortality was slightly higher in those patients undergoing TIPS than in those undergoing HGPCS (26% vs. 13%). Two HGPCS late deaths were due to liver failure and one was caused by colon cancer. Four late TIPS deaths were due to liver failure; two were caused by variceal rehemorrhage; one was due to cholangiocarcinoma; one was due to pneumonia, liver failure, and total-body failure; and one was the result of a motor vehicle accident.

Effects on Nutrient Hepatic Flow

In an attempt to further characterize the effects of shunting on nutrient hepatic blood flow, we measured effective hepatic blood flow by using low-dose galactose clearance. The ability of the liver to clear peripherally injected galactose as a measure of liver function is well established.[45–47] Galactose clearance was determined in 40 patients (20 after each shunt) within 48 hours before shunt placement and again 5 or 6 days after shunting. A 250-mg bolus of 5% galactose is administered IV, and then a constant infusion of 75 mg/min is continued for 1 hour. Peripheral blood collected before and 60 minutes after galactose infusion is measured for galactose levels. The ability to clear galactose was compared in TIPS and HG-PCS patients. Patients who underwent TIPS demonstrated a significant impairment in their ability to clear galactose by this method, whereas HGPCS patients' ability remained unchanged despite reductions in portal flow. H-graft portacaval shunting allowed the preservation of total effective hepatic blood flow, whereas TIPS did not. Of particular note, portal flow increases after TIPS; given the decrease in nutrient hepatic flow, the increase in portal flow after TIPS is nonnutrient (Table 5).

Economic Issues

To address the issue of time and resource allocation, we analyzed cost of care and length of stay beginning at the time of initial shunt placement and continuing to the present. This analysis includes the cost of subsequent admissions for the management of ascites, hepatic encephalopathy, and bleeding varices, as well as routine

---

TABLE 5.
Effects of Shunting on Effective Hepatic Blood Flow

Shunt	N	Portal Flow, mL/sec		EHF, mL/min	
		Preshunt	Postshunt	Preshunt	Postshunt
TIPS	20	21 ± 11.9	31 ± 16.9*	1,684 ± 2161.8	676 ± 451.3*
HGPCS	20	14 ± 7.6	11 ± 11.1	1,901 ± 1818.7	1,662 ± 1035.4

*Significantly changed ($P < 0.05$, Student's *t* test) from preshunt value.
Abbreviations: EHF, effective hepatic blood flow; *TIPS,* transjugular intrahepatic portosystemic shunt; *HCPCS,* H-graft portacaval shunt.

TABLE 6.

Cost of Transjugular Intrahepatic Portosystemic Shunting vs. H-Graft Portacaval Shunting

	Length of Hospital Stay, Days		Cost of Therapy, $	
	ICU	Total	Initial	Total, 1 yr
TIPS	4.6 ± 6.8	9.4 ± 10.8	48,188 ± 43,355	69,276 ± 52,712
HGPCS	6.0 ± 8.3	12.7 ± 12.5	61,522 ± 47,615	66,034 ± 49,110

shunt studies. The results of this analysis, including the length of hospital stay, are summarized in Table 6. These data indicate that although wide variation in patient cost for the initial procedure renders TIPS and HGPCS statistically no different, the less expensive cost associated with an average TIPS patient quickly reaches and surpasses that of HGPCS patients when the cost of keeping that TIPS patent is considered (Table 6).

CLOSING REMARKS

After nearly 100 years of clinical and basic science research, surgical management of the complications of portal hypertension is still not defined. A veritable infant by comparison, TIPS is readily accepted by many as an appropriate or even superior substitute for surgical shunts to achieve portal decompression. Enthusiasm regarding TIPS stems from large series showing results comparable to those of historical surgical shunt controls.[48] Unfortunately, the basis for many of these encouraging reports may lie more in a selection bias rather than true efficacy of the individual procedures. Most centers with enough experience to meaningfully report outcomes have successfully negotiated the learning curve and are recognized centers of excellence in their chosen procedure—a degree of excellence that stems from an unrelenting pursuit to perfect not only the procedure but also the means by which these patients are monitored and cared for. Proponents of both TIPS and HGPCS are equally prone to such compulsivity, and it is for these reasons that carefully controlled head-to-head comparisons of TIPS to other modalities of therapy are so vitally important. Without such data, we run the risk of relegating our patients to a particular therapy based on availability, convenience, or someone else's success with it and not on what is most appropriate for the patient.

The patients enrolled in this study thus far are generally older male alcoholics with moderate to advanced cirrhosis of the liver who are undergoing elective portal decompressive procedures. Because the primary endpoint for any portal decompressive procedure is prevention of life-threatening rehemorrhage from esophagogastric varices, we first set out to determine the efficacy of each procedure in accomplishing this end. Slightly fewer than one third of the TIPS patients rebled within 1 year of having their shunt placed, which is consistent with other investigators' findings.[37, 49–52] Also consistent with other published reports is the efficacy of small-diameter HGPCS in preventing rehemorrhage from esophagogastric varices in our hands.[25, 53] In our total experience of over 110 HGPCS procedures since 1986, the incidence of rehemorrhage is only 3%, with none occurring in patients enrolled in this study. Rehemorrhage in this study accounted for 15% of the total TIPS deaths and none of the HGPCS deaths, although no difference in overall early or late mortality could be demonstrated.

Stenosis and/or occlusion in TIPS remains a significant obstacle and is reported to occur in 18% to 31% of patients.* Our experience is not different from the national experience, with 33% of the TIPS patients in this study requiring some type of intervention for stenotic or occluded shunts, many returning two, three, and four times for revisions. These rates of stenosis are mirrored in our total population of 60 patients who have undergone TIPS since 1993. In this experience, 26 (43% patients underwent a total of 46 shunt revisions because of stenosis or occlusion. Thirty-three of these revisions involved balloon dilation of stenosed shunts, 12 had additional shunts placed to extend foreshortened TIPS, and 3 could not be revised.

Maintenance of shunt patency through more intensive follow-up protocols may preclude potential complications associated with loss of portal decompression, but it is important to note that the procedural savings purported to occur with TIPS[56–58] are soon forfeited when the cost of maintaining adequate function is taken into consideration. Meanwhile, HGPCS continues to demonstrate impressive short- and long-term patency rates, with only a 3% incidence of shunt thrombosis or occlusion in 120 shunts placed in our institution since 1986.

Although encephalopathy was a considerable problem preoperatively in each group, it has been virtually nonexistent long-term

*References 38, 40, 49, 50, 54, 55.

in patients who survive their procedure. It is difficult to comment on the incidence of encephalopathy after either procedure because most of the perioperative deaths involved those patients with pre-operative encephalopathy. Encephalopathy and ascites clearly predict poor outcome in both groups of patients, and relatively high rates of encephalopathy are an acknowledged occurrence with TIPS.[49, 50, 55, 59] We believe that encephalopathy after TIPS is most likely attributable to significant reductions in nutrient hepatic inflow. In this study, HGPCS maintained effective hepatic blood flow, whereas it was significantly reduced after TIPS, and this is consistent with earlier reports from our institution examining HGPCS alone.[60, 61] Additionally, we have noted inflow compromise to be of further consequence when TIPS is applied to palliate patients with intractable ascites, a cirrhotic subpopulation with more advanced liver disease. Our institution's experience in this subgroup of patients indicates that early deaths from hepatic decompensation after TIPS placement for refractory ascites are more than twice those seen in patients with bleeding varices.[62]

Because TIPS will become increasingly available in centers that do not offer surgical shunting or liver transplantation to patients with life-threatening bleeding varices, head-to-head comparisons such as this are critical to accurately define the relative indications for each procedure. It is our belief that the inability to undertake surgical shunting or transplantation does not equate with an ability to undertake TIPS and care for patients with complicated cirrhosis. At this time, patients with advanced cirrhosis and variceal hemorrhage should be cared for in centers offering TIPS, surgical shunting, and transplantation. Physicians practicing in centers not offering these options should prepare patients for transfer and undertake only temporizing measures at their facility. Patients with complications of advanced cirrhosis and inadequate hepatic reserve, which is occasionally difficult to define, should undergo liver transplantation. Patients with adequate hepatic reserve, generally defined as patients with Child's A or B class, should undergo HGPCS unless they are poor operative candidates, for example, those with a history of multiple celiotomies, poor cardiac reserve (especially aortic stenosis and mitral regurgitation), and other organ systems in failure. Because of high rates of occlusion, rebleeding, and shunt failure, TIPS should be reserved for patients not candidates for HGPCS. As a bridge to transplantation, TIPS warrants more mention. Although the concept is a good one, TIPS in many patients may make the need for transplantation a self-fulfilling prophecy. Because TIPS decreases portal nutrient flow so significantly, patients with otherwise adequate hepatic function will be pushed into inadequate liver function by TIPS. H-graft portacaval shunting should not be viewed as a contraindication to hepatic transplantation. Although adhesions associated with previous HG-PCS procedures may increase blood transfusion requirements at transplantation, outcomes of liver transplantation after portacaval shunting are statistically indistinguishable from those occurring after TIPS.[63]

REFERENCES

1. Child CG: Eck's fistula. *Surg Gynecol Obstet* 96:375–376, 1953.
2. Donovan AJ, Covey PC: Early history of the portacaval shunt in humans. *Surg Gynecol Obstet* 147:423–430, 1978.
3. Cates HB: Surgical treatment for cirrhosis: Prognosis subsequent to omentopexy. *Arch Intern Med* 71:183–205, 1943.
4. White S: Discussion on the surgical treatment of ascites secondary to vascular cirrhosis of the liver. *BMJ* 2:1287–1296, 1906.
5. Whipple AO: The problem of portal hypertension in relation to the hepatosplenopathies. *Ann Surg* 122:449–475, 1945.
6. Linton RR, Ellis DS, Geary JE: Critical comparative analysis of early and late results of splenorenal and direct portacaval shunts performed in 169 patients with portal cirrhosis. *Ann Surg* 154:446–459, 1961.
7. Warren WD, Zeppa R, Fomon JJ: Selective transsplenic decompression of gastroesophageal varices by distal splenorenal shunt. *Ann Surg* 166:437–455, 1967.
8. Henderson JM, Gong-Liang J, Galloway J, et al: Portaprival collaterals following distal splenorenal shunt: Incidence, magnitude and associated portal perfusion changes. *J Hepatol* 1:649–661, 1985.
9. Belghiti J, Grenier P, Nonel O, et al: Long term loss of Warren's shunt selectivity: Angiographic demonstration. *Arch Surg* 116:1121–1124, 1981.
10. Drapanas T: Interposition mesocaval shunt for the treatment of portal hypertension. *Ann Surg* 176:435–448, 1972.
11. Drapanas T, Locicero J, Dowling JB, et al: Hemodynamics of the interposition mesocaval shunt. *Ann Surg* 181:523–533, 1975.
12. Fulenwider JT, Nordlinger BM, Millikan WJ, et al: Portal pseudoperfusion: An angiographic illusion. *Ann Surg* 189:257–268, 1979.
13. Dennis MA, Monson RC, O'Leary JP, et al: Interposition mesocaval shunt: A less than ideal procedure. *Am Surg* 44:734–738, 1978.
14. Cameron JL, Harrington DP, Maddrey WC, et al: The mesocaval C shunt. *Surg Gynecol Obstet* 150:401–403, 1980.
15. Paquet K, Lazar A, Koussouris P, et al: Mesocaval interposition shunt with small-diameter polytetrafluoroethylene grafts in sclerotherapy failure. *Br J Surg* 82:199–203, 1995.
16. Sarfeh IJ, Carter JA, Welch HF: Analysis of operative mortality after

portal decompressive procedures in cirrhotic patients. *Am J Surg* 140:306–311, 1980.

17. Sarfeh IJ: Comparison of the major variceal decompressive operations. *Am Surg* 48:261–263, 1982.

18. Bismuth H, Franco D, Hepp J: Portal-systemic shunt in hepatic cirrhosis—Does the type of shunt decisively influence the clinical result? *Ann Surg* 179:209–218, 1974.

19. Marion P, Dumurgier C, Vacca C, et al: Treatment of portal encephalopathy by reduction of porto-caval flow in the bypass. *Chirurgie* 103:279–285, 1977.

20. Sarfeh IJ, Rypins EB, Mason GR: A systematic appraisal of portacaval H-graft diameters: Clinical and hemodynamic perspectives. *Ann Surg* 204:356–363, 1986.

21. Rypins EB, Rosenberg KM, Sarfeh IJ, et al: Computer analysis of portal hemodynamics after small-diameter portacaval H-grafts: The theoretical basis of partial shunting. *J Surg Res* 42:354–361, 1987.

22. Sarfeh IJ, Rypins EB, Mason GR: A systematic appraisal of portacaval H-graft diameters. *Ann Surg* 204:356–363, 1986.

23. Sarfeh IJ, Rypins EB: Partial versus total portacaval shunt in alcoholic cirrhosis: Results of a prospective, randomized clinical trial. *Ann Surg* 219:353–361, 1994.

24. Rosemurgy AS, Goode SE, Camps M: The effect of small diameter H-graft portacaval shunts on portal blood flow. *Am J Surg* 171:154–157, 1996.

25. Adam R, Diamond T, Bismuth H: Partial portacaval shunt: Renaissance of an old concept. *Surgery* 111:610–616, 1995.

26. Darling CR, Shah DM, Chang BB, et al: Long term follow up of poor risk patients undergoing small diameter portacaval shunt. *Am J Surg* 164:225–228, 1992.

27. Johansen K: Partial portal decompression for variceal hemorrhage. *Am J Surg* 157:479–482, 1989.

28. Rosch J, Hanafee WN, Snow H: Transjugular portal venography and radiological portosystemic shunt: An experimental study. *Radiology* 92:1112–1114, 1969.

29. Colapinto RF, Stronell RD, Gildiner M, et al: Formation of an intrahepatic portosystemic shunt using balloon dilatation catheter: Preliminary clinical experience. *AJR Am J Roentgenol* 140:709–714, 1983.

30. Gordon JD, Colapinto RF, Abecassis M: Transjugular intrahepatic portosystemic shunt: A nonoperative approach to life threatening variceal bleeding. *Can J Surg* 30:45–50, 1987.

31. Richter GM, Palmaz JC, Noeldge G: The transjugular intrahepatic portosystemic stent-shunt (TIPSS): Results of a pilot study. *Cardiol Intern Radiat* 13:200–207, 1990.

32. Ring EJ, Lake JR, Roberts JP, et al: Using transjugular intrahepatic portosystemic shunts to control variceal bleeding before liver transplantation. *Ann Intern Med* 116:304–309, 1992.

33. Laberge JM, Ring EJ, Lake JR: Transjugular intrahepatic portosystemic shunts (TIPS): Preliminary results in 25 patients. *J Vasc Surg* 16:258–267, 1992.
34. Richter GM, Noeldge G, Palmaz JC, et al: The transjugular intrahepatic portosystemic stent-shunt (TIPSS): Preliminary clinical results. *Radiology* 174:1027–1030, 1990.
35. Zemel G, Katzen BT, Becker GJ, et al: Percutaneous transjugular portosystemic shunt. *JAMA* 266:390–393, 1991.
36. Garcia-Villarreal L, Zozaya JM, Quiroza J, et al: TIPS for portal hypertension and liver cirrhosis. *J Hepatol* 16:91S, 1992.
37. Jalan R, Redhead DN, Hayes PC: Transjugular intrahepatic portosystemic stent shunt in the treatment of variceal hemorrhage. *Br J Surg* 82:1158–1164, 1995.
38. Laberge JM, Sonberg KA, Lake JR, et al: Two year outcome following transjugular intrahepatic portosystemic shunt for variceal bleeding: Results in 90 patients. *Gastroenterology* 108:1143–1151, 1995.
39. Crecelius SA, Soulen MC: Transjugular intrahepatic portosystemic shunts for portal hypertension. *Gastroenterology* 24:201–219, 1995.
40. Martin M, Zajko AB, Wright H, et al: Transjugular intrahepatic portosystemic shunt in the management of variceal bleeding: Indications and clinical results. *Surgery* 114:719–726, 1993.
41. Ring EJ, Lake JR, Roberts JP, et al: Using transjugular intrahepatic portosystemic shunts to control variceal bleeding before liver transplantation. *Ann Intern Med* 116:304–309, 1992.
42. Rosemurgy AS, McAllister EW, Kearney RE: Prospective study of a prosthetic H-graft portacaval shunt. *Am J Surg* 161:159–164, 1991.
43. Rosemurgy AS, McAllister EW: Small diameter prosthetic H-graft portacaval shunt, in Nyhus LH (ed): *Surgery Annual.* E Norwalk, Conn, Appleton & Lange, 1994, pp 101–113.
44. Rosemurgy AS: Small diameter interposition shunt, in Nyhus L, Baker R, Fischer J (eds): *Mastery of Surgery,* vol II. Boston, Little, Brown, 1997, 1301–1307.
45. Henderson JM, Fales FW: Continuous-flow fluorometry of low galactose concentrations in blood or plasma. *Clin Chem* 26:282–285, 1980.
46. Tygstrup N, Winkler K: Galactose blood clearance as a measure of hepatic blood flow. *Clin Sci* 17:1–9, 1958.
47. Schirmer WJ, Townsend MC, Schirmer JM, et al: Galactose clearance as an estimate of effective hepatic blood flow: Validation and limitations. *J Surg Res* 41:543–556, 1986.
48. Coldwell DM, Ring EJ, Rees CR, et al: Multicenter investigation of the role of transjugular intrahepatic portosystemic shunt in management of portal hypertension. *Radiology* 196:335–340, 1995.
49. Helton WS, Belshaw A, Althaus S, et al: Critical appraisal of the angiographic portacaval shunt (TIPS). *Am J Surg* 165:566–570, 1993.
50. Lind CD, Malisch TW, Chong WK, et al: Incidence of shunt occlusion or stenosis following transjugular intrahepatic portosystemic shunt placement. *Gastroenterology* 106:1277–1283, 1994.

51. Maynar M, Cabrera J, Pulido-Duque JM, et al: Transjugular intrahepatic portosystemic shunt: Early experience with a flexible trocar/catheter system. *AJR Am J Roentgenol* 161:301–306, 1993.
52. Spiess S, Matalon T, Jensen D, et al: Transjugular intrahepatic portosystemic shunt in non–liver transplant candidates: Is it indicated? *Am J Gastroenterol* 90:1238–1243, 1995.
53. Rypins EB, Sarfeh IJ: Small diameter portacaval Hgraft for variceal hemorrhage. *Surg Clin North Am* 70:395–404, 1990.
54. Ochs A, Rossle M, Haag K, et al: The transjugular intrahepatic portosystemic stent-shunt procedure for refractory ascites. *N Engl J Med* 332:1192–1197, 1995.
55. Catchpole RM: Transjugular intrahepatic portosystemic shunt (TIPS): Diagnostic and therapeutic technology assessment (DATTA). *JAMA* 273:1824–1830, 1995.
56. Polak JF: Transjugular intrahepatic portosystemic shunt: Building on experience. *Comment Radiol* 196:306–307, 1995.
57. Hermann RE, Henderson JM: Lessons and prospects. *Ann Surg* 221:459–468, 1995.
58. Conn HO: Transjugular intrahepatic portal-systemic shunts: The state of the art. *Hepatology* 17:148–158, 1993.
59. Radosevich PM, Laberge JM, Gordon RL: Current status and future possibilities of transjugular intrahepatic portosystemic shunts in the management of portal hypertension. *World J Surg* 13:785–789, 1994.
60. Rosemurgy AS, McAllister EW, Godellas CV, et al: The effect of partial portal decompression on portal blood flow and effective hepatic blood flow in man: A prospective study. *J Surg Res* 59:627–630, 1995.
61. Godellas CV, Fabri PJ, Knierim TH, et al: Hepatic function after portosystemic shunt. *J Surg Res* 52:157–160, 1992.
62. Zervos E, Goode S, Rosemurgy AS, et al: A prospective randomized trial comparing TIPS and peritoneovenous shunt in patients with intractable ascites. *Gastroenterology* 110:1368S, 1996.
63. Freeman RB, FitzMaurice SE, Greenfield AE, et al: Is the transjugular intrahepatic portacaval shunt procedure beneficial for liver transplant recipients? *Transplantation* 58:297–300, 1994.

CHAPTER 6

Current Surgical Management of Hepatic Cyst Disease

Bryce R. Taylor, M.D., F.R.C.S.(C.)

Professor of Surgery, University of Toronto; Chairman, Division of General Surgery; Associate Chair, Department of Surgery, University of Toronto; Head, Division of General Surgery, The Toronto Hospital, Toronto, Canada

Bernard Langer, M.D., F.R.C.S.(C)

Professor of Surgery, University of Toronto; Director, Hepatobiliary Program, Division of General Surgery, The Toronto Hospital and University of Toronto, Toronto, Canada

H epatic cysts often pose interesting problems for the general surgeon related to their widely divergent causes, varying manifestations, and the different interventional maneuvers available to treat them. Because of this variability, an understanding of the pathophysiology of hepatic cyst disease is mandatory for the general surgeon to act appropriately.

Cysts may be true or false, depending on the presence or absence of an epithelial lining (see Table 1). The most common lesion encountered is the simple or sporadic cyst, which presumably has similar origins to the lesions seen in adult and childhood polycystic disease. The second most common is the hydatid cyst, which must be handled in specific ways (to be detailed subsequently). The unusual neoplastic cysts can be either primary, e.g., cystadenoma, cystadenocarcinoma, cystic sarcoma, and occasionally squamous cell carcinoma, or secondary from any site, with primary tumors of the ovary or pancreas being most common.

Cystic dilatations may also occur in and around intrahepatic bile ducts, e.g., cases of Caroli's disease and its variants, duplication of the bile duct, or the more recently described peribiliary cysts.[1, 2] False cysts, that is, those without an identifiable epithe-

TABLE 1.
Classification of Hepatic Cysts

True
  Congenital
    Simple (sporadic)
    Polycystic disease
  Parasitic
    Hydatid (echinococcal)
  Neoplastic
    Primary
      Cystadenoma, cystadenocarcinoma, cystic sarcoma, squamous
        cell carcinoma
    Secondary
      From ovary, pancreas, colon, kidney, neuroendocrine
  Duct related
    Caroli's disease and variants
    Bile duct duplication
    Peribilirary cysts
False
  Spontaneous intrahepatic infarction/hemorrhage
  Posttraumatic hematoma
  Intrahepatic biloma

---

lial lining, may arise as a result of spontaneous hemorrhage within
the liver substance, from the development of posttraumatic hematoma, or secondary to intrahepatic bilomas as a complication of surgery.

TRUE CYSTS

CONGENITAL HEPATIC CYSTS

Congenital cysts are epithelial-lined structures that are benign, may
be single or multiple, and range in size from tiny to large. They
may occur either sporadically or as a component of adult or childhood polycystic disease. Their prevalence varies up to 0.3% in autopsy series[3] and up to 17 per 100,000 abdominal explorations according to a Mayo Clinic surgical report in 1974.[4] The theories of
pathogenesis of these cysts are many and include failure of
intralobular bile ducts to fuse with interlobular bile ducts (as a result of failure of normal degeneration of embryonic bile duct-
ules[5, 6] or obstruction of aberrant bile ducts[7]), malformations of

foregut epithelial cells,[8] and more recently, the so-called vascular disruption phenomenon[9] in which cysts may develop because of anomalies of perfusion to developing organs.

The Simple Cyst

In the past, general surgeons have frequently encountered simple cysts at surgery for other reasons and have usually wisely left them untouched; this incidental surgical finding has now been transferred to the ambulatory care setting in which abdominal US examination has too often become part of the primary physician's physical examination. Consequently, asymptomatic cysts are discovered, and surgeons are consulted about their possible surgical treatment.

The majority of simple cysts, regardless of size, are asymptomatic and require no treatment. Because complications are more frequent in larger cysts (greater than 8 cm in diameter), it may be prudent to periodically monitor them with US because growth even in the absence of symptoms may mandate surgical intervention because of increasing concerns about either complications or the presence of a cystadenoma. It is uncommon, however, to note increasing size of an asymptomatic cyst. Such cysts usually contain clear colorless fluid, and occasionally the fluid may be bile stained and point to a biliary communication with cystic contents.

Larger cysts may become symptomatic because of their size and thus cause upper abdominal pain, aching, discomfort, early satiety, or obstructive symptoms such as nausea and vomiting. In these cases, the examining physician and frequently the patient will note hepatomegaly and an accompanying mass. Even previously asymptomatic cysts may become complicated as a result of spontaneous hemorrhage,[10, 11] secondary bacterial infection,[10, 12] torsion of a pedunculated cyst, rupture into the peritoneal cavity, or biliary obstruction.

Diagnosis in asymptomatic cases is generally made initially by US examination. A reliable ultrasonographer will usually distinguish a cyst from other important hepatic space-occupying lesions such as hemangioma, adenoma, focal nodular hyperplasia, and a variety of tumors. Although US is the most available and useful technique, limitations occur when a large cyst of 12 cm or greater is being monitored for size evaluation. At this diameter, subtle differences are more easily measured by CT scanning. Computed tomography is also very useful in the follow-up evaluation of multiple cysts in the liver. These are seen as low-attenuation, smooth-walled, homogeneous structures that contain fluid demarcated by few or no septations[13] (Fig 1). Calcification is not identified in the walls of the cyst, and any heterogeneity of fluid contents, thickening of the wall, or irregularity of the lining should immediately call into question the diagnosis of a simple cyst and suggest hemorrhage, infection, or neoplasia.[14, 15]

Magnetic resonance imaging appears to be useful in differentiating cysts and hemangiomas larger than 1 cm[16, 17] and, in particular, may identify intracystic hemorrhage.[18] Because US and CT are the simplest and most reliable diagnostic tools, the use of radionuclide liver scanning (cysts appear as "cold" areas) and angiography is limited.

TREATMENT.—Most asymptomatic cysts can simply be monitored radiologically, and if after 2 to 3 years they remain unchanged, they can be ignored. However, those that are increasing in size or cause cyst-related symptoms as described earlier should be actively treated. Many methods have been described, including simple aspiration with or without injection of sclerosing solutions,[19–22] evacuation and external drainage, internal drainage with cyst jejunostomy,[23] wide unroofing, and varying degrees of liver resection.[24]

The fundamental objectives of surgery are decompression of the cyst(s) and prevention of recurrence, and consequently many of these modalities are not used currently; simple aspiration is fre-

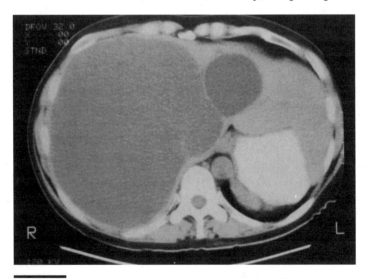

FIGURE 1.
Abdominal CT scan of simple hepatic cysts in a 45-year-old woman.

quently followed by recurrence, external drainage by infection, and internal cyst jejunostomy by closure of the anastomosis and septic complications. Instillation of sclerosing solutions has been enthusiastically adopted in some centers,[19-22, 25] but long-term data regarding recurrence rates are unavailable.

Wide unroofing of a symptomatic cyst with careful oversewing and marsupialization of the edges satisfies the principles of surgery best.[26-28] Seventeen of the 22 patients treated in this way in the Toronto series[27] had excellent results with no complications; however, 4 of the remaining 5 patients treated by either external or Roux-en-Y drainage suffered septic complications. Laparotomies required for such decompressions are usually limited, but in larger cysts and those that are located posterolaterally or superiorly access may necessitate a very long and painful incision; for this reason, laparoscopic methods have been used in recent years because they can achieve the same objectives of wide unroofing or fenestration without the use of a debilitating incision.[29, 30] In fact, some have used laparoscopic US for improved intraoperative clarity,[31] which along with direct examination can identify abnormalities such as epithelial irregularity and biliary communications. Because an experienced laparoscopic surgeon can perform wide unroofing via the minimal-access surgery route, the results should be equal to open surgery. Whichever access is used, the excised cyst wall must be carefully examined pathologically, and that left behind must be visualized in its entirety to rule out neoplasia and biliary communication. The results of wide unroofing are excellent with respect to allaying symptoms and preventing recurrence.

Complicated cysts should be treated by using the same principles, with attention to the specific cause of the complication. If the cyst is infected, temporary external drainage may be required after wide unroofing; if cystic fluid is bile stained, any visible communication with the biliary system can be oversewn with fine sutures.

Polycystic Disease

Childhood polycystic disease occurs in a macroscopically normal liver and consequently has no surgical implications. It affects both the liver and kidneys and consists of thin-walled cysts containing clear fluid that are lined by columnar or cuboidal epithelium. Those children who survive and do not succumb to renal failure frequently eventually contract congenital hepatic fibrosis.

Adult polycystic liver disease, on the other hand, may have significant clinical consequences that require surgical management.

This is an autosomal dominantly transmitted disease that unlike the childhood variety, produces multiple macrocystic lesions throughout the liver. Cysts contain clear fluid secreted by bile duct epithelium, and Von Meyenburg complexes (periportal clusters of rounded biliary channels[32]) are commonly found. Patients with this disease may have cysts in many organs, including the kidneys, spleen, pancreas, ovaries, and lungs.[33] The incidence is higher in women than in men and appears to increase with age. Approximately half those patients with polycystic liver disease have accompanying renal involvement, and about 20% also have intracranial arterial aneurysms.

The clinical picture of patients with adult polycystic disease is initially a painless, enlarged liver with little or no change in liver function. Because the rate of growth of the cysts is slow, patients may be able to carry on relatively normally for years. Eventually, however, they may complain of severe abdominal pain from bleeding into a cyst, or complications may develop from progressive fibrosis, cyst enlargement, parenchymal atrophy, and obstruction to portal and vena caval blood flow.[10] These may include portal hypertension and bleeding esophageal varices, ascites and dependent edema, intracystic hemorrhage, infection, and rupture. Because many patients with polycystic kidneys are now undergoing renal transplantation, more patients with coexisting polycystic livers are surviving into later life and suffering such complications of their liver disease.

Diagnostic modalities are similar to those for simple cysts[34] (Fig 2), but therapeutic maneuvers are more complicated. Patients who have significant symptoms because of a mass effect can improve if enough cystic tissue can be removed. This may be easy if there is one or more very large dominant cyst that can be unroofed. Partial liver resection may also be beneficial if the cyst distribution is asymmetric and the majority of functioning liver tissue can be preserved. The operation of "fenestration," which involves multiple unroofing of small cysts, is often only temporarily effective because of the fibrosis that occurs between cysts and the frequent occurrence of troublesome ascites after that procedure.[35-39] Although eventual symptomatic relief was obtained by Farges and Bismuth[38] in 13 patients, massive ascites developed in 5 postoperatively and recurrence of hepatomegaly in 2, thus emphasizing that positive results are frequently transient.

Other than for unroofing a single large dominant cyst, laparoscopic therapy probably has no role to play in the management of

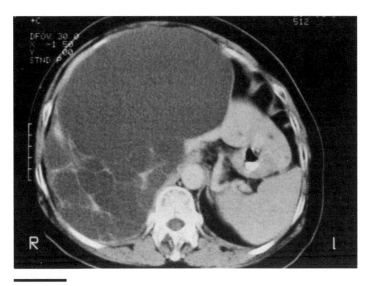

FIGURE 2.

Abdominal CT scan of a 35-year-old patient with polycystic liver disease. Note one dominant cyst overlying many septated cystic areas posteriorly.

polycystic liver disease, even though attempts have been reported.[40]

In those situations in which polycystic liver disease is accompanied by significantly deteriorating liver function or the complications of portal hypertension, orthotopic liver transplantation is the treatment of choice[41, 42] (Fig 3). Results of liver replacement in selected cases are excellent, with good long-term correction of liver function without recurrence of the cystic disease. Klupp et al.[42] described ten patients who had undergone liver transplantation, five of whom had simultaneous kidney transplants. All nine survivors had relief of their debilitating symptoms related to both size of the liver and its deteriorating function.

PARASITIC CYSTS (ECHINOCOCCAL)

Hydatid cysts of the liver are uncommon in North America and Northern Europe, but they are still frequently seen in endemic areas such as the Mediterranean countries. Increased travel and immigration have raised the profile of this unusual problem throughout North America, and physicians need to be aware of its clinical features, appropriate diagnostic methods, and management options. Hydatid disease is caused by one of two types of tapeworm: *Echinococcus granulosus,* which produces the common macrocystic disease, and *Echinococcus multilocularis,* which leads to a particularly aggressive, but fortunately uncommon type of infiltrating disease in humans.

The life-cycle of *E. granulosus* (see Fig 4) begins with the adult worm residing in the intestine of the primary or definitive host, which is usually the dog in the pastoral variety and the wolf or fox in the sylvatic variety. The eggs of the worm are then excreted in the stool by the definitive host and are ingested by an intermediate (or secondary) host, usually sheep or cattle or, in the Northern hemisphere, moose, caribou, or reindeer. The ingested embryo penetrates the small bowel wall and travels via the portal circulation to the liver where it develops into the disease-producing larval form. Most larvae develop into hydatid cysts in the liver,[43] but others occasionally pass through and create cysts in other organs such as the lung, spleen, bone, kidney, muscle, and brain. Cysts may develop over a long period of time, which explains why North American surgeons often see older patients with the initial symptoms of a disease that they acquired years previously. The life cycle of the parasite is completed when a primary host (i.e., dogs or, in the case of the arctic, wolves and foxes) eats organs of an infected secondary host. Humans become infected essentially as an "accidental" secondary or intermediate host when young children contact infected dogs and ingest shed ova, which ultimately cause the same organic cystic development seen in the secondary hosts.[44]

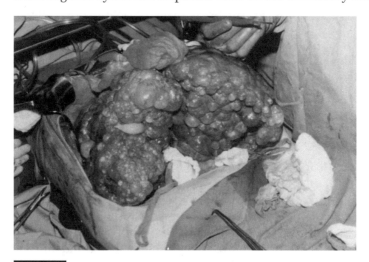

FIGURE 3.
Liver transplant procedure in a young woman with total hepatic replacement by polycystic disease accompanied by deteriorating liver function.

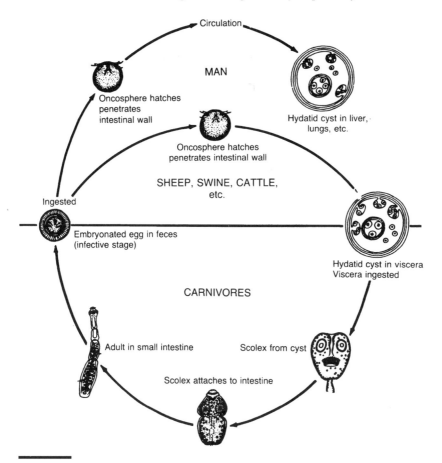

FIGURE 4.
Life cycle of *Echinococcus granulosus.* (Courtesy of McCreery PB, Nelson GS: Larval cestode infections, in Strickland GT (ed): *Hunter's Tropical Medicine,* ed 6. Philadelphia, WB Saunders, 1984, p 774.)

Once in the liver, the larvae and the host together form a hydatid cyst that contains elements of both host and parasite. The outer pericyst is formed by reactive fibrous and compressed liver from the host. The inner parasite-derived layers consist of a laminar membrane and a single-cell layer of germinal epithelium that is responsible for reproduction by the generation of brood capsules, which may separate to form daughter cysts, and the production of protoscolices, which float in the cyst fluid and constitute what is referred to as "hydatid sand." These protoscolices are the embryonic form of the parasite and, if ingested by a primary host, grow into an adult worm in its intestinal lumen. Protoscolices may also develop into new cysts if spilled into the peritoneal or pleural cavities by spontaneous rupture, percutaneous instrumentation, or surgery.

Cysts progressively enlarge to produce symptoms, and sometimes by means of free rupture into the peritoneal cavity or into the biliary tree they cause significant complications. Communication with the biliary tract is found in at least 25% of patients, and this may result in bile staining and/or infection of cyst contents.[45–47] As a result of chronic inflammation, calcification is often noted in the wall of a mature cyst.[48] As cysts enlarge, they become surrounded by large branches of portal and hepatic veins, a situation that has significant implications for surgical approaches.

Clinical Manifestations

Many hydatid cysts may remain asymptomatic, even into advanced age. They produce symptoms either by mass effect similar to simple cysts or by complications such as intraperitoneal leakage, infection, or biliary obstruction. Minor leakage of fluid into the peritoneal cavity may produce little pain and only a mild acute allergic reaction with urticaria. In the case of major rupture, there are often acute peritoneal signs and associated acute anaphylaxis that may be fatal if not treated promptly with adrenaline and steroids. Chronic abdominal discomfort and pain may be related to either the increasing size of the cyst or presumably the inflammatory reaction in adjacent viscera. Some patients have fever when infection develops because of communication with the biliary tract. In others, rupture of daughter cysts into the common bile duct may produce obstructive jaundice.

The diagnosis is often made in asymptomatic patients when US and/or CT scanning is undertaken for other reasons (Fig 5). The radiologic signs are quite typical, and because of calcification seen in the wall, cysts may even be identified on plain films of the abdomen. Ultrasound may identify a cystic structure with contents of variable density caused by daughter cysts and hydatid sand.[49, 50] Computed tomography is very helpful because it details multiple septa and loculations, as well as daughter cysts. Although MRI will adequately demonstrate the cysts, there is no clear advantage to using this particular modality. If a patient has jaundice and the clinical and imaging features of hydatid disease, endoscopic retrograde cholangioportography (ERCP) may be both diagnostic and therapeutic[51] (Fig 6).

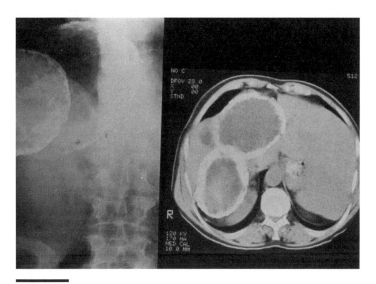

FIGURE 5.

Right, abdominal CT examination of a patient with two calcified hepatic echinococcal cysts. **Left,** plain film of the same patient demonstrating diffuse calcification in the cyst wall.

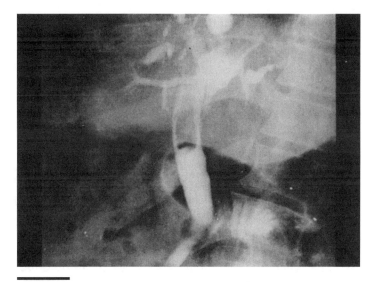

FIGURE 6.

Endoscopic retrograde cholangioportography in a patient with echinococcal disease and jaundice. A large daughter cyst may be noted in the common hepatic duct. This was successfully extracted endoscopically.

Routine bloodwork is not helpful in a specific way, but it may be reflective of a complicated infected cyst when patients demonstrate leukocytosis, abnormal liver test results, and eosinophilia.[46, 47] Serologic studies are useful both for diagnosis and for follow-up after treatment. The indirect hemagglutination test (IHA) is positive in over 80% of patients, and the complement fixation test is also available.[44, 52] Other modalities include the enzyme-linked immunosorbent assay and the latex fixation test. In the past, skin testing (Casoni's test) was also used but has largely been abandoned because it is both inaccurate and potentially dangerous as a result of possible severe local allergic reactions.

Treatment

The objectives of management of hydatid disease are active treatment of major complications if they occur, eradication of the parasite if alive, and protection of the host against dissemination of the parasite.

COMPLICATIONS.—The three significant complications of parasitic cysts are free rupture with or without anaphylaxis, infection of the cyst(s), and biliary obstruction. Free rupture necessitates immediate care of the patient with appropriate measures to combat the allergic reaction, surgical evacuation and sterilization (to be described subsequently), and adequate drainage, as well as supportive care. The same surgical treatment is used for infected cysts, although preliminary percutaneous drainage and antibiotics may be required in an acutely ill patient. Biliary obstruction should be treated with ERCP, with sphincterotomy and evacuation of common bile duct debris and daughter cysts followed later by appropriate treatment of the primary disease in the liver. Shemesh et al.[51] described four patients whose jaundice cleared promptly after endoscopic evacuation of daughter cysts in the common duct. In fact, they suggested that in high-risk patients with biliary obstruction, ERCP may be the only treatment required.

ELECTIVE SETTING.—If the patient is seen in an elective setting, options for treatment include medical, percutaneous, or open surgical.

Medical Treatment of Hydatid Disease.—Many anecdotal reports in the literature have appeared since 1977 and have described effective management of echinococcosis with the anthelmintics mebendazole and albendazole.[15, 53, 54] These medications are effective in only 30% to 50% of patients with liver cysts and have significant gastrointestinal, neurologic, hematologic, and hepatic toxicity. Currently accepted indications for anthelmintic administration include the primary treatment of lung hydatids, which lack a well-developed fibrous capsule and therefore allow better drug penetration. If a liver cyst ruptures spontaneously or spillage occurs during surgical evacuation, the drugs may be useful in preventing the disastrous effects of transcoelomic dissemination. Other groups have suggested that scolices may be effectively killed by these oral medications and, if not used as primary treatment, may be useful as a preoperative measure in decompressing the cyst before intervention.

If the cysts are asymptomatic and have a completely calcified wall, they may in fact be dead and contain no active scolices. In this case, especially if the IHA is negative or low, the cyst should be treated conservatively because the likelihood of complications is minimal.

Percutaneous Aspiration and Alcohol Injection Therapy.—A number of enthusiastic reports have appeared in the radiologic literature in the last 10 years that have described percutaneous aspiration of hydatid cyst contents and immediate instillation of alcohol or other scolicidal agents for sterilization. In one report from Giorgio et al.,[55] 16 patients were treated with percutaneous aspiration and injection of 95% alcohol. Aspirated fluid was replaced with 50% of the aspirated volume, and although viable scolices were found at every first puncture, the second puncture usually performed in approximately 1 week demonstrated live scolices in only 60%. This was accompanied by decreased serologic titers in many of the patients. Follow-up US showed either folded membranes or a solid pattern considered to be "a normalization" of the liver. Before North American physicians treating this disease become overly enthusiastic about nonsurgical injection and aspiration therapy, however, it must be realized that the European reports frequently describe younger patients with unilocular cysts, which are much more amenable to such limited interventions. In the North American setting, especially in complicated patients with many deep-seated cysts, this technique should only be considered when standard surgical approaches are believed to be too risky. The uncommon but serious complication of anaphylaxis during aspiration must be remembered.

Surgery.—Surgery is indicated for the complications of hydatid disease, for symptomatic patients, and for asymptomatic patients in whom attempts at treatment with systemic anthelmintics have failed.

The principles of surgery include eradication of the parasite by complete mechanical removal, followed by sterilization of the cyst

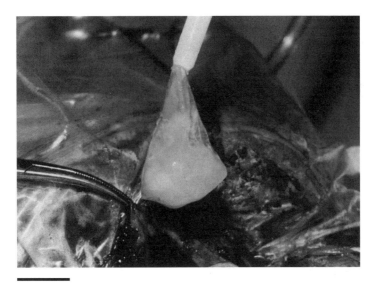

FIGURE 7.

With protection of the peritoneal cavity by using a sterile polyethylene drape sutured to the fibrous pericyst, a large daughter cyst is suctioned from the hydatid cyst during open surgery.

and at the same time meticulous protection of the peritoneal cavity. The specific techniques include cyst aspiration and evacuation, cystopericystectomy, and liver resection.

The first technique requires that all cyst contents, including free fluid, laminar membrane, germinal epithelium, daughter cysts, and biliary sand, be removed with care. After a careful laparotomy identifies the exact location of the hepatic cyst disease and correlates it with the CT and US findings, the peritoneal cavity is protected by suturing a polyethylene drape to the fibrous pericyst.[46] The tough pericyst is then incised, and mechanical removal is achieved by suction (Fig 7). We use a high-powered suction machine designed for therapeutic abortions, which will easily aspirate thick laminar membrane and daughter cysts that would otherwise clog conventional suction machines. The opening is then enlarged, and direct examination of the cyst wall allows more complete removal of the laminar membrane. A variety of scolicidal agents have been recommended for use in sterilizing the remaining cavity; however, complications have been reported with almost all scolicidals, including formalin,[56, 57] hydrogen peroxide,[58] silver nitrate, hypertonic saline,[59] and absolute alcohol.[57, 60, 61] We use only a simple cetrimide solution instilled for 10 minutes, followed by irrigation with normal saline. A meticulous search for biliary communications in the wall of the cyst must be made in every case, and if found, they must be oversewn. If the cyst is deep seated, it can be filled with saline and closed without drainage. If present on the surface, it should be unroofed, carefully oversewing the edges to control any compressed bile ducts or vessels.

Most patients require no drainage, but if a significant biliary communication is identified or the cyst is infected, a temporary closed suction drain should be used. Omentum is rarely required to help fill in a residual cavity. Of the 18 patients with uncomplicated hydatid cysts treated surgically in our series, 11 had simple evacuation, sterilization, and closure, and only 1 suffered a postoperative complication.[46] On the other hand, 4 of the 5 patients treated in the initial part of the series by external drainage (who later would have had sterilization and closure) went on to septic complications and longer hospital stays. We therefore concluded that only infected cysts or those containing bile-stained material require drainage.

Other operations have been described for the treatment of symptomatic hydatid cyst disease. Hepatic resection may be the treatment of choice if the cysts are in an area of the liver easily amenable to resection and considerable liver replacement has occurred (such as segments 2/3, [see Fig 8,A and B]). Formal liver resection, however, is not usually necessary. Another radical surgical approach is cystopericystectomy,[62–64] an operation designed to remove not only the parasite and its germinal epithelium but also the host-derived fibrous pericyst as well. Because a developing and growing cyst often becomes intimate to underlying large intrahepatic venous branches, this particular operation may lead to significant intraoperative bleeding, particularly with deep-seated cysts. Elhamel[63] reported that radical removal was achieved in two thirds of the 45 cysts he found in his 23 patients, but he emphasized that the correct plane of clearage must be found to avoid bleeding. Belli's group[62] found that use of the Pringle maneuver facilitated safe removal of 49 cysts in their 31 patients. Although some have reported this operation enthusiastically, it has not been widely adopted.

If biliary communications persist, bile collections or chronic bile fistulas may develop postoperatively. These can be treated by endoscopic stenting or sphincterotomy to decrease resistance to bile flow and promote ultimate closure of the fistula, which may form from the base of the cyst through a drain site. Postoperative complications include sepsis, biliary leak, and late recurrence of the hepatic and/or intraperitoneal cysts.

Hydatid disease may recur many years after treatment. Patients should be monitored for possible recurrence of cysts by serologic testing and imaging studies if serologic findings suggest recurrence.

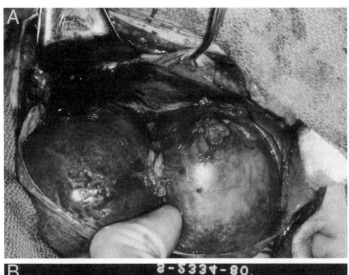

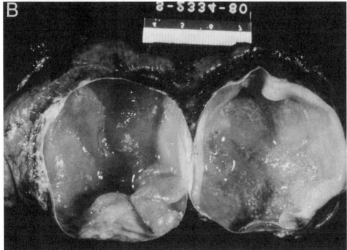

FIGURE 8.

A, bilobed hydatid cyst in segments 2 and 3 of the liver seen at laparotomy. **B,** resected (via a left lateral segmentectomy) specimen with cysts opened.

NEOPLASTIC CYSTS

Benign cystadenomas of the liver, although uncommon, are seen most often in young or middle-aged women.[65-68] Although they produce the same mass-related symptomatology as congenital cysts, they may contain clear or turbid mucinous fluid or blood and may demonstrate on CT scanning the warning signs of irregularities or septations within the cyst wall. An otherwise innocuous-looking cyst that is multiloculated should raise suspicion.

Pathologic diagnosis is made by section of the interior of the suspicious cyst. This may prove difficult inasmuch as polypoid projections from the cyst wall may be subtle and are not found in all cystadenomas. Characteristic microscopic findings are cuboidal or low columnar lining cells on a deeper layer of dense mesenchymal stroma,[67] but these may not be present in all parts of the cyst wall. Careful inspection of the whole wall of any cyst is therefore required. The appropriate surgical treatment of a cystadenoma is complete removal of the wall of the cyst, which can usually be accomplished by enucleating the cyst from surrounding liver after the appropriate plane is developed. The Lahey Clinic group used this technique in four patients[69] and found it particularly useful in large, centrally placed lesions. If cystadenocarcinoma is suspected, treatment should be formal liver resection.[70, 71]

On occasion, squamous cell carcinomas have been reported to develop in congenital cysts lined predominantly by stratified squamous epithelium.[72, 73] From the limited literature available, it appears that these lesions have a particularly bad prognosis.

In addition to these primary neoplastic cysts, malignant cystic tumors from the ovary and pancreas may produce secondary cystic lesions in the liver. Spread from other intra-abdominal carcinomas or sarcomas may degenerate and produce "cavitating" lesions that mimic cysts. Good-quality imaging studies should allow the identification of solid components in the wall.

DUCT-RELATED CYSTS

Various forms of choledochus cyst, including the more generalized Caroli's disease, may produce cystic-like lesions in the liver. In addition, duplication of the bile duct, a rare congenital abnormality, may produce confusing radiologic findings. More recently, peribiliary cysts in the liver have been reported to be associated with an interesting US finding known as "hilar multicystic echo complex."[1] These peribiliary cysts are thought to arise from cystic dilatation of pre-existing intrahepatic peribiliary glands and occur in livers with portal hypertension (related to cirrhosis, hepatocellular carcinoma, portal vein obstruction, etc), adult polycystic disease, and systemic infection. These findings do not appear to have any surgical significance but may draw attention to one of the associated causes.

FALSE CYSTS OF THE LIVER

Collections of cysts in the liver that are not lined by identifiable epithelium are by definition "false" cysts.[7] They may be caused by spontaneous intrahepatic infarction and/or hemorrhage or, more commonly, by trauma. No specific treatment is required for posttraumatic intrahepatic hematomas unless the hematoma enlarges. Although bile collections occur postoperatively or posttraumatically outside the liver, intrahepatic bilomas arising after cholecystectomy have been reported.[74]

REFERENCES

1. Baron RL, Campbell WL, Dodd GD: Peribiliary cysts associated with severe liver disease: Imaging-pathologic correlation. *AJR Am J Roentgenol* 162:631–636, 1994.
2. Terada T, Minato H, Nakanuma Y, et al: Ultrasound visualization of hepatic peribiliary cysts; a comparison with morphology. *Am J Gastroenterol* 87:1499–1502, 1992.
3. Feldman M: Polycystic disease of the liver. *Am J Gastroenterol* 29:83, 1958.
4. Sanfelippo PM, Beahrs OH, Weiland LH: Cystic disease of the liver. *Ann Surg* 179:922, 1974.
5. Lathrop DB: Cystic disease of the liver and kidney. *Pediatrics* 24:215, 1959.
6. Longmire WP, Mandiola SA, Gordon HE: Congenital cystic disease of the liver and biliary system. *Ann Surg* 174:711, 1971.
7. Jones WL, Mountain JC, Warren KW: Symptomatic non-parasitic cysts of the liver. *Br J Surg* 61:118, 1974.
8. Dardik H, Glotzer P, Silver C: Congenital hepatic cyst causing jaundice. *Ann Surg* 159:585, 1964.
9. Avni EF, Rypens F, Donner C, et al: Hepatic cysts and hyperechogenicities; perinatal assessment and unifying theory on their origin. *Pediatr Radiol* 24:569–572, 1994.
10. Grunfeld JP, Albouze G, Jungers P, et al: Liver changes and complications in adult polycystic kidney disease. *Adv Nephrol* 14:1, 1985.
11. Wilcox DM, Weinreb JC, Lesh P: MR imaging of a hemorrhagic hepatic cyst in a patient with polycystic liver disease. *J Comput Assist Tomogr* 9:183, 1985.
12. Bourgeois N, Kinnaert P, Vereerstraeten P, et al: Infection of hepatic cysts following kidney transplantation in polycystic disease. *World J Surg* 7:629, 1983.

13. Levine E, Cook LT, Grantham JJ: Liver cysts in autosomal dominant polycystic kidney disease: Clinical and computed tomographic study. *AJR Am J Roentgenol* 145:229, 1985.

14. Hattner RS, Englestad BL: Diagnostic imaging and quantitative physiological function using radionuclide techniques in gastrointestinal disease, in Sleisinger MD, Fordtran JS (eds): *Gastrointestinal Disease.* Philadelphia, WB Saunders, 1983, p 1667.

15. Schroder R, Robotti G: New aspects in the management of alveolar echinococcosis involving the liver. *World J Surg* 10:968, 1986.

16. Li W, Nissenbaum MA, Stehling MK, et al: Differentiation between hemangiomas and cysts of the liver with nonenhanced MR imaging: Efficacy of T2 values at 1.5T. *J Magn Reson Imaging* 3:800–802, 1993.

17. Goldberg MA, Hahn PF, Saini S, et al: Value of T1 and T2 relaxation times from echoplanar MR imaging in the characterization of focal hepatic lesions. *AJR Am J Roentgenol* 160:1011–1017, 1993.

18. Vilgrain V, Silbermann O, Benhamou JP, et al: MR imaging in intracystic hemorrhage of simple hepatic cysts. *Abdom Imaging* 18:164–167, 1993.

19. Andersson R, Jeppsson B, Lunderquist A, et al: Alcohol sclerotherapy of non-parasitic cysts in the liver. *Br J Surg* 76:254, 1989.

20. Bean WJ, Rodan BA: Hepatic cysts: Treatment with alcohol. *AJR Am J Roentgenol* 144:237, 1985.

21. Kairaluoma MI, Leiononen A, Stahlberg M, et al: Percutaneous aspiration and alcohol sclerotherapy for symptomatic hepatic cysts. *Ann Surg* 210:208, 1989.

22. Trinkl W, Sassaris M, Hunter FM: Nonsurgical treatment for symptomatic nonparasitic liver cyst. *Am J Gastroenterol* 80:907, 1985.

23. Wittig JH, Burns R, Longmire WP: Jaundice associated with polycystic liver disease. *Am J Surg* 136:383, 1978.

24. Fernandez M, Cacioppo JC, Davis RP, et al: Management of solitary nonparasitic liver cyst. *Am Surg* 50:205, 1984.

25. Guglielmi A, Veraldi GF, Fulan F, et al: The Echo-guided percutaneous therapy of dysontogenetic liver cysts. *Ann Ital chir* 62:13–17, 1991.

26. Belcher HV, Hull NC: Non-parasitic cysts of the liver: Report of three cases. *Surgery* 65:427, 1969.

27. Litwin DEM, Taylor BR, Greig P, et al: Nonparasitic cysts of the liver: A case for conservative surgical management. *Ann Surg* 205:45, 1987.

28. Henne-Brins D, Klomp HJ, Kremer B: Non-parasitic liver cysts and polycystic liver disease. Results of surgical treatment. *Hepatogastroenterology* 40:1–5, 1993.

29. Ooi LL, Cheong LH, Mack PO: Laparoscopic marsupialization of liver cysts. *Aust N Z J Surg* 64:262–263, 1994.

30. Watson DI, Jamieson GG: Laparoscopic fenestration of giant posterolateral liver cyst. *J Laparoendosc Surg* 5:255–257, 1995.

31. Marvik R, Myrvold HE, Johnsen G, et al: Laparoscopic ultrasonogra-

phy and treatment of hepatic cysts. *Surg Laparosc Endosc* 3(3):172–174, 1993.

32. Ishak KG: Fibropolycystic diseases of the liver, in *Hepatic Pathology Review Course,* vol 2. Washington, DC, Armed Forces Institute of Pathology, 1987.

33. Sherlock S: Cysts and congenital biliary abnormalities, in Sherlock S, Dodey J (eds): *Diseases of the Liver and Biliary System,* Oxford, England, Blackwell, 10th ed. Science, 1997, p 579.

34. Fred HL, Siddique I: Images in clinical medicine. Polycystic liver and kidney disease. *N Engl J Med* 333:31, 1995.

35. Lin TY, Chen CC, Wang SM: Treatment of non-parasitic cystic disease of the liver. A new approach to therapy with polycystic liver. *Ann Surg* 168:921, 1968.

36. Newman KD, Torres VE, Rakela J, et al: Treatment of highly symptomatic polycystic liver disease. *Ann Surg* 212:30, 1990.

37. Vauthey JN, Maddern GJ, Kolbinger P, et al: Clinical experience with adult polycystic liver disease. *Br J Surg* 79:562, 1992.

38. Farges O, Bismuth H: Fenestration in the management of polycystic liver disease. *World J Surg* 19:25–30, 1995.

39. Blyth H, Ockenden BG: Polycystic disease of kidneys and liver presenting in childhood. *J Med Genet* 8:257, 1971.

40. Jeng KS, Yang FS, Kao CR, et al: Management of symptomatic polycystic liver disease: Laparotomy adjuvant with alcohol sclerotherapy. *J Gastroenterol Hepatol* 10:359–362, 1995.

41. Uddin W, Ramage JK, Portmann B, et al: Hepatic venous outflow obstruction in patients with polycystic liver disease: Pathogenesis and treatment. *Gut* 36:142–145, 1995.

42. Klupp J, Bechstein WO, Lobeck H, et al: Orthotopic liver transplantation in therapy of adjuvant polycystic liver disease. *Chirurg* 67:515–521, 1996.

43. McGreevy PB, Nelson GS: Larval cestode infections, in Strickland GT (ed): *Hunter's Tropical Medicine,* ed 6. Philadelphia, WB Saunders, 1984, p 771.

44. Weller PF: Case records of the Massachusetts General Hospital: Case 45-1987. *N Engl J Med* 317:1209, 1987.

45. Howard RJ, Hanson RF, Delaney JP: Jaundice associated with polycystic liver disease. *Arch Surg* 111:816, 1976.

46. Langer JC, Rose D, Keystone JS, et al: Diagnosis and management of hydatid disease of the liver. *Ann Surg* 199:412, 1984.

47. Pitt HA, Korzelius J, Tompkins R: Management of hepatic echinococcosis in Southern California. *Am J Surg* 152:110, 1986.

48. Grabbe E, Kern P, Heller M: Human echinococcosis: Diagnostic value of computed tomography. *Tropenmed Parasitol* 32:3, 1981.

49. Beggs I: The radiology of hydatid disease. *AJR Am J Roentgenol* 145:639, 1985.

50. Hussain S: Diagnostic criteria of hydatid disease on hepatic sonography. *J Ultrasound Med* 4:603, 1985.

51. Shemesh E, Klein E, Abramowich D, et al: Common bile duct obstruction caused by hydatid daughter cysts—management by endoscopic retrograde sphincterotomy. *Am J Gastroenterol* 81:280, 1986.
52. Chemtai AK, Bowry TR, Ahmad Z: Evaluation of five immunodiagnostic techniques in echinococcosis patients. *Bull World Health Organ* 59:767, 1981.
53. Davis A, Pawlowski ZS, Dixon H: Multicentre clinical trials of benzimidazolecarbamates in human echinococcosis. *Bull World Health Organ* 64:383, 1986.
54. Bekhti A, Schaaps J-P, Capron M, et al: Treatment of hepatic hydatid disease with mebendazole: Preliminary results in four cases. *BMJ* 2:1047, 1977.
55. Giorgio A, Tarantino L, Francica G, et al: Unilocular hydatid liver cysts: Treatment with US-guided, double percutaneous aspiration and alcohol injection. *Radiology* 184:705, 1992.
56. Aggarwal AR, Garg RL: Formalin toxicity in hydatid liver disease. *Anaesthesia* 38:662, 1983.
57. Meymerian E, Luttermoser GW, Frayha GJ, et al: Host-parasite relationships in echinoccosis X: Laboratory evaluation of chemical scolicides as adjuncts to hydatid surgery. *Ann Surg* 158:211, 1963.
58. Belghiti J, Perniceni T, Kabbej M, et al: Complications of peri-operative sterilization of hydatid cysts of the liver. *Chirurgie* 117:343, 1991.
59. Wanninayake HM, Brough W, Bullock N, et al: Hypernatremia after treatment of hydatid. *British Medial Journal Clinical Research Edition* 284:1302–1303, 1982.
60. Pissiotis CA, Wander JV, Condon RE: Surgical treatment of hydatid disease. *Arch Surg* 104:454, 1972.
61. Polo JR, Garcia-Sabrido JL: Sclerosing cholangitis associated with hydatid disease. *Arch Surg* 124:637, 1989.
62. Belli L, Aseni P, Rondinara GF, et al: Improved results with pericystectomy in normothermic ischemia for hepatic hydatidosis. *Surg Gynecol Obstet* 163:127, 1986.
63. Elhamel A: Pericystectomy for the treatment of hepatic hydatid cysts. *Surgery* 107:316, 1990.
64. Moreno Gonzales E, Rico Selas P, Martinez B, et al: Results of surgical treatment of hepatic hydatidosis: Current therapeutic modifications. *World J Surg* 15:254, 1991.
65. Edmondson HA: Tumors of the liver and intrahepatic bile ducts, in *Atlas of Tumor Pathology,* Section VII, Fascicle 25. Washington, DC, Armed Forces Institute of Pathology, 1958.
66. Ishak KG, Willis GW, Cummins SD, et al: Biliary cystadenoma and cystadenocarcinoma. *Cancer* 38:322, 1977.
67. Akwari OE, Tucker A, Seigler HF, et al: Hepatobiliary cystadenoma with mesenchymal stroma. *Ann Surg* 211:18, 1990.
68. Iemoto Y, Kondo Y, Nakano T, et al: Biliary cystadenocarcinoma diagnosed by liver biopsy performed under ultrasonographic guidance. *Gastroenterology* 84:339, 1983.

69. Pinson CW, Munson JL, Rossi RL, et al: Enucleation of intrahepatic biliary cystadenomas. *Surg Gynecol Obstet* 168:535, 1989.
70. Berjian RA, Nime F, Douglas HO, et al: Biliary cystadenocarcinoma: Report of a case presenting with osseous metastasis and a review of the literature. *J Surg Oncol* 18:305, 1981.
71. Devine P, Ucci AA: Biliary cystadenocarcinoma arising in a congenital cyst. *Hum Pathol* 16:92, 1985.
72. Nieweg O, Slooff MJ, Grond J: A case of primary squamous cell carcinoma of the liver arising in a solitary cyst. *HPB Surg* 5(3):203–208, 1992.
73. Pliskin A, Cualing H, Stenger RJ: Primary squamous cell carcinoma originating in congenital cysts of the liver. Report of a case and review of the literature. *Arch Pathol Lab Med* 116:105–107, 1992.
74. Dasgupta TK, Sharma V: Intrahepatic bilomas—a possible complication of cholecystectomy? *Br J Clin Pract* 46(4):272–273, 1992.

CHAPTER 7

Current Status of Stroma-Free Hemoglobin

A.G. Greenburg, M.D., Ph.D.
Department of Surgery, The Miriam Hospital and Brown University, Providence, Rhode Island

H.W. Kim, Ph.D.
Department of Surgery, The Miriam Hospital and Brown University, Providence, Rhode Island

The perception by the public of an unsafe blood supply has become a major driver in the field of red cell substitutes. Whether the risk of transmission of infectious disease is overexaggerated or overappreciated is unclear. The current level of activity in "red cell substitutes" is a response to the worldwide perception of problems with banked blood. It is tempting to digress and provide an exact historical perspective of the field to note the fascinating evolution of key concepts and their identification and solution relative to the necessary technological developments. The basic concept of a red cell substitute and its benefits and liabilities were identified early, whereas addressing and solving issues and making useful solutions took much longer. One goal of this rather detailed summary of the field is to provide a broad reference framework for comparing and contrasting the various products from any number of vantage points.

Hemoglobin solutions were infused into humans as early as 1918.[1] Although not intended as a red cell substitute, some of the properties of a very crude solution were identified. In no way was this a pure hemoglobin, and it was very likely contaminated with stroma—residual red cell membrane—and bacteria, which could account for most if not all of the reported observations. A wonderful summary[3] of the potential for hemoglobin-based red cell substitutes written in 1937 proposed and demonstrated the potential and efficacy for these solutions. It is a most prophetic piece and provides a very nice perspective on the field. A later history[3] that updates developments after 1937 demonstrates the role of technology in resolving some of the vexing problems and chronicles many of the intellectual contributions brought about by the expanding knowledge base of all aspects of hemoglobin as an oxygen carrier.

INDICATIONS

Hemoglobin-based red cell substitutes, often generically called stroma-free hemoglobins because of the relationship of stroma to early toxicity, come in many forms and compositions and can be used or are proposed for use in many clinical situations. The key properties of blood served by these solutions are maintenance of volume and provision of oxygen to tissues. It is well recognized that most if not all of the clinical "shock states" are essentially poor tissue perfusion; many of the organ dysfunction syndromes after restoration of vascular volume and perfusion relate to a period of absolute or relative hypoxia possibly complicated by the effects of reperfusion. It is not the intent of this review to argue the pros and cons of various resuscitation algorithms in terms of composition and/or volume; if the basic underlying mechanism is one of deficient tissue perfusion, a solution with oxygen-carrying capacity and delivery capability may be effective in resuscitation for hypoperfusion.[4, 5]

Originally considered as field-ready, shelf-storable oxygen-carrying resuscitation fluids, hemoglobin-based red cell substitutes have also been proposed for additional applications. Table 1 is a partial list of possible applications of stroma-free hemoglobin solutions. It is critical to note that most of the applications rely on the oxygen-carrying properties and some on the other physical properties of these solutions that may have a beneficial effect such as acellularity, viscosity, or oncotic pressure.

Whether a single solution could be effective in all applications remains to be seen; the tailoring of a solution's composition for purposes of achieving a specific objective is a reasonable concept. In the current era—various clinical phase I, II, and III proposals and studies—a single solution may be generally applicable; developers are proposing evaluation for a specific application to build on once efficacy and safety are demonstrated.

Acceptance of hemoglobin-based red cell substitutes will in some way offset and perhaps minimize the transfusion of allogeneic or even autologous red cells. This precept is certainly valid inasmuch as "transfusion avoidance" has become a desirable general objective. Many of the current algorithms and paradigms for

TABLE 1.
Areas of Potential Application for Hemoglobin-based Red Blood
Cell Substitutes

Volume resuscitation
   After trauma
   As a result of disease
   As a result of surgical blood loss
Immediate transfusion when no compatible blood is available
Hemodilution
   Exchange or hypervolemic
Ischemic rescue
   Occlusive cerebral vascular accident
   Myocardial infarction, cardioplegia
Unanticipated blood loss
In vivo organ perfusion
Organ preservation
Hematopoietic activity in conjunction with erythropoietin
Improving the tissue Po_2 of tumors to augment radiation
   sensitivity
Microcirculatory research
Culture media
Veterinary use

the use of red cell transfusion should change once these potentially useful solutions have established a record of safety and demonstrated efficacy.[6–8]

GENERAL ISSUES

The general categories of red cell substitutes intended as oxygen carriers are shown in Table 2. Many are still in the laboratory or research phase, have not been clinically tested, and will not be discussed in detail. The perfluorocarbons are now in clinical testing as diluents for hemodilution models and cardioplegia and have shown promise. The liposome models appear to have significant problems, both a short intravascular half-life and significant activation of the host defense system—two areas that if unresolved could limit any widespread application.

Hemoglobin solutions, whether considered pharmaceuticals or biologicals, continue to have problems despite great advances. Efficacy and safety are the primary measures for licensure of a new agent. In the area of safety, many aspects of the manufacturing may be relevant to toxicity or side effects. Failure in the manufacturing process could be responsible for enhancing the product's toxicity when it should be minimized. Some aspects of the production process of concern are shown in Table 3, which is provided as a general reference framework helpful when evaluating data regarding the clinical usefulness and applicability of the proposed solutions.

Many of the areas of concern have been previously detailed.[9] It is important to note that the issues surrounding the ADME—absorption, distribution, metabolism, and excretion—of modified hemoglobin solutions are not clear and, in fact, often quite confusing. The exact mechanisms of some observed toxicity or side effects are neither readily nor generally appreciated. For example, the role of nitric oxide (NO), carbon monoxide, and heme oxygenase in mediating or reflecting the responses to infusions of hemoglobin solutions is not clear. More critically, if any of the factors noted in Table 3 are also operative, these detailed biochemical observations could be secondary to a contaminant and not necessarily the hemoglobin or modified hemoglobin solution.[10, 11]

It is also noted that studies on the microcirculation and microphysiology of hemoglobin-based red cell substitutes may fail to have a relationship to whole-animal models because of scant data relating microcirculatory effects to global oxygen delivery physiology, the clinically necessary reference context. Table 4 lists many of the characteristics that could be used to compare the solutions currently in clinical testing. That so many physical and physical-chemical characteristics are needed and required to describe these unique products is no surprise. The difficulty in comparing prod-

---

TABLE 2.
Candidate Red Blood Cell Substitutes

Hemoglobin based
  Chemically modified tetramers
  Conjugated
  Polymerized, oligomerized
Perfluorocarbon emulsions
Modified red blood cells
Encapsulated hemoglobin-liposome
Liposome-embedded heme
Metalloporphyrins

TABLE 3.

Areas of Potential Concern for Hemoglobin-based Red Blood Cell Substitutes

Source
  Synthetic
  Biological
    Outdated red cells
    Bovine
    Recombinant hemoglobin
      Bacteria
      Yeast
      Mammal
Purity of starting material
Sterilization of starting product
Storage modality
Storage stability
Contaminants
  Bacteria
  Virus
  Endotoxin
  Antigens
  Proteins
Chemical modification
  Toxicity: side effects of
    Modified hemoglobin molecule
    Modifier and its metabolism
    Iron overload
    Residuals in solution
    Physiology of the distribution and metabolism of modified
      molecule

ucts at all levels with respect to product characteristics becomes an enormous and complicated task even before consideration of model differences.

"Models" in this context refer to the experimental design applied to the reported phase I and II studies. "Top load" or replacement infusions in escalating doses and at various rates have been used. These variables add new dimensions and thereby increase complexity and complicate interpretation for differences when trying to evaluate and compare the various solutions. Additionally,

TABLE 4.
Physical Properties and Characteristics of Hemoglobin-based Red
Blood Cell Substitutes

Hemoglobin source
P_{50}
Cooperativity
Viscosity
Hemoglobin concentration
   Oxygen-carrying capacity
Methemoglobin concentration
pH
Electrolytes
  Excipient
  Ca^{2+}
  Mg^{2+}
Molecular distribution
  <64 kd
   64 kd
  >64 kd
Oncotic pressure
Additives
Metabolites
No binding
Oxygen radicals
"Purity"

---

sorting out the model characteristics as causative for side effects
or toxicity is further complicated by the physiology. An obvious
example would be the physiologic response to a top load of an on-
cotically active solution: some effects will be due to the volume
expansion and some to the product itself. Separating these effects
is critical and indeed most difficult.

PRECLINICAL ISSUES

Concern about iron overload continues with regard to hemoglobin-
based red cell substitutes. The concern is perhaps overly perceived,
for the amount of iron in 500 mL of a 10% hemoglobin solution
should be that of a unit of red cells. If the ADME is truly different
for these substitutes and more free iron is available, the concern is
probably valid. The interaction of iron and bacteria in sepsis is

also noted; there is little doubt of the relationship of iron in infection.[12] What can be questioned is the relevance of this information to hemoglobin-based red cell substitutes and their use in septic subjects.

Hemoglobin-based solutions have been used as adjuncts in the management of the hypotension of sepsis. It has been demonstrated that a small amount of purified and unmodified stroma-free hemoglobin—not a likely candidate for red cell substitute use because of a short half-life and poor oxygen delivery capability—can effectively reverse the hypotension of endotoxic shock in a rat model.[11, 13] Moreover, addition of the NO synthase inhibitor L-NAME to the model results in improved survival. The mechanism of action appears to be NO scavenging by hemoglobin, which allows a small dose of NO synthase inhibition to be very effective.[14] This interaction is both interesting and intriguing for it opens new pathways for application as well as a means of exploring the physiology in detail.

An intriguing corollary of this observation rests in the possibility that red cells also scavenge NO when infused in a septic patient, thereby effecting a positive hemodynamic response. In recent observations (unpublished), this appears to be the case. Septic patients transfused with red cells improve their overall hemodynamic state without evidence of change in preload that could result from the volume load given. Although only a preliminary observation for now, appreciating this physiology could have a long-term benefit in the design of new therapies.

It has been reported by some groups that solutions in testing exert a significant vasoactive effect by increasing peripheral vascular tone and thus an increase in blood pressure. This chapter is not the forum for arguing the efficacy of increased systemic blood pressure as part of the treatment of hypovolemia and poor tissue perfusion. A beneficial effect may actually be associated with blood pressure elevation in the treatment of some forms of hypovolemia. At the present time it is not a generally accepted paradigm, especially because the debate over resuscitation now includes minimal volume options. Elevated blood loss is associated with increased blood pressure during resuscitation, and the need for supplemental transfusion after definitive therapy is likely to be increased. If the observed increase in mean arterial pressure is real, it is necessary, by experimental design criteria, to have models in which pressors have been used in a reference group to differentiate the volume, oxygen delivery, and pressure effects of the delivered agent. Perhaps complex models to operationalize them are essential if the source of efficacy is to be defined. It must be recalled that improving systemic oxygen delivery is at the cost of increased cardiac work, and one would like to optimize cardiac efficiency without pushing it beyond an acceptable level.[15]

The mechanism of vasoconstriction remains a mystery. It has been proposed that NO interacts with hemoglobin in the endothelial cell–smooth muscle cell interface. This hypothesis assumes that the hemoglobin solution leaks to the interstitium and permits this to occur. There are many interesting aspects of this hypothesis, not the least of which is the fact that not all solutions have this effect nor are the doses at which the effect is seen necessarily equal with all solutions. In some products the effect is seen with doses as low as 50 mg/kg, and in others it is not observed at 500 mg/kg.[16–20]

To these investigators, long in the field, the basic physiologic issues are of great importance. The real challenge is to explain why the effects occur and to design a solution to prevent them. This is, of course, the essential problem of safety for any new agent. That NO is involved in the process is accepted—NO is so ubiquitous, it must be. How the NO mechanism is activated and mediated is the essential problem. It is recognized that combination therapy in the management of shock and resuscitation (e.g., adding an NO synthase blocker) may have unintended consequences that should be considered.

In summary, hemoglobin-based red cell substitutes have many beneficial aspects. In addition, there are some very interesting questions concerning physiology and mechanisms of toxicity and side effects. The limiting factor for approval will of course be the frequency and intensity of these events balanced against the efficacy or benefit that is provided.

EFFICACY

How is the efficacy of a substitute for red cells defined? The easy answer would refer to the models that established the effectiveness of transfusion with red cells and repeat those studies. Alas, that would be a futile exercise, for there is scant solid scientifically based literature to support or document the efficacy of red cell transfusions.[6, 7] Direct or surrogate measures of efficacy will need to be invoked, and as yet they have not appeared, nor are those that have appeared been universally accepted. This poses both a challenge and a dilemma for the field in general and investigators in particular. Absent a universally accepted end point, how can the solutions be assessed and eventually compared? One acceptable end point for defining the efficacy of these solutions could be transfusion avoidance. This generally accepted goal is based on the widely held perception of complications and toxicity associated with both allogeneic and autologous red cell transfusions. These complications include not only minor reactions, major incompatibilities resulting in death, and the transmission of infectious disease, but also an immunosuppressive effect associated with transfusion. The latter may be involved in increased infectious complications in surgical interventions and, as seen in some studies, earlier recurrence of cancer.[21, 22] Whether the red cell substitute solutions will have the same immunosuppressive effects is not yet known. Their use could obviate many of the logistic and tactical aspects of transfusion and thus minimize—but not eliminate—some of the current difficulties.

Efficacy in terms of oxygen delivery, avoidance of ischemic events, and decreased morbidity and mortality will, of necessity, be more difficult to establish. Large randomized trials, multi-institutional, would have to be mounted. These are frequently a nightmare to implement, and as the number of institutions grows, the risk of dilution in data collation and loss of adherence to protocol becomes a factor. These dangers are not unique to red cell substitute studies; they are really universal to all significant major clinical trials and could obfuscate the generation of a real answer.

Sham or no-treatment controls are perceived as ethically unacceptable in this general area. The standard reference solution for oxygen-carrying solutions is packed cells, and that must be the comparator. As red cell transfusions have become more specific and the transfusion decision more sophisticated, the general use of red cells has decreased. The concept of transfusion avoidance and other methods of ensuring safe tissue perfusion has caused shifts in practice. This is not to imply that the use of red cell transfusion is by any means standardized. One look at the Safe and Good Use of Blood in Surgery study[23] reveals a wide pattern of use for red cells and blood and blood products in different Western European countries for different surgical procedures. That such wide variation in product use persists implies that the underlying principles are not appreciated. At this point one could speculate that an available red cell substitute or even its testing would alter clinical behavior and bring about a more standardized approach. That desirable goal will require significant re-education to attain its end.

All the red cell substitutes currently in clinical evaluation will also require pharmacoeconomic analysis as a major part of the efficacy and benefit interpretation. If transfusion avoidance is the objective, this becomes a vital aspect of the data analysis.

It is not clear what the cost to manufacture red cell substitutes is or what the market cost will be. Once these unknowns are defined, a comparison to the cost of transfusion or transfusion avoidance in terms of morbidity, mortality, or other outcome measures is required. The "cost" of some of these adverse outcomes is also not apparent at this time, although some effort is being made to identify and quantitate them for comparison purposes.[24-26]

CURRENT STATUS

The real challenge here is to write a summary of the current status of the field as a balanced scientific discourse and not an analysis of the field from an investor viewpoint. That is no easy task, for few hard data and little information are readily available. Over the past few years, many international symposia dealing with "blood substitutes" have been the focus of attention. The most recent, the "VI International Symposium on Blood Substitutes," took place in Montreal in August 1996. With over 350 attendees and a combination of scientific presentations and posters, the field was rather broadly reviewed. This effort will be published in a special issue of *Artificial Cells, Blood Substitutes, and Immobilization Biotechnology* (Volume 25, 1997) and represents, I believe, a realistic update on developments in the field. The details of the interesting and intriguing research findings on the basic molecular structure and function of hemoglobin, its site-specific modification to enhance specific functionality, the basic physiology of oxygen delivery, and a host of other issues are discussed in these proceedings. Clearly there are future generations and variation in products that are being visualized and studied.

Intriguing among the various options are hemoglobin-based solutions that serve functions other than oxygen delivery and intravascular volume maintenance. These new molecules, and even liposomes, carry a host of enzymes and other active agents that may permit treatment of many of the associated biochemical defects of shock, hypoperfusion, hypoxia, and superoxide radical/free radical generation. Grounded in a more detailed and explicit understanding of the cellular and molecular biological basis of these events in sequence or isolation, these newer complex hemoglobin solutions are directed at correcting, mediating, or even modulating some of the detrimental aspects of the aforesaid conditions. These future-generation products are based on understanding the underlying physiologic mechanisms and could be significant advances in therapy.

Currently, six major companies are involved in various stages of testing hemoglobin-based red cell substitutes. They are listed in Table 5, along with brief product descriptions and an assessment of the state of clinical testing as of this writing (July 1997). Once the safety testing in escalating doses, phase I, has been achieved, each group has taken on a slightly different approach. Not all solutions are equal in hemoglobin concentration, and thus they will not have the same potential efficacy if efficacy is measured in oxygen delivery terminology. Somatogen, which is using a recombinant human hemoglobin produced by *Escherichia coli,* provides a 5% solution, whereas most of the others use 10% solutions. Approximately 50 g of hemoglobin is in a unit of packed red cells, and 500 mL of a 10% solution could be considered the oxygen-carrying equivalent of a unit of red cells. Of particular note is a report showing increased efficacy of an infused hemoglobin solution in comparison to lactated Ringer's control in normal subjects

TABLE 5.
Hemoglobin-based Solutions in Clinical Trial

Company	Product	Phase of Clinical Trial
Baxter	Human Hb 64 kd, α-α cross-link	Completed multiple I and II Approved for III in trauma
Northfield	Human Hb 128–526 kd, PLP modification and gluteraldehyde cross-link	Completed phase I and II, is in phase III
Enzon	Bovine Hb 64 kd, PEG	Phase I completed, some phase II
Biopure	Bovine Hb 64 kd, polymerized	Phase I completed, some phase II
Somatogen	Recombinant human Hb 64 kd	Phase I, phase II
Hemosol	Human Hb Oligimer, *O*-raffinose modification and cross-link 64–526 kd	Phase I, phase II

Abbreviations: Hb, hemoglobin; *PLP;* proteolipid protein; *PEG,* polyethylene glycol.

and doses to 45 g. The diffusion capacity of oxygen was increased in the subjects receiving hemoglobin solution, perhaps indicating better tissue perfusion.[27, 28] A similar study of efficacy in an animal shock resuscitation model showed the 5% solution of Somatogen to be more effective in restoring oxygen delivery physiology than was transfusion of fresh red cells.[29] These observations must be taken seriously, for they appear to reflect improvement in tissue perfusion with a solution less viscous than red cells and with a lower hemoglobin concentration. Whether these observations represent improved microcirculation perfusion or some other mechanism is not clear; in both cases, greater efficacy and efficiency are shown for the hemoglobin solutions than for lactated Ringer's solution or blood—a desirable physiologic outcome. Extrapolation to the clinical situation as potentially relevant must be guarded, for similar data will be most difficult to obtain in large clinical trials.

Some recent clinical trials have begun to look at hemoglobin solutions to increase tissue oxygenation and thus radiation sensitivity for hypoxic tumors.[30] This is a useful model, for the vascular autoregulation of a tumor may be different from that of normal tissue, and should the hemoglobin solution deliver oxygen to the tumor, it would become more radiosensitive. The key element of this model is the circulating half-life of the hemoglobin solution inasmuch as it may affect the timing of the radiation therapy. Such a paradigm shift, even if the trials are shown to be effective, could pose additional logistic problems for the care delivery system. Enzon is primarily involved in this area.

Northfield is in an extended phase II trial with increasing volumes of hemoglobin solutions.[31] Their end point has been transfusion avoidance or deferral, and the solution appears to be effective in decreasing transfusion requirements in the first 24 to 36 hours, but many of these patients subsequently receive transfusions before leaving the hospital. The real issue here is the efficacy measure of transfusion avoidance as compared with decreased transfusion exposure. Much of the outcome, of course, hinges on the indications for transfusion and what the trigger for a transfusion really is. In most studies it is a clinical judgment and not very scientifically defined. Absent that critical piece of data, the end points will still be viewed as "soft" and thus subject to interpretation. Absent low oxygen delivery—oxygen consumption data and measures of aerobic and anaerobic metabolism—this may be the best possible outcome measure.

Hemosol has completed a phase I trial with reasonable safety data and good pharmacokinetic data. At the higher doses, 40 g, abdominal pain was seen as a problem.[32] Although reversible with the use of smooth muscle relaxants, it remains a persistent and pesky side effect. Somatogen and Baxter have seen a similar problem[33, 34] and by further investigation traced the source to an NO phenomenon.[33] This primarily descriptive study sheds little light on the underlying physiologic mechanisms. Exactly how the esophagospasm is mediated and why NO modulation helps decrease it are still unanswered. That this problem, esophagospasm, has been reported for at least three products indicates a commonality of mechanism, even with hemoglobin solutions of different composition, source, and concentration. Hemosol is proceeding with an early phase II study in orthopedic patients, the goal being transfusion avoidance using a variation of autologous predeposit and hemodilution.

The proposed Baxter phase III trial for DCLHb is based in part on 71 patients who received doses up to 285 mg/kg in hemorrhagic states. The proposed study will compare 500- and 1,000-mL infusion of DCLHb with saline controls early in the intervention (within 30 to 60 minutes of emergency room arrival). In this trial, extrapolation from the previous study shows that some of the benefit will be attributed to the pressor effect and some to the low volume of resuscitation fluid used.[16, 34, 35] The end points are 28-day mortality primarily and a reduction in mortality, 48-hour mortality, and 24-hour lactate levels as secondary markers. This is an ambitious study and could yield useful data and information of general application. It is not clear whether the study is sufficiently large to address the end points sought. Differentiating the pressor and volume effects will be most difficult in this model and is perhaps vital to the end point analysis.

Historically, the "brass ring" for the application of red cell substitutes has been their potential for use in trauma and resuscitation; a solution useful in this area would have an impact and could potentially save lives and decrease trauma morbidity generally. For the commercial developers, this is a broad market area and certainly a legitimate goal from a business vantage. Attaining the ring is less easily accomplished than it is stated. Many developers have staked out segments of application that permit gradually increased doses until the amount/volume needed for trauma resuscitation is attained and will then begin testing and evaluating in this critical area. This is a solid, measured approach in view of the imponderables of the many issues previously noted.

Establishing valid end points for safety and efficacy remains a debatable topic. At this time, decreasing or eliminating transfusion of allogeneic blood is a reasonable goal but could be associated with as yet undefined morbidity in terms of altered oxygen delivery and tissue ischemia.

Another issue is the use of experimental blood replacement volume-expanding agents in the trauma victim/subject and the question of obtaining informed consent. This is really a difficult ethical issue and one that has been referred back to local institution review boards for adjudication. Absent specific federally defined guidelines, the local boards can approve the use of these agents if they are comfortable with the product and the protocol. Although a generally positive move to advance the field, there are issues regarding the ability of the local board to assess the information provided when even many experts in the field disagree.

As the transfusion paradigm changes and pressure for the use of more autologous red cells mounts, exploring hemoglobin-based substitutes in models of hemodilution begins to make sense. Hemodilution may be the more cost-effective mode of autologous blood harvest, and it provides whole blood for reinfusion in the postoperative period. Use of a hemoglobin-based red cell substitute is most reasonable, for it provides adequate oxygen delivery, improves microcirculatory flow, and could prevent various ischemic events that surround surgical procedures and contribute to morbidity.

The use of hemoglobin solution as ischemic rescue or organ preservation is also under investigation. As a mechanism of ensuring adequate tissue support in warm ischemia (e.g., angioplasty, organ revascularization) or as part of futuristic resuscitation models for myocardial infarction or occlusive cerebral vascular insults (salvage of the penumbra tissue), these solutions hold great promise. Indeed, ischemic rescue is really a variation of resuscitation inasmuch as the underlying mechanisms of tissue injury are very similar.

SUMMARY

Hemoglobin-based red cell substitute solutions continue to advance and stride toward application in many areas. Closely linked to issues of the undesirable effects of red cell transfusion is the pressure to have a useful shelf-storable red cell substitute for application in trauma or other areas of acute blood loss or the need to improve tissue oxygenation. Despite difficulties in demonstrating or even defining efficacy and proving and establishing safety, a number of products are moving through the regulatory rigors.

This exposition has covered many of the relevant issues the modern clinician should be aware of when evaluating the literature and potential application of these interesting and intriguing solutions.

The future for red cell substitutes is bright. Obviously, there are other competing technologies, and as the medical transfusion paradigm changes—avoidance being a primary objective and autologous red cells a major consideration—the use of these options could influence the acceptance of red cell substitutes. Clearly, all approaches will need full evaluation. In a recent work exploring in a preliminary fashion the potential areas of application of red cell substitutes in surgery, it was established that fully 60% of the current use of allogeneic or autologous blood could be replaced with one of the current solutions.[8]

Expanded clinical trials will bring new information and a depth of understanding and appreciation of problems heretofore unrecognized. The need to address the interface issue for routine laboratory tests is just one other area in which a multidisciplinary approach is required to solve what could be a limiting factor. As molecular engineering of hemoglobin molecules yields proteins with specific function, more specific applications can be identified and subsequently tested. Coupled with an ever-expanding knowledge base of the physiology of the shock state, additives can be included to create more specifically defined treatment options coupled with the oxygen-carrying capacity and volume-expanding characteristics of these fluids. With the perspective of over a quarter-century involvement in the area, it is safe to say that the goal of a hemoglobin-based red cell substitute is in sight and will be realized.

REFERENCES

1. Sellards AW, Minot GR: Injection of hemoglobin in man and its relation to blood destruction with special reference to the anemias. *J Med Res* 34:469–494, 1916.
2. Amberson WR: Blood substitutes. *Biol Rev* 12:48–86, 1937.
3. Winslow RM: *Hemoglobin-Based Red Cell Substitutes.* Baltimore, Johns Hopkins University Press, 1992, pp 7–15.
4. Barber AE, Shires GT: Cell damage after shock. *New Horizons* 4:161–167, 1996.
5. Cornwell EE, Kennedy F, Rodriguez J: The critical care of the severely injured patient—I, assessing and improving oxygen delivery. *Surg Clin North Am* 76:959–969, 1996.
6. Spence RK: Surgical red cell transfusion practice policies. *Am J Surg* 170:2S–15S, 1995.

7. American Society of Anesthesiologists Task Force on Blood Component Therapy: Practice guidelines for blood component therapy. *Anesthesiology* 84:732–747, 1996.
8. Greenburg AG, Kim HW: Use of donor blood in the surgical setting: Potentials for applications of blood substitutes. *Artif Cells Organs Immobil Biotechnol,* 25:25–29, 1997.
9. Greenburg AG: Alternatives to conventional uses of blood products. *Crit Care Med* 14:325–351, 1992.
10. Morterlini R: Interactions of hemoglobin with nitric oxide and carbon monoxide, in Winslow RM, Vandegriff KD, Intaglietta M (eds): *Blood Substitutes, New Challenges.* Boston, Birkhauser, 1996, pp 74–98.
11. Greenburg AG, Kim HW: Nitrosyl hemoglobin formation in-vivo after intravenous administration of a hemoglobin based oxygen carrier in endotoxemic rats. *Artif Cells Blood Substit Immobil Biotechol* 23:271–276, 1995.
12. Ward CG, Bullen JJ, Rogers HJ: Iron and infection: New developments and their implications. *J Trauma* 41:356–364, 1996.
13. Kim HW, Hughes JK, Breiding PS, et al: Nitric oxide scavenging: An alternative therapeutic approach to nitric oxide synthesis inhibition in nitric oxide mediated hypotension of sepsis. *Surg Forum* 45:67–69, 1994.
14. Kim HW, Brieding PS, Greenburg AG: Enhanced modulation of hypotension in endotoxemiatry: Concomitant nitric oxide synthesis inhibition and nitric oxide scavenging. *Artif Cells Blood Substit Immobil Biotechol,* 25:153–162, 1997.
15. Greenburg AG: A physiologic basis for red blood cell transfusion decisions. *Am J Surg* 170:44S–48S, 1995.
16. Malcom DS, Hamilton IN, Schultz SC, et al: Characterization of the hemodynamic response to intravenous diaspirin cross linked hemoglobin solution in rats. *Artif Cells Blood Substit Immobil Biotechnol* 22:91–107, 1994.
17. Katsuyama SS, Cole DJ, Drummond JD, et al: Nitric oxide mediates the hypertensive response to a modified hemoglobin solution (DCLHb™) in rats. *Artif Cells Blood Substit Immobil Biotechnol* 22:1–7, 1994.
18. Maiar RV, Bulger EM: Endothelial changes after shock and injury. *New Horizons* 4:211–223, 1996.
19. Simoni J, Simoni G, Lox CD, et al: Evidence for the direct inhibition of endothelin-1 secretion by hemoglobin in human endothelial cells. *ASAIO J* 41:641–651, 1995.
20. Gulati A, Sharma A, Singh G: Role of endothelin in the cardiovascular effects of diaspirin cross linked and stroma reduced hemoglobin. *Crit Care Med* 24:137–147, 1996.
21. Klein HG: Allogeneic transfusion risks in the surgical patient. *Am J Surg* 170:21S–26S, 1995.
22. Greenburg AG: Benefits & risks of blood transfusion in surgical patients. *World J Surg* 20:1189–1193, 1996.

23. Sircia G, Giovanetti AM, McClelland B, Fracchia GN et al (eds): *Safe & Good Use of Blood in Surgery (SANGUIS).* Luxembourg, European Commission, Office of Publications of the European Communities, 1994.

24. AuBuchon JP: Cost-effectiveness of preoperative autologous blood donation for orthopedic and cardiac surgeries. *Am J Med* 101:38S–42S, 1996.

25. D'Ambra MN, Kaplan DK: Alternatives to allogeneic blood use in surgery: Acute normovolemic hemodilution and preoperative autologous donations. *Am J Surg* 170:49S–52S, 1995.

26. DeAndrade JR: Prudent strategies for red blood cell conservation in orthopedic surgery. *Am J Med* 101:16S–21S, 1996.

27. Hughes GS, Antal EJ, Locker PK, et al: Physiology and pharmacokinetics of a novel hemoglobin based oxygen carrier in humans. *Crit Care Med* 24:756–764, 1996.

28. Hughes GS, Yancy EP, Albrecht R, et al: Hemoglobin-based oxygen carrier preserves submaximal exercise capacity in humans. Clin Pharmacol Ther 53:434–443, 1995.

29. Siegel JM, Fabian M, Smith JA, et al: The use of recombinant hemoglobin solution in reversing lethal hemorrhagic hypovolemic oxygen debt shock. *J Trauma,* 42:199–212, 1997.

30. Suit H: Tumor oxygenation and radio sensitivity in blood substitutes: Physiologic basis of efficacy, in Winslow RM, Vandegriff KD, Intaglietta M (eds): *Blood Substitutes: Physiological Basis of Efficacy.* Boston, Birkhauser, 1995, pp 187–199.

31. Gould SA, Noon EE, Moore FA, et al: The clinical utility of human polymerized hemoglobin as a blood substitute following trauma and emergent surgery. *J Trauma* 39:157A, 1995.

32. Greenburg AG, Magnin AA, Pliura DH, et al: Human hemoglobin based blood substitutes (abstract). Presented at the Consensus Conference on Autologous Transfusion, Edinburgh, 1995.

33. Murray JA, Ledlow A, Launspach JE, et al: The effects of recombinant human hemoglobin on esophageal motor function in humans. *Gastroenterology* 109:1241–1248, 1995.

34. Przybelski RJ, Daily EK, Kisicki JC, et al: Phase I study of the safety and pharmacologic effects of diaspirin cross linked hemoglobin solutions. *Crit Care Med* 24:1993–2000, 1996.

35. Swan SK, Halsterson CE, Collins AJ, et al: Pharmacologic profile of diaspirin cross linked hemoglobin in hemodialysis patients. *Am J Kidney Dis* 26:918–923, 1995.

CHAPTER 8

Current Management of Acute Respiratory Distress Syndrome

Joseph P. Minei, M.D.

Associate Professor, Department of Surgery, The University of Texas–Southwestern Medical Center, Director of Trauma and Surgical Critical Care, Parkland Health and Hospital Systems, Dallas, Texas

Philip S. Barie, M.D.

Associate Professor, Department of Surgery, Cornell University Medical College, Director, Ann and Max A. Cohen Surgical Intensive Care Unit, The New York Hospital–Cornell Medical Center, New York

A cute respiratory distress syndrome (ARDS) is the stereotypical response of the lung to injury from many disparate causes rather than a collection of discrete entities.[1, 2] The incidence of ARDS varies depending on the risk factors involved, but it ranges from 1.5 to 5.3 cases per 100,000 population per year.[3] Many conditions have been associated with ARDS in surgical patients, some of which are direct insults to the pulmonary parenchyma whereas others are the pulmonary response to a systemic insult. However, the risk of ARDS developing from a discrete insult is difficult to define. Garber et al.[3] undertook a systematic literature overview to evaluate the risk factors associated with ARDS. In the articles reviewed, a definition of ARDS was given in only 49%, whereas a definition of the potential risk factor was provided in only 64% of the reports. Twenty-three percent of the published papers provided neither a definition of ARDS nor a definition of risk factors. It is difficult to draw inferences from such pervasive poor descriptions of large clinical series. Moreover, epidemiologic associations do not prove causation. Despite this, the strongest evidence supporting a cause-effect relationship between ARDS and individual risk factors was identified for sepsis, major trauma, multiple transfusions, aspiration of gastric contents, pulmonary contusion, pneumonia, and smoke inhalation. Substantially weaker evidence exists for an association between ARDS and disseminated intravascular coagulation, fat embolism, and cardiopulmonary bypass. Virtually all of the analyzed studies failed to report a relative risk (odds ratio), and furthermore, they failed to control for confounding variables. In a recent review[4] the aforementioned high-risk criteria accounted for almost 80% of ARDS cases. Sepsis appears to be the most prevalent risk factor and accounts for 30% to 40% of all cases of ARDS.[5-7] Conversely, the risk of ARDS developing in patients with sepsis has been variably reported to be between 10% and 25%.[8-10]

Whatever the causal relationship between a risk factor and ARDS might be, the result is the same: pulmonary edema despite low or normal pulmonary microvascular pressures, hypoxemia caused by intrapulmonary shunting and alveolar flooding, and markedly decreased lung compliance. The spectrum of injury is broad, and the injury itself is heterogeneous. Not every patient will have severe disease or progress to the chronic, fibroproliferative form of the syndrome.[11] Because of this variability, the diagnosis is usually based on clinical criteria, but the enormous variability of definitions used in the literature makes comparisons among studies difficult.

Diagnostic criteria for ARDS have historically been arbitrary[11] (hypoxemia, variously defined as a partial pressure of oxygen in arterial blood [Pao_2] of less than 70 mm Hg on an inspired oxygen fraction [Fio_2] of 0.4 or greater or an alveolar-arterial oxygen gradient [$Pao_2 - Pao_2$] greater than 300; radiographic evidence of pulmonary edema; pulmonary wedge pressure less than 18 mm Hg; reduced lung compliance, usually less than 30 mL/cm H_2O) and not reflective of the disparate causes and variable symptoms now recognized as characteristic of ARDS. The lack of descriptive detail in the literature also extends to definitions and the underlying severity of illness. The lung injury score,[12] which can be calculated for every patient (Table 1), describes pulmonary injury reproducibly and accurately. A score greater than 2.5 defines ARDS, whereas a score of 2.5 or less reflects less severe forms of acute lung injury. The development of ARDS is rarely subtle from the clinician's perspective. The patient should have a clearly defined clinical risk factor and is almost always in severe respiratory distress or overt respiratory failure. Hypoxemia may precede clinically apparent pulmonary edema, and treatment to reduce edema (diuretics, ultrafiltration) may not improve hypoxemia. Derangements in gas exchange may occur in the absence of radiologic changes. Tachypnea

TABLE 1.
Lung Injury Score for the Diagnosis of Acute
Respiratory Distress Syndrome

Parameter	Points
Chest radiograph	
No infiltrate	0
One quadrant	1
Two quadrants	2
Three quadrants	3
Four quadrants	4
Hypoxemia: Pao_2/Fio_2	
>300	0
225–299	1
175–224	2
100–174	3
<100	4
PEEP	
≤5	0
6–8	1
9–11	2
12–14	3
≥15	4
Static compliance (when available)	
≥80	0
60–79	1
40–59	2
20–39	3
≤19	4

Note: The lung injury score (LIS) is obtained by dividing the sum of the points scored by the number of components used. Adult respiratory distress syndrome is defined as LID greater than 2.5.
Abbreviation: PEEP, positive end-expiratory pressure.
(Courtesy of Sessler CN, Bloomfield GL, Fowler AA: Current concepts of sepsis and acute lung injury. *Clin Chest Med* 17:213–235, 1996.)

is often the first sign, particularly in nonventilated patients. As the injury progresses, dyspnea develops as interstitial edema progresses to alveolar flooding, with resultant atelectasis and decreased functional residual capacity (FRC). Shunt (the proportion of pulmonary artery blood flow that perfuses unventilated parenchyma) develops from progressive loss of functional alveolar units as a result of loss of surfactant, atelectasis, and alveolar flooding. The acute hypoxic pressor response (hypoxic vasoconstriction) decreases perfusion of the underventilated alveoli in an attempt to restore abnormal ventilation-perfusion ($\dot{V}_A/\dot{Q}$) matching toward normal. In compensation, substantial diversion of blood flow from underventilated units to areas with higher $\dot{V}_A/\dot{Q}$ matching can result in overperfusion of these "normal" units relative to their ventilation, paradoxically producing poor $\dot{V}_A/\dot{Q}$ matching (low $\dot{V}_A/\dot{Q}$ areas or venous admixture).

Simultaneously, as a result of activation of the systemic inflammatory response, adherence of neutrophils to pulmonary capillary endothelium results in microvascular occlusion of significant portions of the pulmonary vascular bed.[3] Microvascular occlusion can also occur from microembolization of particulate debris if hepatic reticuloendothelial host defenses are impaired or as a consequence of fibrin deposition in coagulopathy. This results in significant increases in areas of lung that are being ventilated but not perfused. This "dead-space" ventilation (V_{DS}) is routinely expressed as a fraction of tidal volume (V_T, i.e., V_{DS}/V_T), and is typically about 0.3. Thus in normal ventilation, approximately 30% of each breath goes to filling dead space, most of which (about 2 mL/kg) is the anatomical dead space of the large airways. In ARDS, because of the pathophysiology just noted, V_{DS}/V_T can rise to 0.7 to 0.8, and hence 70% to 80% of each breath goes to filling dead space. This increase in V_{DS}/V_T results in a geometric increase in the work of breathing and rapid venilatory failure with a need for mechanical ventilatory support.

Hypoxemia associated with ARDS does not respond to supplemental oxygen because of these deranged $\dot{V}_A/\dot{Q}$ relationships. Microvascular injury leads to pulmonary hypertension, loss of hypoxic vasoconstriction, and further derangements in $\dot{V}_A/\dot{Q}$ matching. Although pulmonary edema is the hallmark of ARDS, gas exchange abnormalities often do not correlate with the degree of edema and may be unrelated to fluid accumulation. Alterations in lung mechanics tend to be marked in comparison to those characteristic of hydrostatic edema. Although peribronchial edema can cause bronchoconstriction, the release of humoral mediators has a direct effect on airway tone. Increased airway reactivity can persist long afterward in survivors.

A decreasing Pa_{O_2} or increasing $P_{A_{O_2}} - Pa_{O_2}$ is not a good marker of worsening lung injury in ARDS. In the setting of shunt, the partial pressure of oxygen in mixed venous blood ($P\bar{v}_{O_2}$), which may be low, can subsequently lower Pa_{O_2} because there is direct admixture of venous with arterial blood through shunt units and O_2 extraction from ventilated alveoli is already maximal and cannot compensate. A low $P\bar{v}_{O_2}$ may result from low Pa_{O_2}, low hemoglobin concentration, low cardiac output, or increased oxygen consumption (V_{O_2}). Therefore, mixed venous gas tensions are an indicator of ongoing tissue hypoxia and/or hypoperfusion. This is a critical issue because death in patients with ARDS is usually associated not with respiratory failure but with multiple organ dysfunction syndrome, which has been linked to hypoperfusion.

TREATMENT OF ACUTE RESPIRATORY DISTRESS SYNDROME WITH POSITIVE END-EXPIRATORY PRESSURE

Mechanical ventilation with high levels of positive end-expiratory pressure (PEEP) has been the mainstay of therapy for ARDS for nearly 30 years.[13] Positive end-expiratory pressure increases FRC by alveolar recruitment. As FRC rises above critical closing volume (CCV), a greater percentage of perfused lung is being ventilated, which yields a decreased shunt fraction. Oxygenation can usually be supported, but the morbidity—barotrauma (pneumothorax or pneumomediastinum, with a reported incidence of about 5%), reduced cardiac output,[14] difficulty supporting renal function, and pneumonia—has been perceived to be high. The situation was reluctantly accepted for many years because the lesion was incompletely understood, mechanical ventilators were unsophisticated, support of gas exchange was the overriding concern, and there was little else to offer. Mortality remained high (at least 60%).[15]

Therapy with PEEP may cause physiologically significant decreases in cardiac output that must be avoided[14] because there is no clinical advantage to therapy if overall oxygen delivery (D_{O_2}) is reduced. The effect of PEEP on cardiac output may occur at a number of levels. First, PEEP may decrease preload by increasing intrathoracic pressure, thereby decreasing venous return. Second, PEEP may affect cardiac contractility by altering ventricular septal mechanics and anatomy. This effect is in part the result of the pulmonary hypertension and increased afterload on the right heart. Because the use of PEEP can lead to cardiac and pulmonary complications, many strategies have been used to "optimize" PEEP. Reports abound that advocate "maximal," "least," "best," and "optimal" PEEP.[11] "Optimal" PEEP can be variously defined as the least amount of PEEP that will achieve oxygenation, the maximal amount of PEEP that can be tolerated without compromised hemodynamics,[1, 2] or the amount of PEEP that maximizes Do_2. Others have described optimal PEEP as maximized total lung compliance, decreased dead-space ventilation, or decreased shunt fraction. No method has been proved superior. The therapeutic end point should be achievement of adequate oxygenation—Pao_2 greater than 60 mm Hg (90% hemoglobin O_2 saturation, assuming a normal saturation curve)—on an Fio_2 of 0.5 or less without a "significant" reduction in cardiac output. The latter is difficult to define because a diminution in cardiac output of 20% may be devastating in a patient with a perioperative low–cardiac output state but inconsequential in a patient with hyperdynamic gram-negative sepsis. Most large series suggest that 95% of the patients can be supported with 20–cm H_2O PEEP or less.

NEW PERSPECTIVES IN THE PATHOPHYSIOLOGY AND MANAGEMENT OF ACUTE RESPIRATORY DISTRESS SYNDROME

It is now recognized that pulmonary injury in ARDS may be patchy rather than diffuse[16] and that ventilatory therapy may be injurious to the lung.[17] Damage may be heterogeneous, or increased vascular pressures in dependent lung units may magnify fluid accumulation in those regions after a diffuse injury. Many cases of acute lung injury may be exacerbated by injudicious fluid management, thereby compounding diagnostic and management problems. A potential iatrogenic injury from PEEP may relate to alveolar overdistension from the application of high airway pressures to the relatively small population of distensible (nonflooded, nonatelectatic) alveoli. This has been postulated to cause an insidious form of barotrauma that is inapparent clinically but deleterious nonetheless,[17] perhaps via damaged local host defenses and an increased incidence of pneumonia. However, the advantages of PEEP—adequate oxygenation at lower (and therefore less toxic) inspired oxygen concentrations, re-expansion of collapsed alveoli with increased FRC, and improved lung compliance—decrease the work of breathing and appear to promote pulmonary parenchymal repair. This divergence of thought is an active issue—should the lung be "rested" by using lower peak airway pressures accomplished by pressure-controlled, inverse-ratio ventilation (PC-IRV) with "permissive" hypercapnia, or should the lung be "worked" by using high airway pressures to recruit alveoli before fibrosis makes it impossible and exposure to high concentrations of oxygen produces a synergistic injury?[18] Although studies are ongoing, there are few comparative data of the two modalities, and the difficulty is compounded further by recent observations that the overall mortality of ARDS is decreasing, thus making comparison to historic controls problematic.[15]

GUIDELINES FOR MANAGING ACUTE RESPIRATORY DISTRESS SYNDROME WITH HIGH-LEVEL POSITIVE END-EXPIRATORY PRESSURE

Positive end-expiratory pressure therapy is optimized for each patient with the use of a formal "PEEP trial."[1, 2] When adequate oxygenation cannot be achieved with mechanical ventilation, an FIO_2 of 0.5, and 5–cm H_2O PEEP, the patient is sedated and given pure oxygen, and PEEP is increased in 2.5–cm H_2O increments (Fig 1). Intermittent mandatory ventilation (IMV) is preferred over controlled ventilation because of enhanced effects on FRC (increased transpulmonary pressure) and reduced detrimental effects on cardiac output (decreased intrapleural pressure). Cardiac output, Pao_2, and $P\bar{v}o_2$ (or saturations) are monitored after brief stabilization (10 to 20 minutes) at each level of PEEP. Compliance is not monitored because the initial effects are unpredictable unless the patient is paralyzed, which is rarely necessary. Increments of PEEP (up to 20 cm H_2O) are added until cardiac output decreases by 20% from baseline. If PEEP is tolerated hemodynamically, the highest tested level is maintained so that a margin exists to decrease FIO_2 rapidly. When oxygenation ($Pao_2/FIO_2[P:F]$, ≥200) and hemodynamics are stable on an FIO_2 of 0.5, PEEP is weaned in 2.5–cm H_2O decrements down to 5.0 cm H_2O before FIO_2 is reduced further. Slow weaning of PEEP (every 12 hours) is important if the patient is fluid overloaded inasmuch as concomitant diuresis may be required to prevent recurrent pulmonary edema as venous return is increased. Slow weaning of PEEP is also necessary to prevent alveolar collapse and recurrent hypoxemia, which may require the subsequent reapplication of PEEP.

The critical need to monitor cardiovascular parameters makes the use of a Swan-Ganz catheter mandatory in these patients, but interpretation of the data can be problematic because airway pressures can be transmitted to the catheter tip. Accurate hemodynamic data can be ensured if the position of the catheter tip is in a de-

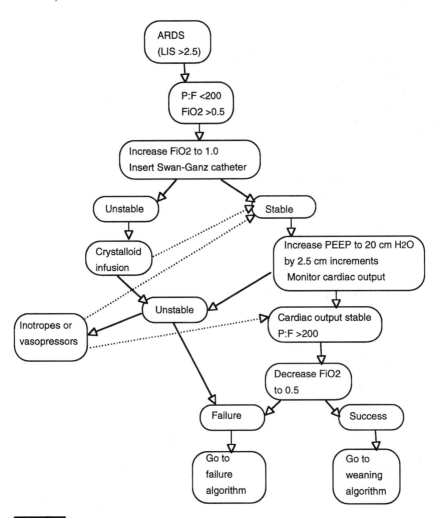

FIGURE 1.
Algorithm for the application of high levels (>10 cm H$_2$O) of positive end-expiratory pressure *(PEEP)* in the management of acute respiratory distress syndrome *(ARDS). Abbreviations: LIS,* lung injury score; *P:F,* Pao$_2$/Fio$_2$.

pendent portion of the lung (zone III) in a euvolemic patient in whom both pulmonary arterial and venous pressures exceed alveolar pressure. Alveolar pressure may exceed pulmonary venous pressure under conditions of high alveolar pressure (PEEP) or low pulmonary venous pressure (hypovolemia) or when the tip of the catheter is above the left atrium, all of which create zone II lung (where pulmonary arterial pressure exceeds airway pressure, which in turn exceeds pulmonary venous pressure) at the expense of zone III. Volume expansion can restore good correlation in a hypovolemic patient even if the catheter tip is not in a good position. Under most conditions, zone III lung will have the greatest blood flow; therefore, Swan-Ganz catheters will preferentially float to these areas. In rare circumstances when questions arise, a cross-table lateral chest radiograph can be performed to verify that the catheter tip is in a dependent portion of the lung.

If cardiac output decreases after PaO_2 has increased but before 20 cm H_2O is reached, a level of PEEP 2.5 cm H_2O below the point where the cardiac output decreased is selected and maintained. If cardiac output decreases before acceptable oxygenation is achieved, additional cardiovascular support is required before the PEEP trial is resumed. Initial support consists of a crystalloid fluid infusion undertaken with caution. If fluid infusion does not stabilize the patient, inotropic support (dopamine or dobutamine) is indicated. The PEEP trial is then resumed from the point of interruption. However, inotropes must also be used with caution. Vasodilator inotropes abolish hypoxic vasoconstriction and can counteract compensatory changes in regional pulmonary perfusion. On balance, it is ideal to keep pulmonary vascular pressures low to minimize edema formation.

Weaning is initiated when oxygenation is stable, at a time before the lesion has resolved by compliance or radiographic criteria (Fig 2). First, FIO_2 is reduced to 0.5 in increments of 0.05 to 0.2 as rapidly as possible to minimize the potential for oxygen toxicity. If the $PaCO_2$ and minute ventilation are stable, arterial oxygen saturation (SaO_2) may be used to assess progress. Once P:F is greater than 200 while $P\bar{v}O_2$ is 35 mm Hg or greater on an FIO_2 of 0.5 in a hemodynamically stable patient, PEEP is decreased in a stepwise fashion 2.5 cm every 12 hours as indicated. As PEEP is reduced, fluid mobilization from the periphery will ensue. The volume of fluid may be very large, depending on the fluid requirement of the disease originally complicated by the ARDS and the amount of fluid administered to support the PEEP trial, and diuretics are often necessary. In rare circumstances, pulmonary edema as a result of fluid mobilization may delay weaning or require restoration of support. Once the patient is ready to resume the work of breathing, the respiratory rate can be decreased to maintain the desired minute ventilation (VE). Reduction in the level of sedation may also be appropriate at this time. Once PEEP is reduced to 5 cm H_2O, conventional weaning continues with IMV and pressure support.

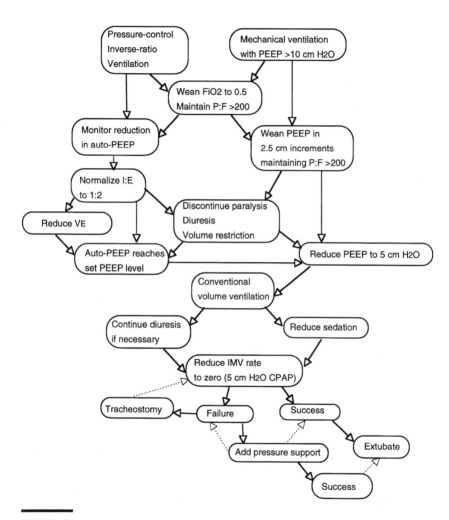

FIGURE 2.

Algorithm for weaning from aggressive ventilatory support in the management of acute respiratory distress syndrome. Note that once the inspiratory/expiratory time ratio *(I:E)* is normalized (i.e., expiration is longer than inspiration), the pressure-control mode is returned to volume control and further weaning proceeds identically. *Abbreviations: PEEP,* positive end-expiratory pressure; *P:F,* Pao_2/Fio_2; *IMV,* intermittent mandatory ventilation; *CPAP,* continuous airway pressure.

GUIDELINES FOR MANAGING ACUTE RESPIRATORY DISTRESS SYNDROME WITH PRESSURE-CONTROL VENTILATION MODES

In the management of patients with evolving ARDS, pressure-controlled (PC) modes of ventilation are increasingly popular.[19-21] In our initial experience, we used conventional-volume ventilation modes with high PEEP until the patient was believed to be maximized. If the patient remained hypoxemic (P:F, ≤200; F_{IO_2}, >0.5), a switch was made to PC ventilation using an inverse inspiratory-to-expiratory time (I:E) ratio (PC-IRV). The switch was time-consuming and often difficult in an unstable patient. A physician with experience in PC-IRV had to be at the bedside making minute-to-minute adjustments in PEEP, respiratory rate, I:E, and PC settings. Because of the instability of the switch-over period, an algorithm has evolved.

The routine mode of ventilation in an uncomplicated patient without ARDS is standard-volume ventilation. When a patient manifests early signs of ARDS, PEEP is added as indicated to no more than 10 cm H_2O (Fig 3). As respiratory failure progresses, compliance worsens, and peak inspiratory pressure (PIP) rises to greater than 35 to 40 cm H_2O, a changeover is made to a PC ventilation mode. Pressure-control ventilation depends on the set inflation pressure, inspiratory time, and respiratory rate, with tidal volume (V_T) and thus V_E dependent on the patient's total (lung and chest wall) compliance. Pressure is applied to the airway in a square-wave pattern. Pressure is therefore applied more evenly throughout the ventilatory cycle, and higher inspiratory gas flow can be delivered, but care must be taken to ensure adequate V_E and consistent V_T. Also, by using a decelerating gas flow at relatively low pressures, less shear force is placed on the airway epithelium. This may result in decreased barotrauma. Although the patient's ventilatory status is not usually severely compromised at this point, it is much easier to convert to a PC mode of ventilation at an early stage. The initial PC setting used is a setting that is adequate to maintain a V_T of no greater than 5 to 7 mL/kg. The respiratory rate is increased to maintain V_E, and PEEP is maintained at the preconversion level. The I:E ratio is maintained at 1:2. If the patient requires further ventilatory support at this point, particular attention must be paid to the patient's volume and hemodynamic status. Although a PC mode of ventilation can limit PIP, it results in significantly higher mean airway pressures. This decreases venous return to the heart and is not well tolerated in a hypovolemic patient. Therefore these patients also require a pulmonary artery catheter for optimization of volume status and cardiac performance.

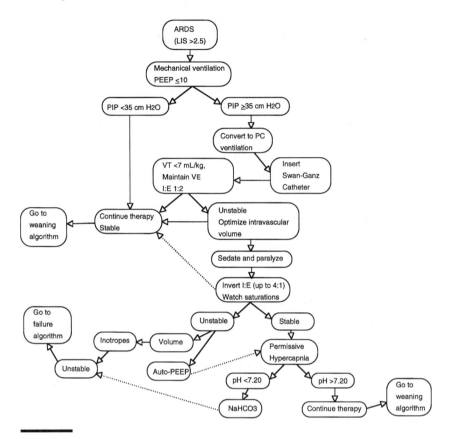

FIGURE 3.

Algorithm for the application of pressure-controlled *(PC)* inverse-ratio ventilation (PC-IRV) in the management of acute respiratory distress syndrome *(ARDS)*. The algorithm is very complex compared to that provided for the management of positive end-expiratory pressure (PEEP) in patients with ARDS (Fig 1). Moment-to-moment adjustments are sometimes necessary, especially when making the switch-over to PC-IRV, and the continuous presence of a physician and respiratory therapist is recommended until experience accrues. *Abbreviations: LIS,* lung injury score; *PIP,* peak inspiratory pressure; *I:E,* inspiratory-to-expiratory time ratio.

If the patient remains hypoxic, PC ventilation is first maximized to a PIP no higher than 35 to 40 cm H_2O. The next maneuver is to invert the I:E ratio (prolong the inspiratory phase, up to 4:1). The rationale for inverse-ratio ventilation is the hypothesis that a longer duration of inspiratory positive pressure will open atelectatic alveoli and the consequently shorter expiratory time will prevent alveolar collapse. Increased Pao_2 may therefore be achieved at lower mean airway pressure and PEEP, but gas trapping may be accentuated in susceptible patients, such as those with chronic obstructive pulmonary disease (COPD). Inverse-ratio ventilation is an uncomfortable sensation, so patients are paralyzed and heavily sedated. The extent of inverse I:E is determined by the response to this maneuver and the resulting Pao_2 and Sao_2. A Pao_2 high enough to maintain Sao_2 greater than 90% is acceptable. The use of oximetric pulmonary artery catheters allows close attention to be paid to $S\bar{v}o_2$ during these maneuvers as a window to cardiac output during rapid ventilator setting changes. If cardiac output is depressed from the added pulmonary pressure and the patient's volume status is optimal, inotropic agents are initiated. Incremental increases in I:E inversion, i.e., balancing alveolar recruitment with the lowest possible airway pressure, are an attempt to minimize cardiac dysfunction and alveolar overdistension. Oxygen exposure is again minimized.

Care must be taken when using PC-IRV. Even though the set PEEP may be about 10 cm H_2O, the use of inverse I:E ventilation with a rapid respiratory rate has potential detrimental effects. First, breath "stacking" occurs at high I:E ratios. This leads to gas trapping under pressure and the generation of "auto-PEEP," which can easily be higher than 20 cm H_2O. The level of auto-PEEP can be estimated by occlusion of the expiratory port of the ventilator in a relaxed patient. Ventilator settings that worsen auto-PEEP (particularly a shortened expiratory time) must be avoided because increased intrathoracic pressure risks the development of diminished venous return and hypotension; patients with COPD are at particular risk. Because auto-PEEP usually increases during acute exacerbations of COPD, resolution during ventilator therapy can be used in such patients as a parameter for weaning. Second, rapid ventilation (20 to 40 breaths per minute) with pressures that give relatively small V_T values leads to an increase in V_{DS}/V_T. It is quite common to have substantial elevations in $Paco_2$ when using PC-IRV. In addition, methods that are typically used to decrease $Paco_2$, such as increasing the respiratory rate, make the hypercapnia greater by shortening the expiratory time of each breath cycle. In patients who have normal renal function, this elevation in $Paco_2$ is well tolerated and acceptable. This "permissive hypercapnia"[22] is routine practice during PC-IRV in this group of patients. Sodium bicarbonate is given only when the pH is less than 7.20 and is rarely needed after the first 24 hours.

Once the patient starts to resolve the ARDS, weaning is initiated (see Fig 2). First, I:E is normalized and then PEEP is decreased. Once P:F is greater than 200; I:E is reduced in a step-wise fashion every 8 to 12 hours as indicated. As I:E is normalized, reductions in mean airway pressure must be monitored closely. For reasons similar to those noted for weaning high levels of PEEP, mean airway pressure should not decrease by more than 2 cm H_2O for every incremental change in I:E. Auto-PEEP will begin to decrease until it reaches the set PEEP. The proximal airway pressure will increase gradually to the level of auto-PEEP as gas continues to empty from alveoli. Pressure-control levels must be watched carefully as the compliance of the lung improves. Weaning often requires a decrease in the PC setting to maintain the desired V_T. Likewise, the respiratory rate can be decreased to maintain the desired V_E. Once I:E is normalized and PEEP is set to 5 cm H_2O, conversion back to normal-volume ventilation and conventional weaning continues with IMV and pressure support.

STRATEGIES FOR REFRACTORY ACUTE RESPIRATORY DISTRESS SYNDROME

Fewer than 20% of patients with ARDS will not be supportable with mechanical ventilation alone. Additional modalities may be attempted in such patients, depending on the likely cause of the problem (Fig 4). The security of the airway should always be confirmed. Some patients will not be able to tolerate the cardiovascular embarrassment associated with increased intrathoracic pressure and reduced cardiac output and may require inotropic drug therapy. Other patients will be embarrassed by fluid overload as a result of massive fluid resuscitation and may require aggressive diuresis, if not ultrafiltration. Occasional patients with a pleural effusion will be intolerant of the additional loss of lung volume because positive airway pressure cannot increase FRC to a sufficient degree because of extrinsic compression. Insertion of a chest tube can dramatically increase oxygenation in selected patients.[23] Similarly, loculated pneumothoraces can produce a picture very similar to that of patients with a pleural effusion.[24] This condition can be very difficult to see on routine chest radiographs and is usually detected only by CT of the chest. A high degree of suspicion must be held to diagnose and appropriately treat this occult pneumothorax.

For truly refractory cases, a number of modalities (both pharmacologic and nonpharmacologic) have had preliminary evaluation. Pharmacologic therapy includes the use of inhaled nitric oxide (INO), partial liquid ventilation, and exogenous surfactant replacement. The most promising pharmacologic therapy in the treatment of ARDS appears to be INO. Pulmonary vasodilation induced by INO is limited to the pulmonary vasculature that is receiving fresh alveolar gas. The use of INO should improve hypoxemia by decreasing shunt through a mechanism that increases blood flow to ventilated alveoli, thus acting to "steal" blood from low-$\dot{V}_A/\dot{Q}$ lung units. Secondary effects of INO occur because of a reduction in pulmonary vascular resistance and improved right heart function. Clinical studies[25-27] evaluating INO in the treatment of ARDS have had variable results, with only about 50% of the patients experiencing an improvement in oxygenation and right heart function. It is possible that most of the benefit in responders may be due to the improved right ventricular function that results from decreased right ventricular afterload. Moreover, improvement may be transitory and last only for the duration of inhalation

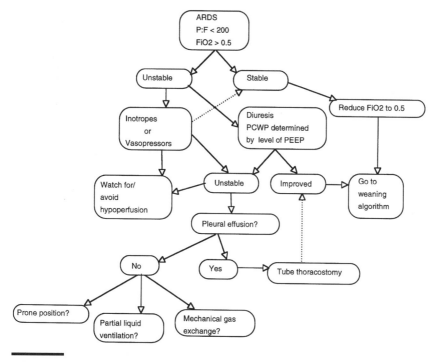

FIGURE 4.

Algorithm for the management of acute respiratory distress syndrome *(ARDS)* when the patient cannot be stabilized and oxygenation cannot be supported (the "failure algorithm"). *Abbreviations: P:F,* Pao$_2$/Fio$_2$; *PCWP,* pulmonary capillary wedge pressure; *PEEP,* positive end-expiratory pressure.

therapy. Phase III prospective trials are under way to definitively evaluate the role that INO will play in the treatment of ARDS.

Partial liquid ventilation is experimental but promising.[28] This mode of ventilation is based on the properties of a volatile liquid fluorocarbon (perflubron), a noncompressible liquid that has high affinity for oxygen and CO_2 in addition to surfactant-like properties. Alveolar recruitment is obtained by filling the lungs with perflubron to FRC. Conventional mechanical ventilation then allows oxygen and CO_2 exchange between air and liquid and subsequently between liquid and alveolar capillary blood. Two recent studies, one in adults[29] and one in children,[30] revealed that partial liquid ventilation decreased physiologic shunt and increased static pulmonary compliance in patients receiving extracorporeal life support and may lead to improved survival. The fluorocarbon evaporates rapidly and requires replenishment during prolonged therapy. Prospective randomized studies are currently under way. It remains unknown whether partial liquid ventilation influences the incidence of pneumonia or its microbiologic diagnosis. However, chest radiographic surveillance becomes impossible because the fluorocarbon is radiopaque and the chest radiograph becomes a "whiteout."

Acute respiratory distress syndrome is also associated with surfactant deficiency. Preliminary studies of surfactant replacement in patients with ARDS suggested a beneficial effect. However, two recent randomized, placebo-controlled studies evaluating aerosolized surfactant in sepsis-induced ARDS found no significant differences in 30-day survival, length of stay in the ICU, duration of mechanical ventilation, or physiologic function.[31, 32] The future of surfactant use in patients with ARDS awaits demonstration of efficacy.

Nonpharmacologic therapies used to treat ARDS include prone positioning and newer ventilatory techniques. It is now recognized that the distribution of edema fluid in patients with ARDS is heterogeneous and accentuated in dependent positions (i.e., dorsally in a supine patient). By placing the patient in the prone position, edema fluid is redistributed to the previously "nondependent" ventral area of the lung. This acts to restore $\dot{V}/\dot{Q}$ relationships, thereby improving oxygenation substantially.[16, 17] Computed tomographic scanning has confirmed the shifting of lung densities by prone positioning.[16] In two small series of ARDS patients,[33, 34] prone-position ventilation resulted in improved oxygenation in approximately 75% of the patients. Improvement can be nearly immediate but is relatively short-lived because the newly dependent lung units become atelectatic and edematous. It may be necessary to re-position the patient every few hours to maintain any benefit.

Newer techniques of ventilation have been tested recently. Tracheal gas insufflation by constant flow through a thin catheter placed through the endotracheal tube entrains a portion of the exhaled tidal volume and may increase airway pressures, augment tidal volume, decrease "wasted" ventilation, and enhance CO_2 removal,[35] especially during PC-IRV. Airway pressure release ventilation (APRV)[36] is a mode of ventilation that alternates two different levels of continuous positive airway pressure (CPAP) to determine and maintain V_T. The pressure curve generated by the ventilator settings is very similar to that of PC-IRV in that the higher level of CPAP is longer (similar to inspiration) and allows for alveolar recruitment and subsequent increased FRC. The lower level of CPAP is usually of short duration (similar to expiration) and allows for ventilation and enhanced CO_2 removal. The presumed advantage with APRV is that the patient can breathe spontaneously during the alternating CPAP levels as opposed to being totally controlled (i.e., sedated heavily and paralyzed) as in PC-IRV.

RESULTS

Few direct comparative data are available to indicate whether PC-IRV provides meaningfully better outcomes in patients with ARDS, although randomized trials are under way. Some nonrandomized studies suggest that mortality is decreased,[22] but other reports that rely on historic controls must be discounted because the overall mortality of ARDS appears to be decreasing.[15] Although our own data are not directly comparable (Table 2) and one center advocates high levels of PEEP and the other uses PC-IRV extensively, the results are quite similar. In addition, the available randomized trial suggests that the outcomes are similar,[37] which is plausible given the increasing body of literature that relates mortality in ARDS to the magnitude of the underlying biological response.[38] It follows that ARDS-associated mortality may be related to the risk factor that initiated the response. When a systemic insult such as sepsis—which is associated with multiple organ dysfunction—induces ARDS, the mortality caused specifically by respiratory failure is difficult to quantitate but probably accounts for no more than 20% of the deaths. Recent epidemiologic studies suggest that sepsis-induced ARDS carries a higher mortality rate than does ARDS associated with other risk factors.[7] However, one study showed the survival rate to be threefold higher for septic patients without ARDS vs. those with ARDS.[39]

TABLE 2.
Results of Ventilatory Support Guidelines in the Management of
Acute Respiratory Distress Syndrome (Lung Injury Score, >2.5)

	High-Level PEEP: New York Hospital	PC-IRV: Parkland Memorial Hospital
Number of patients	177	25
Average age	67	35
Average LIS	3.1	3.2
Mortality	47%	40%
Pneumothorax	6%	8%

Note: These results are only comparable on a limited basis because the age and case mix (the Parkland data reflect mostly trauma patients, and The New York Hospital data include several octogenarians) are different between the groups. Despite this, similarities are readily apparent.
Abbreviations: PEEP, positive end-expiratory pressure; *PC-IRV,* pressure-control inverse-ratio ventilation; *LIS,* lung injury score.

NOSOCOMIAL PNEUMONIA AND ACUTE RESPIRATORY DISTRESS SYNDROME

The diagnosis of nosocomial pneumonia poses both clinical and microbiologic challenges in patients with ARDS. It may be very difficult to confirm the presence of pneumonia in a ventilated patient.[40] The classic findings of fever, cough, purulent sputum, leukocytosis, and a new pulmonary infiltrate are caused by pneumonia in fewer than half of the cases.[41] Recent bronchoscopic surveillance data suggest that nosocomial bacterial pneumonia complicates fewer than 20% of the cases of ARDS.[42] Misdiagnosis results in overuse of antibiotic therapy, which is expensive and potentially morbid and promotes the resistance of resistant pathogens. The analysis of tracheal sputum aspirates collected via a conventional suction catheter is unreliable because such specimens are often contaminated with upper airway flora. The protected specimen brush circumvents many of these difficulties, with sensitivity rates for the diagnosis of pneumonia reported to be between 70% and 90% in patient studies, provided that the patient is not taking antibiotics at the time of specimen collection. Accuracy has been enhanced by the use of quantitative bacteriology to distinguish colonization from invasive infection. The finding of 10^3 colony-forming units per milliliter or greater by quantitative microbiology is a reasonable indicator of invasive infection. The overall accuracy of the protected-brush technique is also limited by the very small sample size obtained.

Bronchoalveolar lavage has increased the overall accuracy of bronchoscopic diagnostic techniques. Instillation of 10 mL saline into a pulmonary segment distal to a "wedged" bronchoscope may sample as many as 10^6 alveoli. The technique has been reported to be 88% sensitive for the diagnosis of bacterial infection of the lower respiratory tract when bacterial counts exceeded 10^4 colony-forming units per milliliter.

CONCLUSION

Since the first description of ARDS in 1967 by Ashbaugh et al.,[43] great progress has been made in understanding the epidemiology, pathophysiology, and underlying mechanisms involved in this disease. This has led to a definition of the clinical criteria to diagnose ARDS, as well as a host of pharmacologic and mechanical ventilatory treatment options. Although reviews are mixed, the overall mortality from ARDS appears to be declining since the beginning of this decade. Until further studies are completed, no one regimen can be supported as the treatment of choice. However, the available literature characterizes ARDS poorly, thereby limiting direct comparability of the data. Consensus definitions of ARDS and quantitative indices such as the lung injury score must become part of the accepted "minimal data set" for future published studies of ARDS; otherwise, problems with interpretation will persist and answerable questions will remain enigmatic.

REFERENCES

1. Barie PS: Acute respiratory failure, in Barie PS, Shires GT (eds): *Surgical Intensive Care.* Boston, Little, Brown, 1993, pp 227–283.
2. Barie PS: Organ-specific support in multiple organ failure: Pulmonary support. *World J Surg* 19:581–591, 1995.
3. Garber BG, Hebert PC, Yelle JD, et al: Adult respiratory distress syndrome: A systematic overview of incidence and risk factors. *Crit Care Med* 24:687–695, 1996.
4. Sessler CN, Bloomfield GL, Fowler AA: Current concepts of sepsis and acute lung injury. *Clin Chest Med* 17:213–235, 1996.
5. Moss M, Goodman PL, Heining M, et al: Establishing the relative accuracy of three new definitions of the adult respiratory distress syndrome. *Crit Care Med* 23:1629–1637, 1995.
6. Hudson LD, Milberg JA, Anardi D, et al: Clinical risks for development of the acute respiratory distress syndrome. *Am J Respir Crit Care Med* 151:293–302, 1995.

7. Milberg JA, Davis DR, Steinberg KP, et al: Improved survival of patients with acute respiratory distress syndrome (ARDS): 1983–1993. *JAMA* 273:306–309, 1995.

8. Rangel-Frausto M, Pittet D, Costigan M, et al: The natural history of the systemic inflammatory response syndrome (SIRS): A prospective study. *JAMA* 273:117–123, 1995.

9. Perl TM, Dvorak L, Hwang T, et al: Long-term survival and function after suspected gram-negative sepsis. *JAMA* 274:338–345, 1995.

10. Fisher CJ, Dhainaut JA, Opal SM, et al: Recombinant human interleukin-1 receptor antagonist in the treatment of patients with sepsis syndrome: Results from a randomized, double-blind, placebo-controlled trial. *JAMA* 271:1836–1843, 1994.

11. Petty TL: Acute respiratory distress syndrome (ARDS). *Dis Month* 36:1–85, 1990.

12. Murray JF, Matthay MA, Luce JM, et al: An expanded definition of the adult respiratory distress syndrome. *Am Rev Respir Dis* 138:720–726, 1988.

13. Shapiro BA, Cand RD, Harrison RA: Positive end-expiratory pressure therapy in adults with special reference to acute lung injury: A review of the literature and suggested clinical correlations. *Crit Care Med* 12:127–136, 1984.

14. Jardin F, Gurdjian F, Desfonds P, et al: Influence of positive end-expiratory pressure on left ventricular performance. *N Engl J Med* 304:387–392, 1981.

15. Weiss SM, Hudson LD: Outcome from respiratory failure. *Crit Care Clin* 10:197–215, 1994.

16. Gattinoni L, Pelosi P, Vitale G, et al: Body position changes redistribute lung computed tomographic density in patients with respiratory failure. *Anesthesiology* 74:15–23, 1991.

17. Marini JJ: Ventilation of the acute respiratory distress syndrome. Looking for Mr. Goodmode. *Anesthesiology* 80:972–975, 1994.

18. Dreyfuss D, Saumon G: Should the lung be rested or recruited? The Charybdis and Scylla of ventilator management (editorial). *Am J Respir Crit Care Med* 149:1066–1067, 1994.

19. Manthous CA, Schmidt GA: Inverse ratio ventilation in ARDS. Improved oxygenation without auto-PEEP. *Chest* 103:953–954, 1993.

20. Papadakos PJ, Halloran W, Hessney JI, et al: The use of pressure-controlled inverse ratio ventilation in the surgical intensive care unit. *J Trauma* 31:1211–1214, 1991.

21. Marcy TW, Marini JJ: Inverse ratio ventilation in ARDS. Rationale and implementation. *Chest* 100:494–504, 1991.

22. Gentilello LM, Anardi D, Mock C, et al: Permissive hypercapnia in trauma patients. *J Trauma* 39:846–852, 1995.

23. Barie PS, Hydo L, Fischer E: Salutary effects of tube thoracostomy drainage of pleural effusion in acute respiratory failure (ARF) refractory to positive end-expiratory pressure (PEEP) ventilation. *Crit Care Med* 23:123A, 1995.

24. Tagliabue M, Casella TC, Zincone GE, et al: CT and chest radiography in the evaluation of adult respiratory distress syndrome. *Acta Radiol* 35:230–234, 1994.
25. Rossaint R, Falke KJ, Lopez F, et al: Inhaled nitric oxide for the adult respiratory distress syndrome. *N Engl J Med* 328:399–405, 1993.
26. McIntyre RC, Moore FA, Moore EE, et al: Inhaled nitric oxide variably improves oxygenation and pulmonary hypertension in patients with acute respiratory distress syndrome. *J Trauma* 39:418–425, 1995.
27. Krafft P, Fridrich P, Fitzgerald RD, et al: Effectiveness of nitric oxide inhalation in septic ARDS. *Chest* 109:486–493, 1996.
28. Hirschl RB, Pranikoff T, Gauger P, et al: Liquid ventilation in adults, children, and neonates. *Lancet* 346:1201–1202, 1995.
29. Hirschl RB, Pranikoff T, Wise C, et al: Initial experience with partial liquid ventilation in adult patients with the acute respiratory distress syndrome. *JAMA* 275:383–389, 1996.
30. Gauger PG, Pranikoff T, Schreiner RJ, et al: Initial experience with partial liquid ventilation in pediatric patients with acute respiratory distress syndrome. *Crit Care Med* 24:16–22, 1996.
31. Anzueto A, Baughman RP, Guntupalli KK, et al: Aerosolized surfactant in adults with sepsis-induced acute respiratory distress syndrome. *N Engl j Med* 334:1417–1421, 1996.
32. Weg JG, Balk RA, Tharratt S, et al: Safety and potential efficacy of an aerosolized surfactant in human sepsis-induced adult respiratory distress syndrome. *JAMA* 272:1433–1438, 1994.
33. Langer M, Mascheroni D, Marcolin R, et al: The prone position in ARDS patients: A clinical study. *Chest* 94:103–107, 1988.
34. Pappert D, Rossaint R, Slama K, et al: Influence of positioning on ventilation-perfusion relationships in severe adult respiratory distress syndrome. *Chest* 106:1511–1516, 1994.
35. Marini JJ: Tracheal gas insufflation: A useful adjunct to ventilation? *Thorax* 49:735–737, 1994.
36. Rasanen J, Cane RD, Downs JB, et al: Airway pressure release ventilation during acute lung injury in a prospective multicenter trial. *Crit Care Med* 19:1234–1241, 1991.
37. Morris AH, Wallace CJ, Menlove RL, et al: Randomized clinical trial of pressure-controlled inverse ratio ventilation and extracorporeal CO_2 removal for adult respiratory distress syndrome. *Am J Respir Crit Care Med* 149:295–305, 1994.
38. Meduri GU, Headley S, Kohler G, et al: Persistent elevation of inflammatory cytokines predicts a poor outcome in ARDS. Plasma IL-1 beta and IL-6 are consistent and efficient predictors of outcome over time. *Chest* 107:1062–1073, 1995.
39. Fein AM, Lippmann M, Holtzman H, et al: The risk factors, incidence and prognosis of ARDS following septicemia. *Chest* 83:40–42, 1983.
40. Winer-Muram HT, Rubin SA, Ellis JV, et al: Pneumonia and ARDS in patients receiving mechanical ventilation: Diagnostic accuracy of chest radiography. *Radiology* 188:479–495, 1993.

41. Meduri GU, Mauldin GL, Wunderink RG, et al: Causes of fever and pulmonary densities in patients with clinical manifestations of ventilator-associated pneumonia. *Chest* 106:221–235, 1994.
42. Sutherland KR, Steinberg KP, Maunder RJ, et al: Pulmonary infection during the acute respiratory distress syndrome. *Am J Respir Crit Care Med* 152:550–556, 1995.
43. Ashbaugh DG, Bigelow DB, Petty TL, et al: Acute respiratory distress in adults. *Lancet* 2:319–323, 1967.

CHAPTER 9

Extracorporeal Life Support for Cardiorespiratory Failure

Harry L. Anderson, III, M.D.
Assistant Professor of Surgery and Anesthesia, University of
Pennsylvania School of Medicine, Philadelphia, Pennsylvania

Extracorporeal membrane oxygenation (ECMO) and extracorporeal life support (ECLS) are terms used to describe prolonged (days to weeks) mechanical support for patients with reversible heart or lung failure. The technology is similar to cardiopulmonary bypass as used during cardiac surgery in the operating room, only modified for prolonged use at the bedside in the ICU. Extracorporeal life support is considered "standard therapy" for neonates in tertiary neonatal centers and can be considered "extraordinary therapy" (*not* experimental) for the treatment of pediatric and adult patients at specialized medical centers throughout the world.

Although ECLS shares much of the same equipment and physiology with cardiopulmonary bypass in the operating room, the extended time of support for an ECLS patient necessitates specialized principles and techniques. This chapter will cover the evolution of ECLS, equipment, techniques and management of extracorporeal perfusion, and the results of ECLS therapy for selected patient populations. Finally, a few innovations in ECLS for respiratory and cardiac support will be presented at the conclusion of the chapter.

BACKGROUND

The concept of circulation of blood outside the body and away from the heart to allow surgery on the heart was described by Gibbon in 1937.[1] This particular system consisted of a vertically mounted cylinder over which blood was pumped by a roller pump to allow gas exchange with ambient air. Return of oxygenated blood to the aorta provided complete support of blood pressure and respiration while the pulmonary artery was occluded at the time of surgery within the chest. It was from this apparatus that cardiopulmonary bypass began.

Technological advances in cardiopulmonary bypass, particularly with regard to blood pumping systems and the oxygenator, have increased the efficiency and safety of extracorporeal perfusion as it is practiced today. The possibility of moving the extracorporeal support system from the operating room to the ICU for long-term support of patients was first successfully accomplished by Hill and colleagues in 1972.[2] Their patient was a motorcycle accident victim who underwent repair of a ruptured thoracic aorta and in whom severe lung dysfunction subsequently developed. This patient, at higher risk of bleeding because of anticoagulation, was successfully weaned and decannulated from ECMO.

Bartlett et al. described the first newborn with neonatal respiratory distress syndrome successfully treated by ECMO in 1976.[3] Extracorporeal membrane oxygenation did not become standard therapy for neonates until studies from three medical centers demonstrated the superiority of ECMO over conventional therapy.[4] Randomized study of ECMO vs. conventional management in neonates was ethically difficult because randomization to conventional management was (as the differences in survival soon became apparent) believed to be essentially randomization to death. Only to stimulate skeptics further, Bartlett was able to achieve statistical significance in a study comparing these two modalities with a technique named "randomized play-the-winner." In this study, additional weighting (favoring the last *successful* modality) is provided for each subsequent randomization, thereby allowing randomization preference to the "winning" modality. A statistical difference in the two modalities was reached when 13 patients treated by ECMO all survived and 1 patient in the conventional management group died.[5, 6]

In 1977, Zapol et al. reported the results of a National Institutes of Health (NIH)-sponsored multicenter comparison of ECMO vs. conventional mechanical ventilation in adult patients with adult respiratory distress syndrome (ARDS).[7] Patients were entered into the study when they had reached a mortality level of 80% based on physiologic parameters. Each patient underwent randomization into either continuing mechanical ventilation or starting therapy with ECMO. It was initially anticipated that 300 patients would be entered into the study; however, the study was stopped when 92 patients had been randomized because of a disappointing 10% survival rate in each group. Bleeding in the ECMO group was approximately 2 L/day per patient. After this report, ECMO was all but stopped for the treatment of respiratory failure in adults.

Gattinoni et al. reported in 1986 a 49% survival rate in the treatment of respiratory failure in adults with the technique of extracorporeal CO_2 removal (ECCO$_2$R).[8] They used entry criteria similar to those used during the NIH-sponsored ECMO trial of the 1970s (predictive of 80% or greater mortality) and designed a modified extracorporeal system that incorporated low flow rates and percutaneous venovenous vascular access. Extracorporeal CO_2 removal is very efficient. Oxygen transfer in these patients was accomplished by "apneic" oxygenation via an intratracheal catheter supplying 100% oxygen and an attached ventilator supplying low-rate, low-pressure inspired breaths. Their approach differed from the venoarterial access and high-pressure mechanical ventilation used during the NIH trial.[8, 9] Shortly thereafter, several other European and U.S. medical centers reported successful treatment of adult respiratory failure with ECMO.[10–20] Refinements in perfusion technology and an improved understanding of the pathophysiology and treatment of cardiac and respiratory failure have contributed to the success of ECMO (or the more modern designation, ECLS). In the modern era, ECLS is a safe and reasonable therapy for patients in whom conventional therapy has failed. It is no longer experimental and is therefore considered *extraordinary* therapy.

EXTRACORPOREAL LIFE SUPPORT TECHNIQUE AND MANAGEMENT

In several aspects, the ECLS circuit is quite similar to the cardiopulmonary perfusion system used in the operating room. Venoarterial bypass (like that provided for cardiac surgery) provides both cardiac (i.e., blood pressure) and respiratory (i.e., oxygenation and ventilation) support, whereas venovenous bypass provides respiratory support only. A schematic of a venovenous ECLS perfusion circuit is depicted in Figure 1. Blood is drained from the vena cava, preferably via the right internal jugular vein (the largest extrathoracic vein with proximity to the heart). However, the femoral vein or right atrium (cannulated directly at the time of sternotomy) can also be used. The blood is pumped through an oxygenator device where oxygen and carbon dioxide exchange take place, it is warmed by a water-jacketed heat exchanger, and then the blood is returned to a major vein (typically the femoral vein) during venovenous bypass. The circuit is essentially the same for venoarterial bypass, the only difference being that warmed and oxygenated

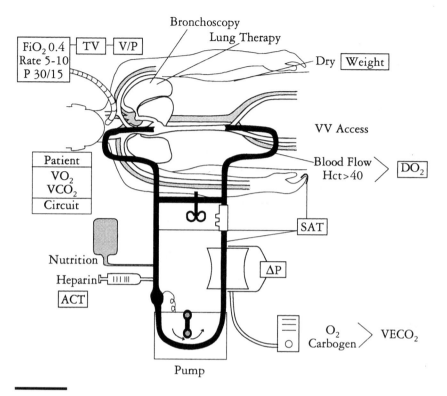

FIGURE 1.

Schematic of a "modern" venovenous extracorporeal life support perfusion circuit. Blood is drained from the right internal jugular vein, oxygenated with CO_2 removed, and reinfused into the right common femoral vein. *Abbreviations: FiO$_2$,* inspired oxygen fraction; *P,* pressure; *TV,* tidal volume; *V/P,* volume/pressure or compliance; *VV,* venovenous; *Hct,* hematocrit; *DO$_2$,* oxygen delivery; *SAT,* hemoglobin saturation by oxygen; *ΔP,* pressure drop across the membrane oxygenator; *VECO$_2$,* percentage of CO_2 in the outlet sweep gas; *ACT,* activated clotting time; *VO$_2$,* oxygen consumption; *VCO$_2$,* CO_2 production. (Courtesy of Anderson HL III, Steimle CN, Shapiro MB, et al: Extracorporeal life support for adult cardiorespiratory failure. *Surgery* 114:162, 1993.)

blood is returned to the aorta by a major artery (carotid, femoral, axillary) or by direct cannulation of the aorta at sternotomy.

Venovenous perfusion is the preferred mode of support for patients with pure respiratory failure because blood does not "bypass" the heart and lungs. Mixing of oxygenated blood (hemoglobin completely saturated with oxygen) from the ECLS circuit with venous blood (saturation usually 60% to 70%) in the vena cava and right atrium raises the oxygen saturation of hemoglobin to 85%

to 90% as it begins to enter the pulmonary circulation. If residual pulmonary function of the native lungs is poor, often the best arterial saturation that can be achieved is 80% to 90% with *full* venovenous support. Nonetheless, there may be a theoretical advantage to venovenous bypass because the lungs and heart continue to receive a full component of native cardiac output of blood with a higher oxygen content than venous blood alone.

Cannulation for ECLS typically occurs at the patient's bedside in the ICU. On occasion it is necessary to cannulate in the operating room and move the patient (while supported by ECLS) to the ICU. The patient is systemically heparinized (heparin, 100 U/kg body weight) before the placement of catheters. Percutaneous cannulation of blood vessels, as described by Pesenti et al., is the preferred method for cannulation of veins. Surgical exposure is not necessary, and bleeding from cannulation sites is less with this technique.[10, 11] Arterial cannulation (for venoarterial bypass) is best performed after direct surgical exposure of blood vessels to allow definite placement of the arterial return cannula within the vessel lumen (Fig 2). Venoarterial and venovenous systems generally use two catheters (one for venous drainage and one for return), although several single-site, single-catheter venovenous perfusion systems have been implemented. One such system incorporates a double-lumen catheter to allow continuous drainage and reinfusion via separate ports on the catheter.[21–23] Several centers have successfully used tidal flow ("push-pull" or "to-and-fro") systems that alternate between drainage and reinfusion cycles through the same catheter lumen.[24–26] Both these systems can provide complete respiratory support for the neonate.

Bypass flow is limited by the rate at which blood can be drained from the patient, and therefore the lowest-resistance configuration is usually assembled on the venous drainage limb of the circuit. Catheters are selected according to the size(s) of the blood vessels and the anticipated blood flow required for support of the patient. Montoya and colleagues have described an indexing system (the "M" number) in which catheters could be categorized on the basis of resistance to flow and therefore the pressure drop to be expected when the catheter was in use.[27–29] Catheters manufactured by the Bio-Medicus Corporation (Division of Medtronic, Inc., Minneapolis) are ideally suited to this application because of their thin, wire-reinforced design and low resistance. Should venous drainage (and therefore pump flow) be inadequate, the patient's bed can be raised higher than the pump to provide additional gravity feed, crystalloid or blood may be transfused, or an additional venous catheter (e.g., in a femoral vein) can be placed and spliced into the venous limb of the circuit.

During venoarterial perfusion, warmed and oxygenated blood is returned to (in order of decreasing preference) the right common carotid artery, the femoral artery, or the axillary artery. The right common carotid artery is usually tied distally at the time of cannulation owing to the generous supply of collateral circulation from the ipsilateral external carotid artery and the vertebrobasilar system through the circle of Willis. Because the femoral and axillary arteries are basically end arteries with minimal collateral supply, cannulation of these vessels necessitates placement of an additional catheter *distally* through the arteriotomy that perfuses the limb via a separate blood return line. During venovenous perfu-

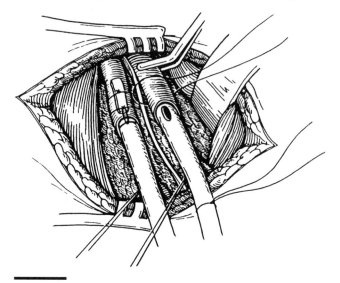

FIGURE 2.

Cannulation of the right common carotid artery and internal jugular vein for venoarterial extracorporeal life support (ECLS) (drawing orientation, right side of the neck with the feet toward the top of the figure). Cannulation is typically performed at the bedside in the intensive care unit. After systemic anticoagulation, vessels are ligated distally and catheters are placed proximally and attached to the ECLS circuit. The vagus nerve is identified within the operative field of the right side of the neck between the vascular structures. (Courtesy of Dembitsky WP, Willms DC, Jaski BE: Peripheral vascular access for organ support, in Zwischenberger JB, Bartlett RH (eds): *ECMO: Extracorporeal Cardiopulmonary Support in Critical Care.* Ann Arbor, Mich, Extracorporeal Life Support Organization, 1995, p 213.)

sion, blood is usually returned through a femoral vein, and a small amount of oxygenated blood is recirculated back through the venous drainage cannula (resulting in lowered efficiency of the perfusion system). Nonetheless, sufficient oxygenated blood travels to the right ventricle and pulmonary artery to provide adequate oxygen delivery and carbon dioxide removal.

Three basic pump designs are used for ECLS perfusion. The servo-controlled roller pump is the most popular for ECLS and probably the most familiar to perfusionists. It has the advantage of having no moving parts in direct contact with blood, is relatively inexpensive, but must be speed-regulated in response to patient venous drainage to prevent cavitation. The centrifugal (vortex) pump has recently become popular for cardiac perfusion and has found use for shorter-term (days) ECLS. The centrifugal pump does not require direct regulation of rotational pump head speed in response to changes in venous drainage. However, this pump also can produce cavitation and air bubbles during inlet occlusion, thus creating the potential for air embolism. The centrifugal pump is more expensive than the roller pump and incorporates a spinning impeller that is in direct contact with blood, which results in hemolysis and thrombosis.[30] A third pump design, manufactured in Europe by Rhone Poulenc (Paris), uses a nonocclusive rotor around which a passively filling bladder is stretched to act as a raceway.[24, 31] Occlusion of the pump outlet is tolerated because the normally ovoid raceway becomes circular, thus overcoming any occlusion and preventing overpressurization. Occlusion of the inlet causes the raceway to flatten, again preventing suction or underpressurization to the inlet. Although not currently approved for use in the United States, this pump may be the ideal system for both short- and long-term operative perfusion. A prototype is currently under testing in the United States in anticipation of Food and Drug Administration clearance for medical use[31] (Fig 3).

The oxygenator is the ECLS component that has undergone the most modification, driven primarily by clinical use for cardiac surgery. Considerations such as maximizing gas transfer, minimizing thrombosis and thromboembolism, and providing low resistance to transoxygenator blood flow have resulted in several designs, of which the spiral coil membrane (Kolobow membrane lung) and hollow-fiber type are the two most popular for ECLS. Anticoagulation is necessary primarily because of areas of blood stagnation in the oxygenator and blood contact with a large nonendothelial surface. The Kolobow membrane lung is the most common type used owing to its excellent gas exchange capability and extensive clini-

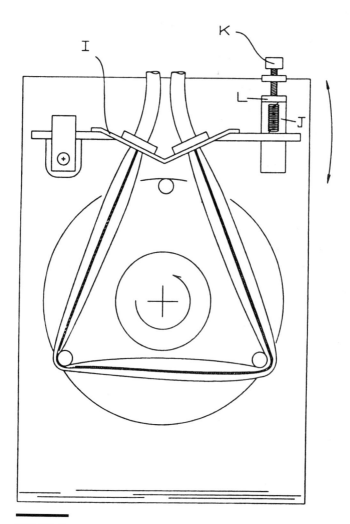

FIGURE 3.

Schematic of a nonocclusive pump (M-pump). Distensible ovoid (in cross section) raceway tubing is stretched over three rollers of a rotor. Occlusion of the blood inlet causes the raceway to collapse, thereby stopping flow (and preventing cavitation). Occlusion of the blood outlet causes the raceway to become round, which overcomes the occlusion of the rollers, decreases flow, and prevents overpressurization (and tubing rupture). (Courtesy of Montoya JP, Merz SI, Bartlett RH: Laboratory experience with a novel, non-occlusive, pressure-regulated peristaltic blood pump. *ASAIO J* 38:M408, 1992.)

cal experience in both cardiac surgery and ECLS. It is also the most prone to thrombosis and has a higher resistance to blood flow. The hollow-fiber oxygenator, designed such that blood flows outside and around hollow fibers carrying oxygen, has lower resistance to blood flow and also has excellent gas exchange capacity. Much effort has been focused on the hollow-fiber oxygenator in an attempt to provide a thromboresistant coating by binding heparin to the hollow-fiber surface in contact with blood. The Duraflo II heparin coating (Baxter Health Care, Inc.) and Carmeda Bioactive Surface (Medtronic, Inc.) are two such processes that use an ionic bond or covalent bond (respectively) to attach heparin molecules to plastic materials.[11, 19, 32, 33] Theoretically, these processes would allow a reduction in the level of anticoagulation necessary for short- or long-term perfusion, although experience with this system in the operating room has provided mixed results.[34–37] The heparin-bonded hollow-fiber system has been used extensively in Europe for prolonged ECCO$_2$R and also in some centers in the United States. Still, it is the unpredictable leakage of plasma across the fiber from the blood phase to the gas phase that limits the usefulness of heparin-bonded hollow-fiber oxygenators for ECLS.[11, 38, 39] Investigation continues in an attempt to provide the most optimal system that minimizes or eliminates the need for anticoagulation.

As the blood leaves the oxygenator, it is warmed to slightly greater than body temperature by a water-jacketed heat exchange before returning to the patient. The heat exchanger is mounted in a vertical orientation, with blood entering the top and exiting the bottom of the cylindric device. In this position, a small reservoir of blood at the top of the heat exchanger also acts to trap small gas bubbles that may pass beyond the oxygenator, thus precluding the need for a special bubble trap.

Systemic anticoagulation during ECLS is necessary after the initial heparin bolus for cannulation. Heparin is infused continuously, and anticoagulation is monitored by bedside measurement of the activated clotting time (ACT). Because the ACT is a measurement of heparin activity on *whole blood,* it is preferred over other measures of heparin activity such as the partial thromboplastin time or the thrombin clotting time, which only measure heparin effect on *plasma.* Normal ACT is 90 to 120 seconds, and heparin infusion is adjusted to maintain the ACT at levels of 160 to 200 seconds, typically 170 to 190 seconds. At higher ACTs, thrombosis of circuit components is reduced, yet bleeding from the patient (endobronchial, cannulation site, or chest tube site bleeding) becomes problematic. For an actively bleeding patient, the target ACT is usually reduced (150 to 170 seconds).[17, 40] Whittlesey et al. have described heparinless bypass for several days; with this clinical approach it is best to plan for oxygenator and circuit thrombosis and failure—a second, primed and readied circuit is kept nearby in anticipation of the need to replace the failed circuit with a new one.[41]

Blood product administration is necessary during ECLS to replace red blood cells, platelets, and coagulation factors that are lost in bulk (because of bleeding, laboratory sampling, etc.), consumed (platelet activation and aggregation, red blood cell hemolysis, clot formation, etc.), and sequestered (platelets trapped in the membrane oxygenator or removed by the spleen or liver). Bleeding occurs in 15% to 80% of cases and is more common in the nonneonatal patients given the greater likelihood of co-morbid disease (gastric ulcer) or other insults (pelvis fracture in trauma patients, two cannulation sites rather than one, etc.). Central nervous system bleeding is more typical in premature neonates and often mandates early cessation of ECLS.[42, 43] Packed red blood cells are transfused to maintain the hematocrit at 40% to 45% (hemoglobin, 130 to 150 g/L) to maximize oxygen delivered per liter of blood reinfused by the ECLS circuit. Concentrated platelets are transfused to maintain the platelet count greater than $100,000/mm^3$ during routine ECLS and greater than $150,000/mm^3$ if bleeding is present. It is useful to remember that although platelet number may be "adequate" during ECLS, the platelets are usually rendered dysfunctional because of extensive blood–foreign surface contact and activation of the many inflammatory cascades within blood. Cryoprecipitate and fresh frozen plasma are transfused to maintain the fibrinogen level at 250 mg/dL (2.5 g/L) and to replace other clotting factors (including antithrombin III) consumed during ECLS.

All fluids and medications are typically administered through the ECLS circuit. These patients are usually fluid-overloaded before going on ECLS, and effort is made early to achieve dry weight within the first few days.[17, 44, 45] Fluids and parenteral or enteral nutrition are concentrated as much as possible, and diuretics (furosemide [Lasix], ethacrynic acid [Edecrine], or mannitol) are given in an effort to force diuresis and achieve a negative fluid balance. Should more rapid fluid removal or hemodialysis be necessary, a small dialyzer/hemofilter can be attached to the ECLS circuit to allow slow continuous ultrafiltration or continuous arteriovenous hemofiltration with dialysis. Parenteral nutrition is used initially but is converted to enteral nutrition through a nasoduodenal tube as soon as practical.

The concept of "lung rest" was introduced by Gattinoni, and it is the primary goal of ECLS to provide sufficient respiratory support such that ventilator support (using high airway pressures and high levels of inspired oxygen) can be decreased to "safe" levels allowing lung healing. "Lung rest" settings typically include a low inspired oxygen fraction (FIO_2, <0.5), pressure-controlled ventilation (peak pressure limited to less than 30 to 40 cm H_2O), moderate positive end-expiratory pressure (less than 5 to 15 cm H_2O), and a low ventilatory rate (ten breaths per minute).[8] Prone positioning, also advocated by Gattinoni, should be used as part of routine ICU respiratory management before ECLS and is carefully continued during therapy with ECLS.[46] A tracheostomy, if not done already, is usually performed early during the ECLS run. We prefer the percutaneous method described by Ciaglia and Graniero because of the possibility of tracheal suctioning and in anticipation of weaning from ECLS and ultimately from the ventilator.[47]

A typical ECLS patient course for treatment of respiratory failure is shown in Figure 4. As pulmonary function improves, the increase in arterial Po_2 allows ECLS pump flow to be decreased until support is about 10% or less of the patient's metabolic requirement (or cardiac output). At this time a "trial off" ECLS is performed by increasing ventilatory parameters to modest settings, clamping the drainage and return catheters, and opening the bridge. Blood within the ECLS circuit is allowed to circulate, thereby preventing thrombosis, and the patient is monitored with noninvasive devices (pulse oximetry and end-tidal CO_2). If return of pulmonary function has been satisfactory and the patient maintains adequate blood gas status, mixed venous oxygen saturation, and hemodynamic parameters, decannulation is performed. Should the patient fail the "trial off," bypass support is resumed and trial off is again performed the next day. For patients undergoing ECLS for cardiac support, preload must be adequate and perfusion sufficient with minimal inotropic support before decannulation can be considered.

Once the decision to decannulate has been made, the indwelling cannulas are clamped and cut from the circuit. Percutaneously placed venous cannulas are removed and the percutaneous skin site closed with a mattress suture. Operatively placed cannulas in vessels are again removed by exposure of blood vessels in the cannulation site. Veins are usually ligated after removal of the surgically placed cannulas, although if possible, repair by simple closure of the venotomy is performed. The common carotid artery is typically ligated after cannula removal because of the risk of distal embolization. Several centers have successfully repaired the carotid arteries of neonates who have undergone ECLS by using vascular end-to-end repair or patch angioplasty.[48–50] Unilateral liga-

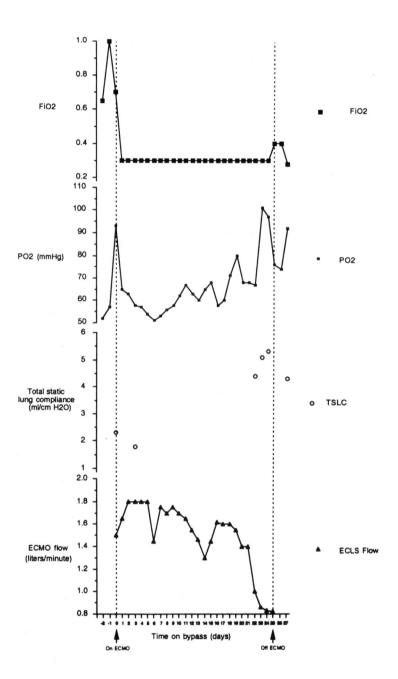

tion of the carotid has been performed safely after decannulation in patients of all age groups with minimal or no morbidity, and any proposed alternative technique (e.g., carotid repair) must be compared with ligation. The long-term result of unilateral carotid ligation in these patients remains unknown; the oldest survivor of therapy with venoarterial ECLS is developmentally normal at 20 years of age.

PATIENT SELECTION

As a technology, ECLS is resource and labor intensive and should be offered as therapy only to those patients who will benefit the most (survive). As the knowledge base for critical care therapy increases, better ventilators are designed, better antibiotics are developed, etc., there will be a change in the population for whom ECLS is used, as well as a change in the indications for ECLS. This has already been seen in the neonatal population, where introduction of the oscillatory ventilator has resulted in greater success of conventional neonatal critical care in treating the neonatal respiratory distress syndrome.[51] Consequently, today the neonates are referred for ECLS are much sicker, and most neonatal ECLS centers are now treating respiratory failure resulting from congenital diaphragmatic hernia more often than other nonsurgical neonatal conditions.

In understanding the spectrum of uses of ECLS for cardiac or respiratory failure, it is helpful to understand the specific criteria used for the selection of patients. In the selection of neonates for ECLS therapy, the entry criteria are relatively standardized, given the fact that ECLS became standard therapy for neonatal respiratory failure in 1984.[4] Small differences in indications between medical centers reflect the variability in neonatal survival from center to center (based on patient population, availability of specialized ventilators, etc.).

The neonatal conditions responsible for respiratory failure during the first 2 weeks of life share similar pathophysiology, and most

---

FIGURE 4.

Extracorporeal life support *(ECLS)* course of a 2-year-old infant with respiratory failure from varicella pneumonia. The inspired oxygen fraction *(FiO₂)*, arterial *PO₂*, total static lung compliance *(TSLC)*, and ECLS pump flow are plotted against time. At day 25, the patient successfully weaned from bypass and was decannulated. This patient was discharged home. (Courtesy of Anderson HL III, Attorri, RJ, Custer JR, et al: ECMO for pediatric cardiorespiratory failure. *J Thorac Cardiovasc Surg* 99:1015, 1990.)

have some component of persistent fetal circulation because of elevated pulmonary vascular resistance resulting in a right-to-left shunt (hypoxemia). Conventional therapy may involve pulmonary vasodilator therapy, alkalinization, a higher inspired oxygen fraction, and higher mean airway pressure on the ventilator. The last two maneuvers may contribute to direct pulmonary injury. Neonates become candidates for ECLS when they reach the 80% mortality threshold, based on certain measured parameters. The postductal alveolar-arterial oxygen gradient is one such measurement, or more commonly, the oxygenation index (OI) is calculated and used:

$$OI = \frac{F_{IO_2} \times [\text{Mean airway pressure (MAP, cm } H_2O)]}{\text{Arterial } P_{O_2} \text{ (mm Hg)}} \times 100$$

Three successive OI calculations of 25 predict a 50% mortality, and an OI consistently greater than 40 predicts an 80% mortality. A neonate consistently at an OI of 25 for 12 hours—or once an OI of 40 is reached despite conventional and maximal therapy—will probably be placed on ECLS should no contraindication to anticoagulation exist. As time allows, each neonatal respiratory failure candidate for ECLS undergoes cranial ultrasound to rule out intracranial or intraventricular hemorrhage, as well as echocardiography to rule out a surgically correctable cardiac anomaly. Any patient with a major chromosomal aberration or estimated to be less than 34 weeks' gestational age is typically excluded from consideration for ECLS therapy.

Although respiratory failure may develop in neonates through a small number of defined disease entities, in the pediatric and adult populations, respiratory failure develops through a much wider range of disease processes and more varied pathophysiology. Selection of these older patients is more complex. The selection criteria used in the 1970s were predictive of 80% or higher mortality, and some of those same criteria (low static compliance, high transpulmonary shunt) are applied today (Table 1). Because of the diversity in disease processes, the survival rate with ECLS treatment is lower; therefore, closer scrutiny of these patients as candidates is appropriate.

The goal of ECLS for pediatric or adult patients is again to provide lung rest from the high levels of oxygen and higher airway pressures that are necessary to support oxygenation and ventilation. Proper selection involves determining in which patient the disease process itself is reversible (with 1 to 2 weeks of ECLS support) and in which patient conventional therapy has not yet contributed to irreversible injury (barotrauma, volutrauma, and "oxytrauma," all of which may appear pathologically as pneumothoraces and fibrosis). In our experience, survival with ECLS drops sharply as the time of intubation and mechanical ventilation before cannulation exceeds 7 days, and mechanical ventilation beyond 10 days is considered an absolute exclusion.[52] Interestingly, Gattinoni and colleagues have successfully treated patients with respiratory failure (with $ECCO_2R$) who had undergone mechanical ventilation more than 6 weeks before bypass support.

Patients with multiple organs failing in addition to respiratory failure are typically not selected for ECLS because the underlying disease process is probably not limited to the lungs alone. In addition, patients with acute onset and deterioration but healthy lungs would be expected to have a more favorable outcome than patients with the same acute process superimposed on some other chronic pulmonary condition (cystic fibrosis, chronic obstructive pulmonary disease, pulmonary hyptertension, etc.). Pure capillary leak syndromes (ARDS), nonnecrotizing pneumonias (both bacterial and viral), and pulmonary contusion are typical disease processes that would be expected to reverse with "lung rest" during 1 to 2 weeks of ECLS support.

Venoarterial ECLS for primary cardiac failure has been largely applied in the pediatric population, but there are limited uses in

TABLE 1.

Selection Criteria for Extracorporeal Life Support (Pediatric and Adult)

Indications
   Reversible respiratory failure
   Time on mechanical ventilation, 7 days or less (10 days absolute maximum)
   Total static lung compliance, <0.5 cc/cm H_2O/kg
   Transpulmonary shunt, >30% on an inspired oxygen fraction of 0.6 or greater
Exclusions
   Potential for severe bleeding
   Time on mechanical ventilation, 11 days or greater
   Necrotizing pneumonia
   Poor quality of life (those patients with metastatic malignancy, major CNS injury, or quadriplegia)
   Age over 60 years

adult patients.[16, 18, 53] A benefit with the use of ECLS (as opposed to right or left ventricular assist devices) is that cannulation can be performed at extrathoracic sites and median sternotomy is not necessary. In the case of cardiac support for "bridging" to cardiac transplantation, this is of obvious benefit because the mediastinum is not violated for cannulation. This is a reasonable application for ECLS, but only when a suitable organ has been identified, and short-term support is necessary while the logistics of harvesting and transportation of the donor organ are being worked out. Open-ended support in the hope of finding an organ is usually met with disappointment (waiting times often are greater than the 1 to 2 weeks that a patient can be *safely* supported with ECLS), and emotional anguish on the part of the family, the ECLS team, and ICU nurses usually results.

Two reversible medical causes of cardiac failure amenable to ECLS support are myocarditis and cardiomyopathy. Indications include a cardiac index less than 2 L/min/m^2 and a mixed venous oxygen saturation ($S\bar{v}o_2$) less than 50% for 2 hours.[16, 40, 53–56] One must carefully ascertain whether the apparent organ dysfunction (anuria, coma, etc.) is due to the low-flow state or whether irreversible organ failure has in fact occurred (thereby excluding the patient). For postoperative cardiac patients requiring ECLS support, the sternum is usually left open and the skin defect closed temporarily with a synthetic patch. Activated clotting times are kept lower (150 to 170 seconds), platelet counts are maintained above 150,000/mm^3, and the fibrinogen level is maintained greater than 200 mg/dL (0.2 g/L). The sternal patch minimizes mediastinal contamination yet allows decompression of the pericardium and easy access to the chest at the bedside for evacuation of hematoma and correction of bleeding.

RESULTS

It is with some surprise that the concept of ECLS as an efficacious and useful technique (using technology that has been continuously refined beginning more than half a century ago and using techniques similar to the first successful adult case nearly a quarter of a century ago) is met with controversy and skepticism by critical care physicians around the world.[14, 15, 57] The technology is expensive in terms of equipment, disposables, hospital resources (blood products, etc.), and personnel time (the ECLS specialist who sits bedside managing the ECLS circuit on a round-the-clock basis). The annual cost of a 20-patient-per-year ECLS program has been esti-

TABLE 2.
Neonatal, Pediatric, and Adult Extracorporeal Life Support Results Compiled by the Extracorporeal Life Support Organization Registry (Ann Arbor, Michigan) as of July 1996

Group	Patients Reported	Number Survived	Survival Rate, %
Neonatal respiratory	11,182	8,994	80
Pediatric respiratory	1,067	567	53
Pediatric cardiac	1,650	705	43
Adult	246	114	46
Totals	14,145	10,380	73

(Courtesy of *ECMO Quarterly Report*. Ann Arbor, Mich, ECMO Registry of the Extracorporeal Life Support Organization, July 1996.)

mated to be $328,100 (range, $185,600 to $437,900).[58] The benefits of supporting an ECLS program include increased referral of patients (some of whom undergo ECLS and some do well with conventional therapy alone), a benefit to society (salvage of moribund patients who return to productivity), higher regard for the medical center as a "tertiary or quaternary" referral center, and a benefit to the nurses, medical students, and physicians in the ICU as new knowledge and techniques are learned.

Does ECLS improve survival (over conventional management) in patients? We believe that the answer across the board is yes, but the available evidence is strongest for neonates. A registry of ECLS cases (now totaling nearly 14,000 patients) has been maintained at the University of Michigan by the Extracorporeal Life Support Organization (ELSO) since 1989 (Table 2).[59] With a membership of 116 centers in the United States and overseas, the data from each patient are reported at the conclusion of the ECLS run to the registry database. The registry is a wealth of information with regard to pre-ECLS care, survival data, time on ECLS, complications, etc. Several multicenter trials have been conducted under direction of ELSO, and thus questions are easily and more rapidly answered with combined efforts of the member ECLS centers and health care professionals.[13, 60, 61]

The survival rate (defined as discharge from the hospital) for neonates is highest (80%), and this figure includes all diagnoses resulting in respiratory failure in the first 2 weeks of life. This higher survival of neonates than pediatric or adult patients reflects the different underlying pathophysiology of respiratory failure. The survival rate from ECLS treatment of meconium aspiration syndrome is 94%, whereas the much lower survival rate of patients with congenital diaphragmatic hernia (58%) reflects the complexity of this truly surgical disease. One must remember that neonatal respiratory failure (at an OI greater than 40) carries a mortality rate greater than 80%, but with ECLS, mortality can at best be reduced to 5% to 8% at the more experienced centers.[40, 59]

Extracorporeal life support for the neonate can be performed safely, and the typical ECLS course for a patient with respiratory failure but no congenital diaphragmatic hernia is relatively short, about 4 to 7 days. Complications related to the patient (e.g., intracranial hemorrhage and infarct, bleeding) are more common than circuit-related complications (e.g., oxygenator failure, tubing rupture), and such complications occur with greater frequency the longer the ECLS run. Schumacher et al. prospectively examined neurologic and pulmonary morbidity, mortality, and charges in patients randomized to early ECLS vs. late initiation of ECLS, where some patients randomized to the "late ECLS" group improved and were not treated with ECLS. Although not reaching statistical significance in 41 patients, "early ECLS" patients had a trend of lower charges and fewer intensive care unit days than all patients who randomized to the "late ECLS" group. The greatest neurologic and pulmonary morbidity, and charge was in those "late ECLS" patients who did not go on to ECLS. The authors concluded that *late initiation* of ECLS had additional risk in terms of morbidity.[62]

Recently, ECLS has been used more commonly for pediatric patients, particularly for postoperative support after cardiac surgery for congenital anomalies. Most medical centers with a neonatal ECLS program have a nearby and functional pediatric ICU, so it is a seemingly logical progression to move up to only slightly larger patients because ECLS on these patients necessitates the same equipment used for the neonate, only instead a larger oxygenator and larger tubing and cannulas are used. What is not apparent at first glance is that the pediatric patients typically undergo ECLS for 10 to 20 days, have more circuit-related complications, and are more likely to bleed and require more blood products than the usual neonate treated with ECLS for meconium aspiration syndrome. The pediatric cases are technically more challenging and, as would probably be expected, have a much lower survival rate. Typical pediatric respiratory diseases successfully treated by ECLS are varicella or aspiration pneumonia, pulmonary contusion, and near-drowning.[53, 63, 64] Venovenous support (two-catheter access) is used for respiratory failure, and venoarterial support (often with cannulation of the common carotid artery through the right side of the neck) can be used for both cardiac and respiratory failure in pediatric patients.

Management and support of adult patients require another increment in hospital resources and personnel time, and ECLS in adults is even more challenging than in pediatric patients because of a wider range of diseases and the general reduction in organ reserve that is inevitable with advancing age. When Zapol reported an equivalent 10% survival rate in both ECMO-treated and conventionally treated groups during the NIH-sponsored multicenter comparison of these two modalities for the treatment of adult respiratory failure, ECMO was no longer considered efficacious.[7] Using percutaneous cannulation and focusing on $ECCO_2R$, Gattinoni et al. achieved 49% survival rate in 43 adult patients with respiratory failure.[8] It was this report in 1986 that sparked renewed interest in ECLS, and several centers returned to using this critical care technique with a greater focus on Gattinoni's concept of "lung rest" (low-pressure, low-rate "apneic oxygenation" applied with $ECCO_2R$). Clemmer and Morris have recently tested the efficacy of $ECCO_2R$ with pressure-controlled, inverse-ratio ventilation vs. conventional mechanical ventilation alone by using randomization upon reaching entry criteria. They found no significant difference in the two protocol arms. What was novel about their study was that ventilator management was "controlled" in the two groups, thereby removing any bias possibly introduced by more attention being focused on the "new-therapy" group ($ECCO_2R$). Criticism of their study centers around the fact that the study was undertaken immediately upon introduction of $ECCO_2R$ to the ICU (and not when the typical "learning curve" of extracorporeal circulation had been surpassed after the treatment of 15 to 20 patients). Bleeding as a complication also resulted in $ECCO_2R$ patients being removed from extracorporeal support. Their study demonstrated that "standardized" control of the mechanical ventilator (with computer-driven monitoring and specific algorithms) is feasible, and such control should be part of testing hypotheses, particularly in the ICU.[14, 15]

We and several other groups have found that modern-day therapy for adult respiratory failure with ECLS can be achieved with low morbidity and a survival rate (discharge to home) of at least 50% (Table 3). In our experience, good prognostic indicators include a pre-ECLS time on mechanical ventilation of 7 days or

TABLE 3.
International and U.S. Centers Performing Extracorporeal Life
Support for Adult Patients

Center	N	Survivors
Paris	64	27 (42%)
Berlin	49	27 (55%)
Freiburg, Germany	31	15 (48%)
Marburg, Germany	165	97 (56%)
Mannheim, Germany	9	4 (44%)
Munich	21	17 (81%)
Milan-Monza, Italy	98	43 (44%)
Kuopio, Finland	6	1 (17%)
Stockholm	26	9 (35%)
Lund, Sweden	3	2 (67%)
Leicester, United Kingdom	18	12 (67%)
Sharpe Memorial Hospital (San Diego, Calif)	9	3 (33%)
University of Michigan (Ann Arbor)	103	57 (56%)
University of Pennsylvania (Philadelphia)	1	1 (100%)
University of Pittsburgh (Pa)	11	7 (64%)
LDS Hospital, University of Utah (Salt Lake City)	21	7 (33%)
Totals	635	329 (52%)

less, a diagnosis of (sterile) ARDS, pulmonary artery pressures less than 50% of systemic levels, and no other organ failure. With some of these caveats borne in mind, the technology of ECLS and critical care resources can be allocated to those patients who will benefit the most.

INNOVATIONS

As ECLS has entered the "modern era," many of the advances have occurred through technological breakthroughs in perfusion equipment and monitoring. One particular focus is to improve the safety and efficacy of ECLS and increase automation of the system.

When ECLS is performed in the ICU, the patient is cared for by both an ICU nurse and an ECLS specialist (who monitors and troubleshoots the ECLS system). One design alternative would be to have the ECLS system sufficiently automated so as to wean pump flow or the oxygenator sweep gas flow or composition by using feedback from specific patient, ventilator, or blood gas parameters. Features such as air bubble detection and a high-pressure system cutoff might provide added safety to the patient and at the same time make the system more self-regulating and user-friendly to the bedside ICU nurse. Merz et al. have described a prototype system for automated ECLS that incorporates many of these same features.[65]

The intravascular oxygenator (IVOX, Cardiopulmonics, Inc., Salt Lake City, Utah) is a device that was designed as a spin-off of ECLS technology. The IVOX (Fig 5) is a surgically implantable device that augments gas exchange. The actual gas exchange membrane resides intracorporeally, where CO_2 is removed and oxygen added to venous blood. The original concept was introduced by Mortensen in 1987, and several refinements in this device led to animal testing and phase I and II testing in 160 humans in the United States and Europe.[66–68]

The IVOX resembles a balloon pump in configuration and is inserted surgically into the vena cava after cutdown over the right internal jugular or femoral veins. The hollow-fiber strands are constructed of siloxane-coated microporous polypropylene and then coated with heparin to provide thromboresistance. The fibers are mounted from the middle to the distal end of the implanted portion of the supporting stalk. The fibers of the device are first tightly twisted around the stalk before insertion and then unfurled after satisfactory placement in the vena cava under fluoroscopic guidance. Oxygen is applied to the central stalk and then carried to the distal end where the fibers transmit the gas flow proximally to the gas outlet by the application of subatmospheric pressure (suction). This mode of bulk gas movement in the device (while residing in the blood path of the vena cava) is rather ingenious in preventing air embolism; fiber breakage results in blood being drawn into the hollow fiber, thereby clotting and occluding it.

The IVOX is more efficient at CO_2 removal than oxygen exchange, and under optimal conditions it is only able to remove about 20% to 30% of metabolically produced CO_2. In its intended design, the IVOX would provide augmentation of CO_2 removal and allow ventilatory support to be decreased. Several factors were found to increase CO_2 exchange and the effectiveness of the device: (1) "crimping" of the hollow fibers, which increases turbulence and thus increases overall contact of venous blood with each fiber; (2) increasing the oxygen gas flow within the system; and (3) raising the level of venous P_{CO_2} (permissive hypercapnia), thus producing a greater gradient for diffusion of CO_2 into the system.[69]

Although the IVOX is only being used experimentally, several investigators are working on a second-generation IVOX that should

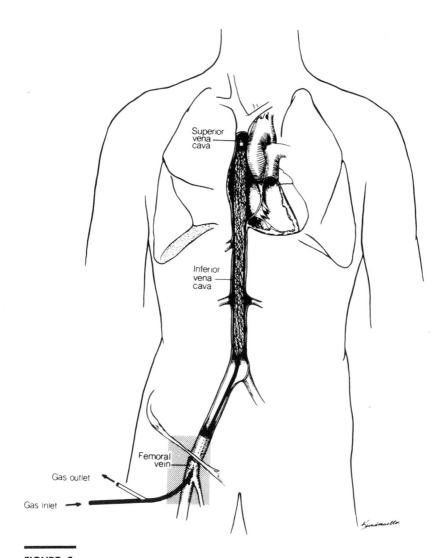

FIGURE 5.

Intravascular oxygenator. After surgical exposure of the right internal jugular or femoral veins, the device is twisted to reduce insertion diameter and placed in the vena cava under fluoroscopic guidance. Unfurling the device allows oxygen sweep gas within the fibers to exchange oxygen and CO_2 with venous blood. (Courtesy of CardioPulmonics, Inc., Salt Lake City, Utah.)

augment CO_2 removal to a greater degree. Snider et al. have designed a miniaturized intravascular lung that resides not only in the vena cava but also in the right atrium, ventricle, and pulmonary artery for added gas exchange.[70] Fazzalari et al. have taken the intracorporeal concept one step further and have developed a small implantable artificial lung that is placed within the chest and anastomosed to the pulmonary artery for short-term lung support.[71]

CONCLUSION

Extracorporeal life support is a critical care technique in which significant advances in the last decade have evolved in both perfusion technology and our understanding of the pathophysiology of respiratory and cardiac failure. The technique is both reasonable and safe and results in survival in about 50% of the patients in the pediatric and adult population after selection for an intrinsic mortality greater than 80% to 90% when treated by conventional means. Survival appears to be highest in patients with isolated organ failure in whom intervention is undertaken *early* during the disease process. In the modern era, ECLS and the related technologies will probably find a greater role for support of salvageable patients in the intensive care setting.

REFERENCES

1. Gibbon JH Jr: Artificial maintenance circulation during experimental occlusion of the pulmonary artery. *Arch Surg* 34:1105, 1937.
2. Hill JD, O'Brien TG, Murray JJ, et al: Extracorporeal oxygenation for acute post-traumatic respiratory failure (shock-lung syndrome): Use of the Bramson membrane lung. *N Engl J Med* 286:629–634, 1972.
3. Bartlett RH, Gazzaniga AB, Jefferies MR, et al: Extracorporeal membrane oxygenation (ECMO) cardiopulmonary support in infancy. *ASAIO Trans* 22:80–88, 1976.
4. Short BL, Pearson GD: Neonatal extracorporeal membrane oxygenation: A review. *J Int Care Med* 1:47–53, 1986.
5. Bartlett RH, Roloff DW, Cornell RG, et al: Extracorporeal circulation in neonatal respiratory failure: A prospective randomized study. *Pediatrics* 4:479–487, 1985.
6. Cornell RG, Landenberger BD, Bartlett RH: Randomized play-the-winner clinical trials. *Communications Statistics Theory Methods* 1:159–178, 1986.
7. Zapol WM, Snider MT, Hill JD, et al: Extracorporeal membrane oxygenation in severe acute respiratory failure: A randomized prospective study. *JAMA* 242:2193–2196, 1979.
8. Gattinoni L, Pesenti A, Mascheroni D, et al: Low-frequency positive-pressure ventilation with extracorporeal CO_2 removal in severe acute respiratory failure. *JAMA* 256:881–886, 1986.

9. Kolobow T, Solca M, Gattinoni L, et al: Adult respiratory distress syndrome (ARDS): Why did ECMO fail? *Int J Artif Organs* 4:58–59, 1981.
10. Pesenti A, Gattinoni L, Kolobow T, et al: Extracorporeal circulation in adult respiratory failure. *ASAIO Trans* 34:43–47, 1988.
11. Pesenti A, Gattinoni L, Bombino M: Long term extracorporeal respiratory support: 20 years of progress. *Intensive Crit Care Dig* 12:15–18, 1993.
12. Morris AH, Menlove RL, Rollins RJ, et al: A controlled clinical trial of a new 3-step therapy that includes extracorporeal CO_2 removal for ARDS. *ASAIO Trans* 34:48–53, 1988.
13. Anderson HL III, Delius RE, Sinard JM, et al: Early experience with adult extracorporeal membrane oxygenation in the modern era. *Ann Thorac Surg* 53:553–563, 1992.
14. Clemmer T, Morris A, Suchyta M, et al: Extracorporeal support does not improve ARDS survival. *Crit Care Med* 20:61S, 1992.
15. Morris AH, Wallace CJ, Menlove RL, et al: Randomized clinical trial of pressure-controlled inverse ratio ventilation and extracorporeal CO_2 removal for adult respiratory distress syndrome. *Am J Respir Crit Care Med* 149:295–305, 1994.
16. Anderson HL III, Steimle CN, Shapiro MB, et al: Extracorporeal life support for adult cardiorespiratory failure. *Surgery* 114:161–173, 1993.
17. Anderson HL III, Shapiro MB, Delius RE, et al: Extracorporeal life support for respiratory failure due to trauma—a viable alternative. *J Trauma* 37:266–274, 1994.
18. Hill JG, Bruhn PS, Cohen SE, et al: Emergent applications of cardiopulmonary support: A multiinstitutional experience. *Ann Thorac Surg* 54:699–704, 1992.
19. Bindslev L, Bohm C, Jolin A, et al: Extracorporeal carbon dioxide removal performed with surface-heparinized equipment in patients with ARDS. *Acta Anaesthesiol Scand Suppl* 95:125–131, 1991.
20. Wagner P, Knoch M, Sangmeister C, et al: Extracorporeal gas exchange in adult respiratory distress syndrome: Associated morbidity and its surgical treatment. *Br J Surg* 77:1395–1398, 1990.
21. Anderson HL III, Otsu T, Chapman RA, et al: Venovenous extracorporeal life support in neonates using a double lumen catheter. *ASAIO Trans* 35:650–653, 1989.
22. Anderson HL III, Snedecor SM, Otsu T, et al: Multicenter comparison of conventional venoarterial access versus venovenous double lumen catheter access in newborn infants undergoing extracorporeal membrane oxygenation. *J Pediatr Surg* 28:530–535, 1993.
23. Perreault T, Mullahoo K, Morneault L, et al: Use of a 12 French double-lumen catheter in a newborn supported with extracorporeal membrane oxygenation. *ASAIO J* 40:100–102, 1994.
24. Durandy Y, Chevalier JY, Lecompte Y: Single cannula venovenous bypass for respiratory membrane lung support. *J Thorac Cardiovas Surg* 99:404–409, 1990.

Moving?

I'd like to receive my *Advances in Surgery* without interruption.
Please note the following change of address, effective:

Name: _____

New Address: _____

_____

City: _____ State: _____ Zip: _____

Old Address: _____

_____

City: _____ State: _____ Zip: _____

Reservation Card

Yes, I would like my own copy of *Advances in Surgery*. Please begin my subscription with the current edition according to the terms described below.* I understand that I will have 30 days to examine each annual edition. If satisfied, I will pay just $69.95 plus sales tax, postage and handling (price subject to change without notice).

Name: _____

Address: _____

City: _____ State: _____ Zip: _____

Method of Payment
O Visa   O Mastercard   O AmEx   O Bill me   O Check (in US dollars, payable to Mosby, Inc.)

Card number: _____ Exp date: _____

Signature: _____

LS-0908

---

*Your Advances Service Guarantee:

When you subscribe to *Advances*, we'll send you an advance notice of future volumes about two months before they publish. This automatic notice system is designed to take up as little of your time as possible. If you do not want *Advances*, the advance notice makes it quick and easy for you to let us know your decision, and you will always have at least 20 days to decide. If we don't hear from you, we'll send you the new volume as soon as it's available. And, of course, *Advances* is yours to examine free of charge for 30 days (postage, handling and applicable sales tax are added to each shipment.).

BUSINESS REPLY MAIL

FIRST CLASS MAIL   PERMIT No. 762   CHICAGO, IL

POSTAGE WILL BE PAID BY ADDRESSEE

Chris Hughes
Mosby-Year Book, Inc.
161 N. Clark Street
Suite 1900
Chicago, IL 60601-9981

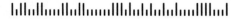

NO POSTAGE
NECESSARY
IF MAILED
IN THE
UNITED STATES

BUSINESS REPLY MAIL

FIRST CLASS MAIL   PERMIT No. 762   CHICAGO, IL

POSTAGE WILL BE PAID BY ADDRESSEE

Chris Hughes
Mosby-Year Book, Inc.
161 N. Clark Street
Suite 1900
Chicago, IL 60601-9981

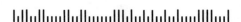

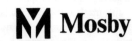

Dedicated to publishing excellence

25. Tsuno K, Terasaki H, Tsutsumi R, et al: To-and-fro veno-venous extracorporeal lung assist for newborns with severe respiratory distress. *Intensive Care Med* 15:269–271, 1989.
26. Chevalier JY, Couprie C, Larroquet M, et al: Venovenous single lumen cannula extracorporeal lung support in neonates. A five year experience. *ASAIO J* 39:M654–M658, 1993.
27. Montoya JP, Merz SI, Bartlett RH: A standardized system for describing flow/pressure relationships in vascular access devices. *ASAIO Trans* 37:4–8, 1991.
28. Sinard JM, Merz SI, Hatcher MD, et al: Evaluation of extracorporeal perfusion catheters using a standardized measurement technique—the M-number. *ASAIO Trans* 37:60–64, 1991.
29. Delius RE, Montoya JP, Merz SI, et al: New method for describing the performance of cardiac surgery cannulas. *Ann Thorac Surg 53:278–281, 1992.*
30. Steinhorn RH, Isham-Schopf B, Smith C, et al: Hemolysis during long-term extracorporeal membrane oxygenation. *J Pediatr* 115:625–630, 1989.
31. Montoya JP, Merz SI, Bartlett RH: Laboratory experience with a novel, non-occlusive, pressure-regulated peristaltic pump. *ASAIO J* 38: M406–M411, 1992.
32. Shanley CJ, Hultquist KA, Rosenberg DM, et al: Prolonged extracorporeal circulation without heparin: Evaluation of the Medtronic Minimax oxygenator. *ASAIO Trans* 38:M311–M316, 1992.
33. Toomasian JM, Hsu L-C, Hirschl RB, et al: Evaluation of Duraflo II heparin coating in prolonged extracorporeal membrane oxygenation. *ASAIO Trans* 34:410–414, 1988.
34. Gorman RC, Ziats NP, Rao AK, et al: Surface-bound heparin fails to reduce thrombin formation during clinical cardiopulmonary bypass. *J Thorac Cardiovasc Surg* 111:1–12, 1996.
35. Videm V, Svennevig JL, Fosse E, et al: Reduced complement activation with heparin-coated oxygenator and tubings in coronary bypass operations. *J Thorac Cardiovasc Surg* 103:806–813, 1992.
36. Barstad RM, Ovrum E, Ringdal M-A, et al: Heparin-coated extracorporeal circuit decreases monocyte procoagulant activity in coronary artery bypass surgery. *J Thorac Cardiovasc Surg* 1996, in press.
37. Borowiec J, Thelin S, Bagge L, et al: Heparin-coated circuits reduce activation of granulocytes during cardiopulmonary bypass. *J Thorac Cardiovasc Surg* 104:642–647, 1992.
38. Mottaghy K, Oedekoven B, Starmans H, et al: Technical aspects of plasma leakage prevention in microporous capillary membrane oxygenators. *ASAIO Trans* 35:640–645, 1989.
39. Montoya JP, Shanley CJ, Merz SI, et al: Plasma leakage through microporous membranes: Role of phospholipids. *ASAIO J* 38:M399, 1992.
40. Bartlett RH: Extracorporeal life support for cardiopulmonary failure. *Curr Probl Surg* 10:627–705, 1990.

41. Whittlesey GC, Kundu SY, Salley SO, et al: Is heparin necessary for extracorporeal circulation. *ASAIO Trans* 34:823–826, 1988.
42. Cilley RE, Zwischenberger JB, Andrews AF, et al: Intracranial hemorrhage during extracorporeal membrane oxygenation in neonates. *Pediatrics* 78:699–704, 1986.
43. Bui KC, LaClair P, Vanderkerhove J, et al: ECMO in premature infants: Review of factors associated with mortality. *ASAIO Trans* 37:54–59, 1991.
44. Heiss KF, Pettit B, Hirschl RB, et al: Renal insufficiency and volume overload in neonatal ECMO managed by continuous ultrafiltration. *ASAIO* 10:54–57, 1987.
45. Anderson HL III, Coran AG, Drongowski RA, et al: Extracellular fluid and total body water changes in neonates undergoing extracorporeal membrane oxygenation (ECMO). *J Pediatr Surg* 27:1003–1008, 1992.
46. Langer M, Mascheroni D, Marcolin R, et al: The prone position in ARDS patients. A clinical study. Chest 94:103–107, 1988.
47. Ciaglia P, Graniero KD: Percutaneous dilational tracheostomy—results and long term follow-up. *Chest* 101:464–467, 1992.
48. Spector ML, Wiznitzer M, Walsh-Sukys MC, et al: Carotid reconstruction in the neonate following ECMO. *J Pediatr Surg* 26:357–359, 1991.
49. Taylor BJ, Seibert JJ, Glasier CM, et al: Evaluation of the reconstructed carotid artery following extracorporeal membrane oxygenation. *Pediatrics* 90:568–572, 1992.
50. Baumgart S, Streletz LJ, Needleman L, et al: Right common carotid artery reconstruction after extracorporeal membrane oxygenation: Vascular imaging, cerebral circulation, electroencephalographic, and neurodevelopmental correlates to recovery. *J Pediatr* 125:295–304, 1994.
51. Clark RH: High-frequency ventilation. *J Pediatr* 124:661–670, 1994.
52. Pranikoff T, Hirschl RB, Steimle CN, et al: Mortality is directly related to the duration of mechanical ventilation before the initiation of extracorporeal life support for severe respiratory failure. *Crid Care Med* 25:28–32, 1997.
53. Anderson HL III, Attorri RJ, Custer JR, et al: Extracorporeal membrane oxygenation (ECMO) for pediatric cardiopulmonary failure. *J Thorac Cardiovasc Surg* 99:1011–1019, 1990.
54. Pennington GD, Swartz MT: Circulatory support in infants and children. *Ann Thorac Surg 55:233–237, 1993.*
55. Delius RE, Bove EL, Meliones JN, et al: Use of extracorporeal life support in patients with congenital heart disease. *Crit Care Med* 20:1216–1222, 1992.
56. Klein MD, Shaheen KW, Whittlesey GC, et al: Extracorporeal membrane oxygenation for the circulatory support of children after repair of congenital heart disease. *J Thorac Cardiovasc Surg* 100:498–505, 1990.
57. Bosken C, Lenfant C: Extracorporeal membrane oxygenation revisited . . . again. *Ann Thorac Surg* 53:551–552,1992.

58. Bartlett RH, Schumacher RE, Chapman RA: Economics of extracorporeal life support, in Zwischenberger JB, Bartlett RH (eds): *ECMO: Extracorporeal Cardiopulmonary Support in Critical Care.* Ann Arbor, Mich, Extracorporeal Life Support Organization, 1995, pp 533–550.
59. ECMO Quarterly Report. Ann Arbor, Mich, ECMO Registry of the Extracorporeal Life Support Organization, July 1996.
60. Meyer DM, Jessen ME: Results of extracorporeal membrane oxygenation in neonates with sepsis. The Extracorporeal Life Support Organization experience. *J Thorac Cardiovasc Surg* 109:419–427, 1995.
61. O'Rourke PP, Stolar CJ, Zwischenberger JB, et al: Extracorporeal membrane oxygenation: Support for overwhelming pulmonary failure in the pediatric population. Experience from the Extracorporeal Life Support Organization. *J Pediatr Surg* 28:523–529, 1993.
62. Schumacher RE, Roloff DW, Chapman RA, et al: Extracorporeal membrane oxygenation in term newborns: A prospective cost-benefit analysis. *ASAIO J* 39:873–879, 1993.
63. Morton A, Dalton H, Kochanek P, et al: Extracorporeal membrane oxygenation for pediatric respiratory failure: Five-year experience at the University of Pittsburgh. *Crit Care Med* 22:1659–1667, 1994.
64. Moler FW, Palmisano JM, Custer JR: Extracorporeal life support for pediatric respiratory failure: Predictors of survival from 220 patients. *Crit Care Med* 21:1604–1611, 1993.
65. Merz S, Montoya PJ, Shanley CJ, et al: Implemenataton of a controller for extracorporeal life support. *ASAIO Trans* 22:69A, 1993.
66. Mortensen JD: An intravenacaval blood gas exchange (IVCBGE) device—preliminary report. *ASAIO Trans* 33:570–573, 1987.
67. Jurmann JM, Demertzis S, Schaefers H-J, et al: Intravascular oxygenation for advanced respiratory failure. *ASAIO J* 38:120–124, 1992.
68. Conrad SA, Eggerstedt JM, Morris VF, et al: Prolonged intracorporeal support of gas exchange with an intravenacaval oxygenator. *Chest* 103:158–161, 1993.
69. Cox CS Jr, Zwischenberger JB, Grave DF, et al: Intracorporeal CO_2 removal and permissive hypercapnia to reduce airway pressure in acute respiratory failure: The theoretical basis for permissive hypercapnia with IVOX. *ASAIO J* 39:97–102, 1993.
70. Snider MT, High KM, Richard RB, et al: Small intrapulmonary artery lung prototypes: Design, construction, and in vitro water testing. *ASAIO J* 40:M522–M526, 1994.
71. Fazzalari FL, Montoya JP, Bonnell MR, et al: The development of an implantable artificial lung. *ASAIO J* 40:M728–M731, 1994.

CHAPTER 10

The Flank vs. the Abdominal Approach for Aortic Surgery: The Abdominal Approach

Michael Belkin, M.D.
Assistant Professor of Surgery, Department of Surgery, Brigham and Women's Hospital, Harvard Medical School, Boston, Massachusetts

Magruder C. Donaldson, M.D.
Associate Professor of Surgery, Department of Surgery, Brigham and Women's Hospital, Harvard Medical School, Boston, Massachusetts

John A. Mannick, M.D.
Moseley Distinguished Professor of Surgery, Department of Surgery, Brigham and Women's Hospital, Harvard Medical School, Boston, Massachusetts

Anthony D. Whittemore, M.D.
Chief, Professor of Surgery, Department of Surgery, Brigham and Women's Hospital, Harvard Medical School, Boston, Massachusetts

M anagement of abdominal aortic aneurysms (AAAs) entered the modern era in 1951 when Charles Dubost performed the first successful repair with an aortic homograft.[1] That remarkable achievement prolonged the patient's life by 8 years and stood in stark contrast to the dismal results of prior methods of repair, including aneurysm ligation, induced thrombosis, and wrapping. The next major advance occurred in 1953 when Voorhees first used a prosthetic graft to repair an aortic aneurysm.[2] Despite these early advances, operative mortality rates approximated 20%.[3] Subsequent advances in anesthetic and operative techniques improved the mortality rates to 4% to 9% by the 1970s.[4] Chief among these was the introduction and adoption of the graft inclusion technique as advocated by Creech.[5] More recently, further refinements in preoperative cardiac evaluation and intraoperative cardiac and fluid management have contributed to further reductions in operative mortality to below 4%.

Ironically, although the initial aneurysm repair performed by Dubost was conducted via the retroperitoneal, thoracoabdominal approach, the standard approach for infrarenal AAA repair became the transabdominal approach familiar to all vascular surgeons. Although several series of retroperitoneal AAA repairs appeared in the 1960s and 1970s, it was not until Williams et al. reintroduced the left flank retroperitoneal approach to AAA repair in 1980 that widespread interest and use of this technique developed.[6] Since that time a number of retrospective and prospective studies promoting the virtues of the retroperitoneal approach to AAA repair have appeared.[7–9]

Although we use the retroperitoneal approach to AAA repair on a selective basis, the transabdominal technique remains our standard approach and is currently used in over 90% of our operations. In this review, we will address the advantages and disadvantages as well as the relative indications for both transabdominal and retroperitoneal AAA repair. We then will review the current technique for transabdominal repair along with the current results that have been achieved on our service and elsewhere.

RELATIVE ADVANTAGES OF THE TRANSABDOMINAL AND RETROPERITONEAL APPROACHES

TRANSABDOMINAL APPROACH

The advantages and disadvantages of the transabdominal surgical approach are reviewed in Table 1. The major obvious benefit of the transabdominal technique is related to the flexible, broad abdominal exposure this approach allows. Careful intraoperative examination of the abdomen will reveal a significant incidence of concomitant pathology, including malignancies in 4% to 12% of the cases.[10] Potentially important benign pathology, including cholelithiasis (4% to 19%) or diverticulitis, may also frequently be identified. Direct evaluation of the left colon for evidence of ischemia is particularly important in patients with compromised mesenteric vessels or collateral perfusion (e.g., patients who have had previous partial colon resections). A major advantage of the transabdominal approach is the ease of exposure and repair of aneurysms extending into the right iliac artery. Although seldom necessary, exposure of the right femoral vessels for thrombectomy or distal

TABLE 1.
Transabdominal Approach to Aneurysm Repair

Advantages
    Familiar anatomy to most surgeons
    Broad abdominal exposure and complete abdominal
      exploration
    Ease of exposure of the right femoral, iliac, and renal arteries
Disadvantages
    Surgery in a "hostile" abdomen: multiple previous operations
    Abdominal wall stomas
    Difficult aortic anatomy: suprarenal aneurysm, recurrent
      aneurysm, inflammatory aneurysm, horseshoe kidney

anastomosis is simple and direct when the transabdominal approach is used. Similarly, exposure of the right renal artery for bypass or endarterectomy, as well as the subsequent evaluation of blood flow, is best performed via the transabdominal approach. Finally, the increased familiarity with the transabdominal exposure for most surgeons will result in an easier, more expeditious repair.

Disadvantages of the transabdominal approach relate to the patient's pathologic anatomy. Patients with multiple past abdominal operations will often have severe adhesions that may complicate and prolong the surgical exposure. True suprarenal aneurysms are difficult to expose and repair via the transabdominal approach and generally require complex modifications such as medial visceral rotation. Similarly, in patients with inflammatory aneurysms or pseudoaneurysms above previous repairs, proximal aortic dissection and control may be difficult to achieve via the anterior transabdominal technique. Patients with aortic aneurysms and horseshoe kidneys are also difficult to repair via the transabdominal approach. Depending on their location and anatomy, bowel or urinary stomas may complicate exposure and repair via the transabdominal approach.

Relative indications for transabdominal AAA repair encompass the majority (90%) of the operations performed on our service and reflect the advantages outlined earlier. They include operations performed for uncomplicated aneurysms of the aorta and aortoiliac arteries. In particular, the transabdominal technique is used when the bowel is at risk for ischemic complications and when surgery on the right iliac, femoral, or renal arteries is anticipated.

RETROPERITONEAL APPROACH

The major advantages of the retroperitoneal approach are related to the pathologic anatomy of the aneurysm (Table 2). The retroperitoneal approach greatly facilitates exposure of the suprarenal aorta and left renal and proximal mesenteric vessels. Safe suprarenal cross-clamping and aneurysmal repair in this segment of the aorta are favored because of the increased control and broadened exposure. Other advantages of the retroperitoneal approach arise when anterior exposure of the aneurysm is complicated. As outlined earlier, these include patients with severe abdominal adhesions, inflammatory aneurysms, recurrent aneurysms, or pseudoaneurysms and patients with horseshoe kidneys. Exposure and repair can be greatly facilitated via the retroperitoneum in these difficult cases.

Disadvantages of the retroperitoneal approach include limited familiarity with this exposure for many surgeons and the resultant increased complexity and operative time. Although the abdominal cavity can be entered if intra-abdominal pathology is suspected, the abdominal contents are generally not inspected. Many proponents of routine application of the retroperitoneal approach contend that exposure of the right iliac and femoral vessels is uncomplicated. In our experience, however, such exposure is cumbersome and often requires counterincisions (for sufficient iliac artery exposure). "Blind" transaortic right renal endarterectomy is simple via the left retroperitoneal exposure; however, subsequent evaluation of renal

---

TABLE 2.
Retroperitoneal Approach to Aneurysm Repair

Advantages
   Improved exposure to the suprarenal aorta and visceral
      segment
   Improved exposure of complex aortic aneurysms: suprarenal
      aneurysm, recurrent aneurysm, inflammatory aneurysm,
      horseshoe kidney
   Avoidance of a hostile abdomen and abdominal wall ostomies
Disadvantages
   Limited familiarity of many surgeons with anatomy
   Limited visualization of abdominal contents
   Difficult/limited exposure of the right femoral, iliac, and renal
      arteries
   Increased incisional pain and long-term wound problems

blood flow for the recognition and repair of technical problems related to the endarterectomy is difficult. Direct surgery on the right renal artery for bypass or open endarterectomy is not usually possible via the left flank exposure.

Another disadvantage of the retroperitoneal approach relates to long-term incisional problems. In our experience, these incisions tend to be more painful beyond the perioperative period than are the midline incisions of the transabdominal approach. Flank incisions are also frequently complicated by a permanent protrusion around the incision. This usually represents weakness of the abdominal wall musculature because of denervation rather than frank herniation.

The relative indications for application of the retroperitoneal exposure reflect the aforementioned advantages. Currently, we perform 10% of our *infrarenal* aneurysm repairs with this approach, with the most common indication being a "hostile" abdomen resulting from multiple previous surgeries. Conversely, the retroperitoneal exposure remains our preferred approach for true *suprarenal* aneurysms. Repair of juxtarenal aneurysms, i.e., those extending close to the renal arteries, is readily performed via the retroperitoneal approach or the transabdominal approach, depending on the surgeon's preference.

TECHNIQUE OF TRANSABDOMINAL AORTIC ANERUSYM REPAIR

PREOPERATIVE EVALUATION AND PREPARATION

All patients undergo preoperative cardiac evaluation. Patients free of significant risk factors for coronary artery disease who are asymptomatic undergo surgery with no further cardiac evaluation.[11] Those with a history of angina, a previous myocardial infarction, or significant risk factors undergo echocardiography and either dipyridamole (Persantine) myocardial scintigraphy or Holter monitoring for silent cardiac ischemia. All patients have preoperative maximization of their medical regimens, and only a small minority undergo coronary arteriography. Only patients with severe ischemic symptoms such as unstable angina are recommended for preoperative coronary artery revascularization.

In the past we performed preoperative arteriography in most patients before AAA repair. With improvements in cross-sectional imaging techniques, in particular, high-resolution spiral CT scanning, we now reserve arteriography for selected patients. These include patients with arterial occlusive disease, suspected renal artery disease, and other more rare indications. Similarly, in the past all patients received preoperative pulmonary artery thermodilution catheters. We have now adopted a more selective strategy, with approximely 50% of our patients receiving only central venous cannulation. All patients receive radial artery cannulation and preoperative epidural catheterization. The epidural catheter has proved to be a helpful adjunct to the intraoperative general anesthetic, as well as to postoperative pain management.

TECHNICAL ASPECTS OF REPAIR

The abdomen is opened and explored through a midline incision extending from the xiphoid to just above the pubis. The small bowel is mobilized superiorly and to the right and packed into the right upper quadrant of the abdomen. Exposure of the operative field is greatly facilitated by a mechanical self-retaining retractor fixed to the operating table. The peritoneum is incised with scissors along the inferior border of the third and fourth portions of the duodenum, and the duodenum is retracted laterally to the patient's right. The peritoneum and areolar tissue overlying the aorta are opened longitudinally with scissors or a cautery to expose the anterior surface of the aneurysm (Fig 1).

The incision is carried superiorly to the level of the left renal vein and inferiorly to a point below the aortic bifurcation. The aorta just above the aneurysm and below the left renal vein is freed from its surrounding tissues by a combination of sharp and gentle blunt dissection anteriorly and laterally. No attempt is made to dissect behind the aorta at this level, nor is the neck of the aneurysm encircled with tape. The dissection along each lateral wall of the aorta is continued far enough posteriorly so that the neck of the aneurysm can be compressed easily by an occluding clamp, which will be applied at this level.

Inferiorly, the anterior and lateral walls of both common iliac arteries are freed by sharp dissection in a similar fashion without separating these vessels from their attachments to the common iliac veins posteriorly. Dissection of the lateral walls of the aneurysm is kept to a minimum to eliminate the necessity for ligating the multiple small vessels that traverse the surrounding lymphatic and areolar tissue. In particular, mobilization of the aneurysm wall from the inferior vena cava is unnecessary and is avoided to reduce the risk of injury.

Heparin is administered to the patient systemically, 4,000 to 5,000 U IV in an average adult. Although it is possible to repair many AAAs successfully without the use of heparin, anticoagula-

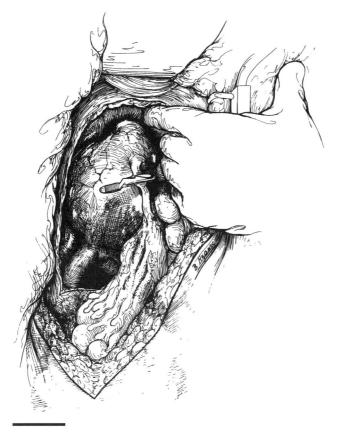

FIGURE 1.
Initial exposure and dissection of an infrarenal aortic aneurysm.

tion is advisable when the aorta and iliac arteries are clamped; otherwise, extensive distal thrombosis can occur in patients who have severe distal arterial occlusive disease and in those instances in which mural thrombus or atherosclerotic debris from the aneurysm is inadvertently embolized distally.

After anticoagulation, large straight Fogarty vascular clamps are applied to both common iliac arteries, and a Fogarty or Debakey reverse-angle aortic clamp is applied to the aorta above the aneurysm. The superficial, adventitial layer of the aneurysm is incised longitudinally with an electrocautery to minimize bleeding from the aortic wall. The aneurysm is then opened with Mayo scissors. Each end of the aneurysm is then "T'ed" laterally to increase exposure to the aneurysm cavity (Fig 2). All mural thrombi and loose

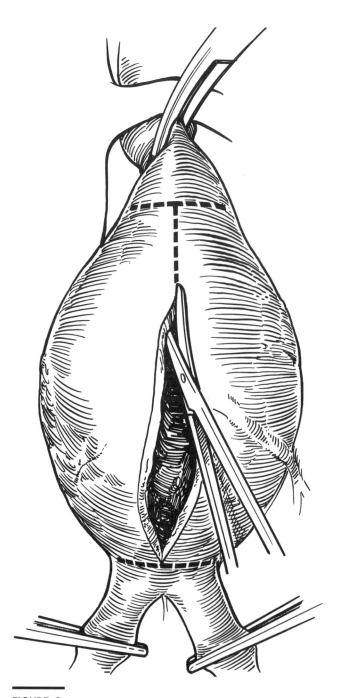

FIGURE 2.

Once the proximal and distal clamps are applied, the aorta is opened longitudinally with lateral "T" extensions to increase exposure.

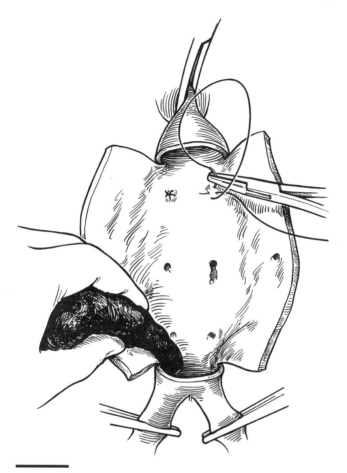

FIGURE 3.

Once the aorta is opened, the mural thrombus is removed while avoiding impaction of debris into the iliac artery origins. Backbleeding lumbar arteries are oversewn.

atherosclerotic debris are evacuated from the lumen of the aneurysm. Special care is taken to avoid impaction of thrombus or atherosclerotic debris into the origins of the iliac arteries.

The origins of bleeding lumbar arteries are oversewn with figure-of-8 sutures of 3-0 polypropylene (Fig 3). The origin of the inferior mesenteric artery is similarly sutured if this vessel is still patent and backbleeding is vigorous. If the inferior mesenteric artery is widely patent and backbleeding is sluggish, reimplantation of the artery into the aortic prosthesis should be considered. The decision to reimplant the inferior mesenteric artery is based on the appearance of the sigmoid colon and the strength of mesenteric Doppler signals after restoration of flow to the pelvis.

In patients with no significant iliac aneurysms, a tube graft of woven or collagen-impregnated knitted Dacron is our preference for aneurysm replacement. Sixty-six percent of the aneurysms on our service are reparable with a tube graft. This is sutured distally to the aortic bifurcation, which usually remains a reasonably normal size even when the aneurysm involves the entire infrarenal abdominal aorta.

The posterior wall of the aorta is not divided either proximally or distally. The posterior aortic wall is often a rather tenuous structure, and we prefer to add strength to the posterior suture line by including the surrounding fascial tissue in the posterior stitches of the anastomosis. A Dacron tube graft of appropriate size is sewn with a double-armed 3-0 polypropylene suture to the posterior wall of the aorta at the neck of the aneurysm. A double thickness of aortic wall is included in each bite posteriorly. The suture is carried around each side of the neck of the aneurysm and tied anteriorly (Fig 4).

The proximal anastomosis is then tested for leaks by clamping the tube graft and releasing the aortic clamp briefly. If any leaks

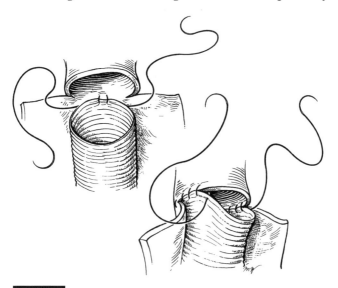

FIGURE 4.

The proximal anastomosis is initiated with a posterior horizontal matress suture of 3-0 polypropylene, which is tied down. The suture is then run anteriorly in a continuous fashion.

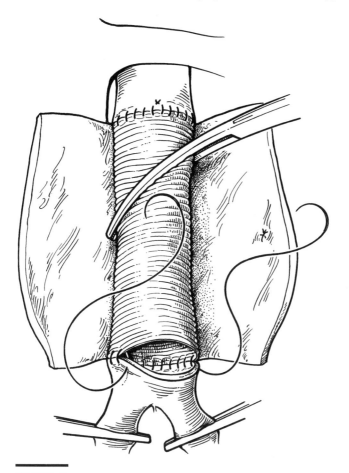

FIGURE 5.

After the proximal anastomosis is completed, the graft is flushed and the clamp transferred down onto the graft. The distal anastomosis is completed as for the proximal anastomosis.

are noted in the anastomosis, they are repaired with simple or figure-of-8 sutures of 3-0 polypropylene. The aortic clamp is then replaced on the graft just distal to the proximal anastomosis. After being evacuated of all blood with a sucker, the graft is placed under slight tension and cut to the appropriate length for anastomosis with the aortic bifurcation. The lower anastomosis is performed by using a double-armed suture of 3-0 polypropylene (Fig 5). In cases in which the aortic bifurcation is densely calcified, judicious endarterectomy of calcified plaque may be required to facilitate suturing of the distal anastomosis.

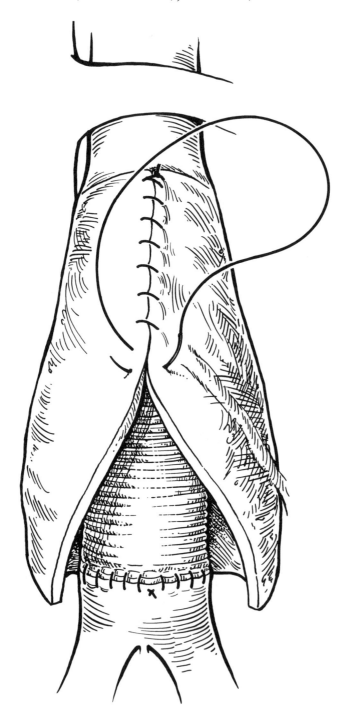

All vessels are flushed before completion of this suture line. The suture line is then completed and tied anteriorly as for the proximal anastomosis. The iliac clamps are released and the lower anastomosis is inspected for leaks, which are repaired as for the proximal anastomosis. The proximal aortic clamp is then gradually released while the anesthesiologist carefully monitors the patient's blood pressure and infuses additional volume IV if needed. After release of the clamps, the iliac arteries are inspected for adequate pulsation, and the presence of good femoral pulses in the groin is determined by palpation. Depending on the duration of aneurysm repair and the appearance of the operative field, we use protamine sulfate on a selective basis for heparin reversal. Any residual bleeding points in the aneurysm wall are sutured, ligated, or electrocoagulated, and the aneurysm wall is sutured back over the prosthesis with a running 3-0 polypropylene suture (Fig 6). This is helpful for both hemostasis and exclusion of the prosthetic graft from the duodenum and other viscera. The posterior peritoneum and periaortic lymphatic tissues are then approximated over the aorta and, if possible, over the resutured aneurysm wall by a running absorbable suture in order to provide further retroperitoneal hemostasis. This also has the advantage of placing yet another layer between the prosthesis and the posterior wall of the duodenum. The abdomen is then closed with a continuous suture of no. 2 polypropylene to the rectus fascia and stapled to the skin.

If common iliac aneurysms are present, a similar operative procedure is followed. However, the iliac clamps are applied to the iliac bifurcations, with care taken to avoid injury to the ureters, which usually cross the common iliac arteries distally. Iliac aneurysms are opened longitudinally. A bifurcation graft of Dacron is used and the upper anastomosis is performed as described. The iliac limbs are sutured on either side to the distal common iliac arteries, again from inside the iliac aneurysms (Fig 7). Limited endarterectomies of the iliac bifurcation to remove dense calcium may be necessary to facilitate the distal anastomosis. The aneurysm walls may also be sutured back over the graft limbs to provide an extra layer of host tissue between the graft and the abdominal viscera. In the case of a large left iliac aneurysm, it may be more con

---

FIGURE 6.

The aneurysmal sac is then sutured back over the graft for hemostasis and to exclude the graft from the duodenum and other viscera.

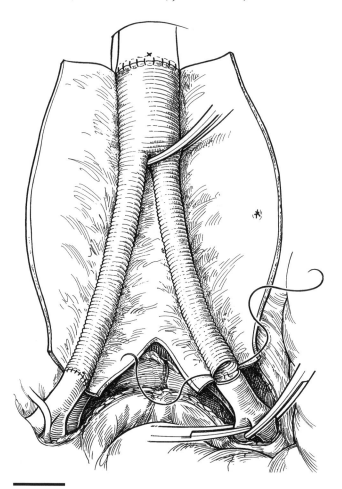

FIGURE 7.

When the aortic aneurysm involves the iliac arteries, a bifurcation graft extending down to the iliac bifurcations is required. Distal control is obtained either by clamping the distal common iliac arteries or by placing separate clamps on the external and internal iliac arteries. Exposure of the left iliac bifurcation usually requires mobilization of the sigmoid colon medially.

venient to exclude the aneurysm and suture the left limb of the graft in an end-to-side fashion to the external iliac artery inferior to the sigmoid mesentery.

In so-called juxtarenal aneurysms, where the abdominal aortic aneurysm extends more proximally than usual and there is little or no neck of normal aorta between the aneurysm and the renal arteries, it is helpful to place the aortic clamp at the level of the diaphragm while the proximal anastomosis is performed.

The aorta at the level of the diaphragm can be exposed by incising the attachments of the left lobe of the liver to the diaphragm and retracting the liver to the right. The lesser sac is entered and the aorta is exposed as it passes underneath the crus of the diaphragm. The crus is incised longitudinally and blunt finger dissection is used to complete the lateral exposure of the aorta at the hiatus (Fig 8). At this level the vessel is usually disease free, of normal caliber, and free of branches.

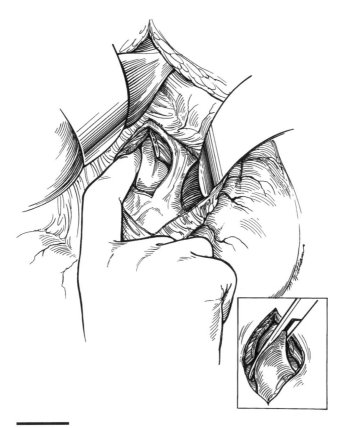

FIGURE 8.

An alternative site of aortic control is the supraceliac aorta. Exposure is obtained by incising the gastrohepatic ligament and retracting the stomach and esophagus to the patient's left. The diaphragmatic crus is incised, and the index finger is used to dissect along each side of the supraceliac aorta posteriorly until the vertebral body is palpable. A cross-clamp can be placed over the fingers onto the supraceliac aorta.

Backbleeding from the celiac axis and superior mesenteric artery can be controlled with an intra-aortic balloon catheter inserted from below, and the graft can be anastomosed proximally with excellent visibility from inside the aneurysm into the normal aorta just distal to the renal artery orifices. After completion of the proximal anastomosis, the aortic clamp is released and the prosthesis is clamped to restore flow to the viscera and to the renal arteries. We believe that this technique is much less hazardous to the kidneys than attempts to clamp the aorta close to the renal artery orifices, which may result in artherosclerotic embolization to one or both kidneys. Some patients with juxtarenal aneurysms have a considerable distance between the renal artery orifices and the origin of the superior mesenteric artery. In such individuals, it may be more convenient to free the aorta just above the renal arteries and left renal vein. The aorta can then be safely clamped below the superior mesenteric artery, thus avoiding even a brief period of visceral ischemia.

RESULTS

CURRENT SERIES

Our own experience with transabdominal AAA repair has previously been reported and is updated herein.[11] From 1972 to 1994, 794 elective transabdominal AAA repairs were performed on our service. Seventy-two percent of the patients were asymptomatic, whereas 24% were symptomatic with back pain and 4% had distal emboli. The mean age was 70 years, with 81% of the patients being male and 19% female. Risk factors included coronary artery disease (49%), hypertension (48%), smoking (52%), chronic obstructive pulmonary disease (24%), chronic renal failure (7%), and congestive heart failure (8%). The mean aneurysm diameter (determined by CT scan) was 6.3 cm and ranged from 3.5 to 15 cm. Sixty-six percent of the repairs were completed with tube grafts, whereas 34% required bifurcation grafts. A concomitant renal artery reconstruction was completed in 9% of the cases.

Overall morbidity was 33% and included myocardial infarction (2.3%), arrhythmia (17.4%), transient renal failure (4.9%), pulmonary complications (5%), and prolonged ileus (3.1%). The overall 30-day operative mortality was 1.8%.

COMPARATIVE SERIES

Most of the series comparing the transabdominal and retroperitoneal approaches to AAA repair are retrospective reviews that are difficult to accurately evaluate. In many series the operative approach was influenced by patient anatomy, and these retrospective reviews are often subject to unintentional, subtle biases. Two large prospective randomized comparisons of the transabdominal and retroperitoneal approaches to routine AAA repair have recently been reported.

In the first study, Cambria et al. compared 59 transabdominal and 54 retroperitoneal operations for AAA repair.[12] No differences were found in operative time, transfusion or fluid requirements, or any other operative parameters. Intensive care unit parameters, including ventilatory and fluid requirements and length of ICU stay, did not differ. Similarly, no differences in respiratory physiology, metabolic parameters, morbidity, or mortality could be detected. The retroperitoneal patients did resume alimentation nearly a day earlier than the transabdominal patients, but this did not result in a decreased length of stay, which was similar for both groups. Most importantly, when the authors compared the results achieved in both the transabdominal and retroperitoneal groups with transabdominal patients operated on during the 2 years before the study, significant advances had been achieved during the study period. This observation points out the pitfalls of using historic controls and emphasizes the continued improvements we are achieving in the management of AAAs. The authors concluded that there is no demonstrable benefit to either the transabdominal or retroperitoneal surgical approaches and that selection should be based on the patient's anatomy and surgeon's preference.

A second recent randomized prospective comparison was reported by Sicard et al.[13] This study was based on a prior retrospective review from the same authors that demonstrated advantages for the retroperitoneal incision.[7] These authors compared 75 transabdominal and 70 retroperitoneal procedures, including both AAA repairs and aortofemoral arterial reconstructions for occlusive disease. The two groups in this study were not strictly comparable because there was a significantly higher incidence of chronic obstructive pulmonary disease (COPD) in the transabdominal patients (28% vs. 11%). The authors found no difference in mortality rate or total length of hospital stay. The incidence of complications was higher after the transabdominal repair, which is explained by the higher incidence of ileus and small-bowel obstruction in the transabdominal group. Despite the higher incidence of COPD in the transabdominal group, the incidence of pulmonary complications did not differ. Long-term incisional pain was a greater problem in the patients operated on via the retroperitoneal approach.

In summary, these two randomized trials confirm a benefit in terms of a reduced incidence of prolonged ileus in patients operated on via the retroperitoneal approach. As our experience has matured with the transabdominal technique, however, we have removed nasogastric tubes earlier and resumed enteral feedings more rapidly without an apparent increase in ileus or gastrointestinal complications. The overall significance of decreased ileus noted in patients operated on via the retroperitoneal approach is unclear.

CONCLUSIONS

Advances in perioperative management and operative techniques have made AAA repair an increasingly safe and effective operation. Successful repair may be accomplished via both the transabdominal and retroperitoneal approaches. We prefer the transabdominal approach for routine AAA repair because of its simplicity, versatility, and safety. We use the retroperitoneal approach on a selective basis when dictated by the patient's pathologic anatomy.

REFERENCES

1. Dubost C, Allary M, Oeconomos N: Resection of an aneurysm of the abdominal aorta; re-establishment of the continuity by a preserved human arterial graft, with result after five months. *Arch Surg* 64:405–408, 1952.
2. Blakemore AH, Voorhees AB: The use of tubes constructed from Vinyon "N" cloth in bridging arterial defects—experimental and clinical. *Ann Surg* 140:324–334, 1954.
3. DeBakey ME, Crawford ES, et al: Aneurysm of the abdominal aorta: Analysis of results of graft replacement therapy one to eleven years after operation. *Ann Surg* 106:622–639, 1964.
4. Hicks GL, Eastland MW, et al: Survival improvement following aortic aneurysm resection. *Ann Surg* 181:863–869, 1975.
5. Creech O: Endo-aneurysmorraphy and treatment of aortic aneurysm. *Ann Surg* 164:935–946, 1966.
6. Williams GM, Ricotta J, Zinner M, et al: The extended retroperitoneal approach for treatment of extensive atherosclerosis of the aorta and renal vessels. *Surgery* 88:846–855, 1980.
7. Sicard GA, Freeman MB, VanderWoude JC, et al: Comparison between the transabdominal and retroperitoneal approach for reconstruction of the infrarenal abdominal aorta. *J Vasc Surg* 5:19–27, 1987.
8. Johnson JN, McLoughlin GA, Wake PN, et al: Comparison of extraperitoneal and transperitoneal methods of aorto-iliac reconstruction. *J Cardiovasc Surg* 27:561–564, 1986.
9. Peck JJ, McReynolds DG, Baker DH, et al: Extraperitoneal approach to the abdominal aorta: Revisited. *J Cardiovasc Surg* 24:529–531, 1986.
10. Weinstein ES, Langsfeld M, DeFrang R: Current management of coexistent intra-abdominal pathology in patients with abdominal aortic aneurysms. *Semin Vasc Surg* 8:135–143, 1995.

11. Golden MA, Whittemore AD, Donaldson MC, et al: Selective evaluation and management of coronary artery disease in patients undergoing repair of abdominal aortic aneurysms. *Ann Surg* 212:415–423, 1990.
12. Cambria RP, Brewster DC, Abbott WM, et al: Transperitoneal versus retroperitoneal approach for aortic reconstruction: A randomized prospective study. *J Vasc Surg* 11(2):314–325, 1990.
13. Sicard GA, Reilly JM, Rubin BG, et al: Transabdominal versus retroperitoneal incision for abdominal aortic surgery: Report of a prospective randomized trial. *J Vasc Surg* 21(2):174–183, 1995.

CHAPTER 11

Flank vs. Abdominal Approach for Abdominal Aortic Surgery: The Flank Approach

R. Clement Darling, III, M.D.
Associate Professor of Surgery, Department of Vascular Surgery, Albany Medical College, Albany, New York

Robert P. Leather, M.D.
Professor of Surgery, Department of Vascular Surgery, Albany Medical College, Albany, New York

Philip S.K. Paty, M.D.
Assistant Professor of Surgery, Department of Vascular Surgery, Albany Medical College, Albany, New York

Benjamin B. Chang, M.D.
Assistant Professor of Surgery, Department of Vascular Surgery, Albany Medical College, Albany, New York

Dhiraj M. Shah, M.D.
Professor of Surgery, Department of Vascular Surgery, Albany Medical College, Albany, New York

E volution of the surgical treatment of aortic disease has been marked by an increasing ability to safely operate on patients with significant co-morbid disease while progressively reducing mortality and morbidity rates. Improvement in perioperative management, operative technique, and anesthetic management have all played significant roles in decreasing the mortality rate of aortic surgery to less than 5% at most vascular surgery centers. Nevertheless, aortic replacement by the conventional midline transperitoneal approach still remains a major undertaking that exposes the patient to significant physiologic stress and a need for prolonged hospital stays and ICU utilization. Conversely, the retroperitoneal approach, which consists of a series of incisions for exposure of the abdominal aorta and its branches, has been shown to lessen some of these physiologic disturbances. And of equal importance, the treatment of many cases of aortic pathology is technically easier through the flank approach.

In the initial reports of aortoiliac reconstruction, Dubost et al. and Oudot and LaGrefe used a retroperitoneal incision to improve exposure of the distal aorta and left iliac artery.[1, 2] They credited this method to Dr. Jean Patel, who had compared transabdominal and retroperitoneal exposures for aortic and iliac embolectomy.[3] In expanding on these initial experiences, Charles Rob in 1963 reported a large clinical series of over 500 procedures performed through an anterolateral retroperitoneal approach.[4] He concluded that this exposure had several physiologic advantages such as decreased pain, decreased ileus, shorter hospital stay, and early resumption of diet. The relatively limited proximal aortic exposure produced by the anterolateral approach made it applicable to only 25% of his patient population with aortic disease. However, he concluded that this approach should be used whenever possible. Later, Williams et al. reported an extended left posterolateral retroperitoneal approach that produces superior exposure of the proximal infrarenal and even visceral aorta and its branches[5].

Although a transperitoneal approach to the aorta was traditionally used in the 1960s and 1970s, an increased appreciation of the advantages of the retroperitoneal approach has evolved over the past several years. Sicard and associates, in a prospective randomized study, re-emphasized that the retroperitoneal approach was associated with a decreased perioperative fluid requirement, fewer perioperative pulmonary complications, less ileus, early resumption of diet, and decreased length of stay in the ICU and hospital.[6] Studies from Johnson et al., Gregory et al., and our group have also outlined the technical and physiologic improvements in perioperative outcome in patients who had undergone retroperitoneal aortic procedures.[7–9] In the only study to dispute these data, Cambria et al., in a prospective randomized trial, demonstrated no improvement in the perioperative hospital course in patients undergoing aortic procedures by the retroperitoneal exposure as compared with the transabdominal approach.[10] It should be noted that they used the more difficult anterolateral retroperitoneal approach, which has the aforementioned limitations, and they included large numbers of patients with aortic occlusive disease, a group whose physiologic disturbances by any technique are less than those seen in patients undergoing surgery for aneurysmal disease. Hudson et al. have reported a reduction in prostacyclin release and a more stable hemodynamic course as measured by mean arterial pressure, systemic vascular resistance, and changes in the heart rate and cardiac index when the retroperitoneal approach was compared with transabdominal exposures.[11] This was attributed to avoidance of mesenteric traction during retroperitoneal exposure. In addition, several authors have reported less disturbance of respiratory mechanics in the immediate postoperative period as measured by pulmonary function studies.

Classically, many surgeons regard the retroperitoneal approach as a technique for "high-risk" patients. However, others have extended this approach to all patients in an effort to minimize operative trauma and shorten the hospital stay.[12]

INDICATIONS

Properly used, the retroperitoneal approach may be applied to virtually all aortic surgeries, often with a superior and more flexible exposure of the aorta than is gained transperitoneally. In turn, this often translates into a much simpler and easier operation. This approach is especially useful in aneurysms involving the juxtarenal and visceral aorta and its branches, patients requiring reoperative aortic procedures, inflammatory aneurysms, aneurysms with an associated horseshoe kidney, and patients with severe pulmonary or cardiac insufficiency.[13–16]

In addition, aortic surgery in obese patients and patients with intra-abdominal adhesions and/or inflammatory processes is greatly facilitated by the use of this exposure. We have even extended this approach to the management of patients with visceral and/or renal artery occlusive disease, ruptured abdominal aortic aneurysms, symptomatic aneurysms, and infected aortic grafts.[17, 18]

PERIOPERATIVE MANAGEMENT

All elective surgery patients undergo biplanar angiography, and those with expected aneurysmal disease undergo CT. Patients with a history of renal or visceral insufficiency are further evaluated by selective angiography.

Preoperative cardiologic evaluation is performed before all elective cases. This consists of a comprehensive history and physical assessment of risk factors and ECG. Thallium persantine stress testing and cardiac catheterization are performed as indicated. All patients undergo general anesthesia with cardiac monitoring.

Twenty-five grams of mannitol is given IV before the incision to promote vigorous diuresis. Subsequently, 5 g/hr of mannitol is administered IV throughout the early postoperative period. Heparin (30 U/kg) is given IV before arterial cross-clamping. Postoperatively, patients are managed in the surgical ICU until extubated and hemodynamically stable. They are usually transferred to the surgical floor the next morning, and once ambulating and tolerating an oral diet, they are discharged home.

By using this algorithm, over the past 5 years the mean ICU stay for elective abdominal aortic aneurysm surgery has been 0.7 days. In more than 87% of these patients, resumption of an oral diet occurred on the first postoperative day. Seventy-four percent of these patients could then be discharged by postoperative day 6.

Every 3 months for the first year and every 6 months thereafter, patients undergo clinical examinations, pulse volume recordings, and duplex or renal flow scans as indicated. Duplex examinations are also used to document patency of the visceral reconstructions. Patients with recurrent symptoms or changes in their noninvasive laboratory tests receive further investigation by angiography. Postoperative complications are considered major if the patient's hospital discharge was delayed, major therapeutic intervention was needed, or the complication compromised the patient's postoperative recovery.

SURGICAL TECHNIQUES

LEFT RETROPERITONEAL APPROACH

After induction of anesthesia, the patient is placed on a suction beanbag (Olympic Vac-Pac) in the right lateral decubitus position with the left shoulder elevated 30 to 60 degrees from the horizontal position. The pelvis is minimally rotated to allow easier access to the groin. The beanbag is then evacuated to hold the patient in this position. The left arm is supported by a cross-arm sling. The left thigh is elevated 12 to 18 inches above the horizontal plane by folded blankets or a second beanbag, thus relaxing the ipsilateral iliopsoas muscle and allowing easier access to the distal aorta and the left iliac arteries. Finally, the table is extended 10 to 30 degrees to open the space between the ribs and the iliac crest. After the patient's skin is prepared and draped, the incision is extended in an oblique fashion, posteriorly and superiorly through the 10th or 11th interspace to the mid to posterior axillary line. The muscle layers of the abdominal wall are divided to the edge of the ipsilateral rectus abdominis, and the retroperitoneal space is entered laterally, thereby avoiding the peritoneum. The posterior layers of Gerota's fascia along with the left kidney and ureter are retracted anteriorly, medially, and cephalad. This exposure is maintained by the use of a self-retaining retractor. Laparotomy pads must be used to pad the contents of the abdomen before placing the retractor blades. In particular, vigorous retraction of the anterior and cephalad margin of the incision may be associated with splenic and/or renal injury. Distal arterial control is obtained before proximal aortic mobilization to prevent embolization. If significant involvement of the right common or external iliac artery is present, a small suprainguinal counterincision may be made on the right side of the abdomen to gain extraperitoneal exposure of these vessels. If necessary, a vertical groin incision may be made to expose the femoral arteries. After the patient is systemically heparinized and the outflow vessels are occluded, the neck of the aneurysm is then approached from its posterolateral aspect. With the left kidney retracted anteriorly and medially, the landmarks for the neck of the aneurysm are the origin of the left crus of the diaphragm, the lumbar branch of the left renal vein, and the left renal artery. Familiarity with finding these landmarks is mandatory before progressing further to prevent injury to surrounding structures such as the left renal artery or vein. After division of the lumbar branch of the left renal vein, the lymphoareolar tissue is dissected and the proximal infrarenal aorta can be identified. The nonaneurysmal portion of the infrarenal abdominal aorta may then be clamped. If a standard endoaneursymorrhaphy with in-line graft replacement of the aneurysm is to be performed, the lumbar arteries may be controlled from outside the aneurysm sac, as may be the inferior mesenteric artery. The aneurysm sac may then be opened and residual bleeding controlled with suture ligatures. An appropriate graft may then be anastomosed proximally and distally with 3-0 propylene suture. If aortic disease extends into the iliacs, a bifurcated graft is used and the limbs are sewn to the appropriate vessel in either an end-to-end or end-to-side fashion.

To minimize the operative dissection necessary for aortic replacement for aneurysmal disease, we have adopted the modification of aneurysm exclusion with bypass.[19] After initial outflow occlusion of the distal vessels to avoid embolization and to place the proximal aortic clamp, a second clamp is placed 2 to 3 cm below the first aortic clamp. The aorta is then divided just slightly cephalad to the distal clamp, and this clamp and the proximal aortic aneurysm are oversewn with a continuous double suture line of 3-0 propylene. The aneurysm sac is then retracted caudad and posteriorly to facilitate performance of the proximal anastomosis. After completion of the proximal anastomosis, the proximal common iliacs are either divided, oversewn, or ligated in continuity to isolate the aneurysmal sac from the direct arterial circulation. Lumbar arteries and the inferior mesenteric artery may be ligated outside the aneurysm to complete the exclusion. The distal iliac or femoral anastomoses may be performed again in an end-to-end or end-to-side fashion as dictated by the anatomy. The right limb of the bifurcated graft may be tunneled anatomically along the iliac artery or anteriorly along the suprapubic space (Retzius) to the recipient iliac or femoral artery. The goal of this exclusion technique is to minimize blood loss and surgical dissection to lessen cardiopulmonary stress.

RIGHT RETROPERITONEAL EXPOSURE

The right retroperitoneal approach to the abdominal aorta may be used in several situations in which a left flank incision may not be optimal. Specific indications for this approach fall into two categories. First, the right-sided approach may be used to gain better access to the structures on the right side, such as the right renal or right common iliac artery or in situations in which the aorta is tortuous and makes exposure from the right side technically more advantageous. Second, it may be used to avoid scar tissue or inflammation in the left retroperitoneal space from previous surgeries or infections.

After the retroperitoneal space is entered, the plane between the peritoneum and Gerota's fascia is identified and developed. Usually, the right kidney and ureter are left in the anatomical position while the peritoneum is mobilized medially. This exposes the aorta from the right renal artery to the aortic bifurcation. The overlying lymphoareolar tissue is divided and small branches of the vena cava are suture-ligated. The vena cava is then gently retracted laterally. This exposes the neck of the aortic aneurysm or the infrarenal aorta. The remainder of the operation may be completed as desired by exclusion or endoaneurysmorrhaphy techniques. This exposure is excellent for patients with occlusive disease or a generous infrarenal neck. It may be more difficult in patients who have large aneurysms that extend to or above the renal arteries. Also, this approach should be avoided in patients who have symptomatic or ruptured aneurysms because proximal control is limited by fixed structures such as the liver and supraceliac control is difficult if not impossible.

BILATERAL RENAL REVASCULARIZATION

A left flank incision is made and carried into the tenth intercostal space for the retroperitoneal exposure. The left crus of the diaphram is divided. The aorta is dissected free of surrounding structures circumferentially to allow visualization of the proximal renal and visceral vessels. Renal artery reconstructions are performed by using endarterectomy, bypass, or both. For endarterectomy, the aorta is clamped above the involved artery(s). If replacement of the aorta is not necessary, a "trapdoor" type of aortotomy is fashioned. An extension of the proximal aortotomy allows intraluminal exposure of the renal and visceral artery orifices. If renal artery bypass is performed, the proximal aortic clamp may be placed above or below the renal arteries depending on the extent of aortic disease. An additional clamp is placed below the level of the renal arteries and the aorta is divided transversely above the lower clamp after controlling the renal arteries and visceral vessels. Anterior and cephalad mobilization of the proximal aorta facilitates right renal artery exposure and control.

If renal bypass is necessary and aortic replacement is to be performed, 6-mm polytetrafluoroeythelene (PTFE) grafts are sewn onto the body of the aortic graft before aortic cross-clamping to minimize the operating and warm ischemia times. The proximal aortic anastomosis is then performed with continuous 3-0 propylene suture. Once this proximal anastomosis is completed, the right renal artery can then be dissected over a distance of about 3 to 4 cm beyond the orifice. A curved Cooley clamp is then used to obtain stable control of the exposed right renal artery. The proximal renal artery just beyond the orifice is then divided and either hemoclipped or oversewn with a continuous suture, and an end-to-end anastomosis is constructed between the 6-mm graft limb and the distal right renal artery with 6-0 polypropylene continuous suture. After completion of this anastomosis, the clamp is then shifted down to allow flow to the right renal artery. The left renal artery anastomosis is then constructed similarly.

One limitation of the left retroperitoneal approach for repair of renal artery lesions involves the extent of disease of the right renal artery. If the extent of disease is beyond 3 to 4 cm from the renal artery ostium, i.e., beyond the point at which the renal artery passes behind the inferior vena cava, the exposure becomes problematic. Close inspection of the preoperative angiogram by the operative surgeon is therefore of paramount importance.

VISCERAL ARTERY RECONSTRUCTION

If visceral artery reconstruction is to be performed, the origins of
the superior mesenteric and celiac arteries are identified at their
origins from the aorta. Each vessel may be further exposed if necessary by dissecting the tissue along the axis of the artery. If further dissection of the superior mesenteric artery is necessary, the
left kidney may be left in its anatomical position, and dissection is
then performed anterior to Gerota's fascia while retracting the peritoneum medially. The dissection thus proceeds between the body
and uncinate process of the pancreas and the duodenum to allow
exposure of approximately 5 to 10 cm of the superior mesenteric
artery beyond its orifice. If further exposure is necessary, the peritoneum may be incised. The celiac axis may be exposed in a similar fashion up to its trifurcation, at which point the left gastric artery continues superiorly and the common hepatic posteriorly and
to the right into the peritoneum. The splenic artery may be
followed along its course by dissecting along the superior of the
body and tail of the pancreas. If endarterectomy is necessary, it can
be performed through a trapdoor-type endarterectomy with clamping of the aorta proximally at the supraceliac level and distally below the renal arteries.

MODIFICATIONS OF THE LEFT RETROPERITONEAL APPROACH FOR EMERGENT REPAIR OF SYMPTOMATIC AND RUPTURED ABDOMINAL AORTIC ANEURYSMS

A left flank incision is made from the edge of the ipsilateral rectus
abdominis muscle to the posterior axillary line along the 11th rib.
The underlying musculature is divided with electrocautery. The
retroperitoneum is entered laterally without exposing the aneurysm. A hand is inserted along the diaphragm until the crus and
the underlying supraceliac aorta are encountered. The aorta is then
manually compressed against the vertebral column (Fig 1). At this
time there is usually a perceptible increase in blood pressure.
Manual control in this fashion can usually be gained reliably
within 5 minutes after intubation. An assistant positioned on the
right side of the patient places a large deep handheld Dever retractor and retracts the peritoneum and its contents at the level of the
supraceliac aorta to provide visualization of this region. The operating surgeon subsequently divides the left crus of the diaphragm
transversely immediately caudal to the area of compression with a
pair of long scissors under direct vision. At this level, the aorta is
not usually adherent to surrounding structures. An aortic clamp is
then used to clamp the supraceliac aorta. These additional steps

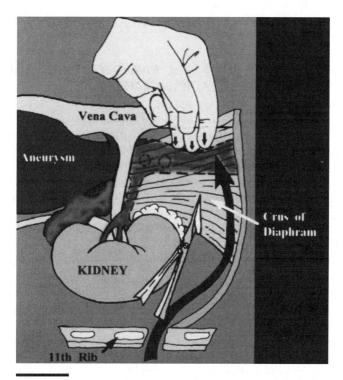

FIGURE 1.

The aorta is manually controlled through the crus of the diaphragm. The crus is then divided to clamp the supraceliac aorta.

usually require an extra 1 to 2 minutes. At this point, the patient is resuscitated and is given fluid by the anesthesiologist to maintain stable blood pressure.

After the aorta is cross-clamped at the supraceliac level, the retroperitoneal space is opened more widely, and the peritoneum and left kidney are retracted medially and cephalad. The position is maintained by a self-retaining retractor. The infrarenal neck of the aneurysm is then identified by using the standard techniques previously mentioned. A second aortic cross-clamp is placed infrarenally at the neck of the aneurysm. The supraceliac clamp is then removed. The remainder of the operation is performed similar to standard elective aneurysm repair through the retroperitoneal approach. The only situation precluding an emergent left retroperitoneal exposure for a ruptured aneurysm is a patient undergoing cardiopulmonary resuscitation with manual chest compression. In such patients, a standard midline transperitoneal incision is made and approach and repair of the aorta performed according to standard techniques.

RETROPERITONEAL IN-LINE AORTIC BYPASS FOR THE TREATMENT OF INFECTED INFRARENAL AORTIC GRAFTS

In patients with a previously placed aortic graft with documented infection established by CT scan of the abdomen or indium-labeled white blood cell scan, the left retroperitoneal approach may be used for the provision of an in-line aortic replacement graft through a noninfected field. Several conditions should be satisfied before the performance of in-line aortic graft replacement in this setting. The left retroperitoneal gutter should be noninfected. The patient should be relatively hemodynamically stable so that the clean part of the operation may be performed first before removal of the infected graft.

A left flank incision is made for an extended retroperitoneal approach through the tenth interspace. The suprarenal aorta is approached first posterolaterally and then controlled temporarily after dividing the crus of the diaphragm. The dissection is continued caudad to identify the renal arteries. If this area is not believed to be infected by clinical criteria or by Gram stain of the periaortic tissue, the aorta is divided just below the renal arteries between two clamps, with sufficient aorta left below the level of the proximal clamp to perform the new proximal anastomosis. As an alternative, the aorta may be divided above the level of the renal arteries and renal revascularization may be performed by means of 6-mm PTFE limbs sewn to the body of the new aortic prosthesis. The distal aorta is then oversewn with a continuous monofilament suture line and then buried in the peraortic tissue. Samples of the fluid and surrounding tissues in this area are next obtained for culture and Gram staining. If possible, a section of the native aorta should be sent for tissue culture. The proximal anastomosis is then performed to a bifurcated PTFE graft with a continuous monofilament suture. The graft limbs are tunneled to the noninfected outflow vessels to avoid the infected area. The right iliac or femoral arteries are approached through separate incisions in either the groin or right flank, and the right graft limb is tunneled through the space of Retzius. The left graft limb may then be tunneled under the inguinal ligament and beneath the sartorius, rectus femoris, or psoas fascia. After completion of the distal anastomosis, flow is restored in the new graft.

The wounds are then closed and covered with sterile plastic drapes. The patient is placed into a supine position for a transperitoneal approach. The field is reprepared and redraped for the contaminated part of the procedure. A midline transperitoneal incision is made. The dissection is performed to identify the proximal and distal suture lines, and the graft is then removed in its entirety. The graft bed is débrided and irrigated copiously with an antibiotic solution. Any involved intestine is débrided and closed primarily, with gastrostomy and feeding jejunostomy tubes placed when appropriate. Wounds in the groin that are infected are packed open. The midline wound is usually closed with drains placed in the infected bed if necessary.

RESULTS

Over a 15-year period, 2,340 retroperitoneal aortoiliac reconstructions were performed in 2,243 patients.[12] Reconstructions for aortic disease were performed in 1,756 cases. Of these, 1,109 were performed for elective abdominal aortic aneurysms, 210 for ruptured and symptomatic aortic aneurysms, and 399 for aortoiliac occlusive disease. In addition, 18 procedures were performed for infected aortic grafts and 20 for various other indications. Iliofemoral occlusive disease accounted for the remaining 584 procedures. This approach was also used in 417 renal and 50 celiac and superior mesenteric artery reconstructions.

The mean age of this population of patients was 67 years, with 1,590 men and 653 women. Fifteen percent of these patients were diabetics and 40% were cigarette smokers. The overall operative mortality for all aortic procedures, elective and emergent, was 5.2%. For elective abdominal aortic aneurysms, the mortality was 2.4% (27/1,109). Forty-one percent of this group (11/27) died of cardiac complications. Nonfatal cardiac complications occurred in 2.6% of the survivors, pulmonary complications developed in 2.1%, 2.1% had worsening renal dysfunction, and 0.7% had colonic ischemia. Two immediate graft occlusions were treated by thrombectomy with continued long-term patency and 7 late occlusions (4 treated by thrombectomy and 3 treated by a redo bypass). Mean intraoperative blood loss for the elective group was 810 ± 800 mL (mean ± SD). Tube grafts were placed in 28% of the patients and bifurcated grafts in the remaining 72%.

Retroperitoneal exclusion of the aorta with bypass was performed in a total of 995 patients. The operative mortality was 2.4% in this group. The estimated blood loss with this procedure was 661 ± 718 mL (mean ± SD). Of the 107 ruptured aneurysms repaired through the retroperitoneal approach, 36% were repaired by using tube grafts and 64% were repaired with bifurcated grafts. The operative mortality in this group was 29% (31/107). Fifty-two percent of these deaths occurred as a result of multisystem organ failure. Seven nonfatal pulmonary complications and 2 cardiac and 2 cerebrovascular accidents occurred. Four patients had worsening of their renal function. Three patients had colonic ischemia and 1 patient had paralysis of the lower extremity. One immediate graft occlusion was revised with no late occlusions. The estimated procedural blood loss was 2,962 ± 1,928 mL (mean ± SD).

One hundred three patients with symptomatic abdominal aortic aneurysms were taken expeditiously to the operating suite and later found to have nonruptured aneurysms. In these patients the operative mortality was 12.6% (13/103). Thirty-one percent of these patients died of cardiac complications. Thirteen nonfatal cardiopulmonary complications occurred in this group.

The operative mortality for patients who underwent surgery for aortoiliac occlusive disease was 4.5% (18/399). The primary cause of mortality was cardiac (39%). Estimated blood loss was 558 ± 569 mL (mean ± SD). The 5-year graft patency rates for aneurysm and occlusive disease were 99% and 95%, respectively.

Of the 417 renal artery reconstructions performed, 255 were performed in concert with abdominal aortic aneurysm repair, 84 were primary procedures for renovascular hypertension, and 78 were performed with other aortic reconstructions. Sixty bilateral renal revascularization procedures were performed, 310 bypasses were performed with 6-mm PTFE graft limbs, 71 transaortic endarterectomies were performed, and 30 renal arteries were repaired by direct implantation. The operative mortality for these reconstructions was 5.7% (20/351). The majority of the operative deaths were, again, a result of cardiopulmonary complications (25%). Seven patients had worsening of their renal dysfunction. Only 1 patient required long-term dialysis. There were 5 early graft renal artery bypass occlusions, 4 of which were revised successfully. Late occlusions have developed in 2 patients. Blood pressure was improved in 27%, stabilized in 70%, and worsened in 3%.

In the 584 procedures performed for iliac occlusive disease, the operative mortality was 1.9%. Nine nonfatal cardiac complications, 2 strokes, and 2 instances of chronic ischemia occurred.

In the visceral artery reconstruction group, 29 reconstructions were performed to the superior mesenteric artery, 17 to the celiac artery, and 2 each to the splenic artery and inferior mesenteric arteries. The operative mortality for elective and emergent operations was 10.9% (5/46). Two late arterial occlusions occurred; in 1 patient the occlusion was repaired at 19 months, and in the other patient, an ischemic bowel developed at 24 months and led to death.

Eighteen patients underwent in-line aortic reconstruction for an infected aortic graft through a left retroperitoneal approach without cross-contamination of the newly placed graft and with subsequent removal of the infected prosthesis transperitoneally. One patient died of myocardial infarction at 2 months (5.6%). Patients have been monitored by indium-labeled leukocyte scans and clinical examination. No evidence of recurrent graft infection or sepsis has been seen in these patients for 4 months to 9 years postoperatively. Seventeen percent of these patients have had major complications (one bleed, one nonfatal myocardial infarction, one graft limb thrombosis).

COMPLICATIONS

As has been described, numerous anatomical and physiologic advantages are conferred by use of the retroperitoneal approach for aortic reconstructions. However, some complications may occur as a result of this approach. The use of a stabilizing self-retaining retractor is necessary for exposure of the aorta through the left retroperitoneal approach. With vigorous cephalad and medial retraction, splenic injury may occur. This is more likely to occur through extension of the incision posteriorly into the tenth intercostal space. In addition, the presence of adhesions of the spleen to the diaphragm may also set the stage for this complication, which may be minimized by the use of laparotomy pads to cushion the retractor and the avoidance of repeated changes in position of these retractors. This complication has occurred in six patients undergoing these procedures.

In addition, with vigorous retraction in patients who have had prior left retroperitoneal exposure, the ureter may be tethered at the pelvic brim. This may put the ureter at increased risk for traumatic disruption. In these cases it may be beneficial to either drop a kidney back to its anatomical location or perform extensive ureterolysis to prevent the ureter from being avulsed. This has occurred three times in over 2,000 cases. Although it did not complicate the aortic surgery, this complication may require further urologic surgery or intermittent stenting to prevent stenosis.

With layered closure of the flank incision, incisional hernias occur in fewer than 1% of the patients. However, approximately 5% of the patients will have some form of an annoying flank bulge on the side of the operative incision. This bulge is usually a consequence of division of the 11th or 12th intercostal nerve with subsequent denervation of the flank musculature. Although it may be perceived by the patient as a hernia, it represents a diastasis. The best form of treatment is to avoid this complication by isolating the nerve and preventing its injury or division during dissection. Symptomatic treatment may be given in the form of an abdominal binder.

In addition, intercostal neuralgia may occur. This usually responds to serial nerve injections. In patients in whom incomplete relief of symptoms is obtained with this treatment, operative resection of the intercostal nerve may be performed with local anesthesia for complete pain relief.

Another complication that can occur in patients undergoing aortic exclusion and bypass has been the persistence of flow in the excluded aneurysm sac. This problem has occurred in 1.8% (18/995) of our patients. Fourteen of these patients have required further surgery to evacuate the sac and ligate the inflow vessels. Two were treated by embolizations of the inflow source to the excluded aneurysm, and the remaining 2 are being observed. This condition can be detected on postoperative surveillance of the excluded aneurysm sac by duplex examination by either persistence of flow in the aneurysm sac or enlargement of the dimensions of the sac. Unfortunately, no preoperative angiographic criteria can predict the occurrence of this complication. In the vast majority of cases, thrombosis of the excluded sac is complete within 3 weeks to 3 months after the operative repair. To minimize the occurrence of this complication, insonation of the excluded sac immediately after performance of this procedure and before closure of the incision should be performed with an intraoperative Doppler probe. Finally, one must be careful when developing a tunnel for the aortic graft to go to the contralateral limb. Two blunt injuries to the bladder were caused by blind tunneling in the space of Retzius. This tunnel should be created manually with a finger or under direct vision, and force should never be used to pass a clamp or tunneling device to retrieve the graft.

CONCLUSION

The extended posterolateral approach to the aorta and its branches is a viable option for reconstruction of the abdominal aorta. This approach provides the surgeon with the ability to easily expose the entire subdiaphragmatic aorta and its branches. In addition, symptomatic and ruptured aneurysms as well as selected infrarenal infected aortic grafts can be repaired without an increase in mortality and morbidity and with optimal results. Charles Rob, in his seminal paper in 1963, stated that most of the advantages of the extraperitoneal approach relate to the fact that the patient's entire postoperative course is made considerably easier and not only are complications much less frequent, but recovery is smoother and faster.[4] This exposure offers not only the physiologic and technical advantages of the retroperitoneal approach but also the flexibility that many think can only be achieved by the transperitoneal approach.

REFERENCES

1. Dubost C, Allary M, Oeconomos N: Resection of an aneurysm of the abdominal aorta. *Arch Surg* 64:405–408, 1952.
2. Oudot J, LaGrefe P: Vasculaire dan les thromboses du carrefour aortique. *Presse Med* 59:234–236, 1951.
3. Patel J: Chirurgie de la fourche aortique. *Presse Med* 58:214–217, 1950.
4. Rob CG: Extraperitoneal approach to the abdominal aorta. *Surgery* 53:87–89, 1963.
5. Williams GM, Ricotta J, Zinner M, et al: The extended retroperitoneal approach for treatment of extensive atherosclerosis of the aorta and renal vessels. *Surgery* 888:846–855, 1980.
6. Sicard GA, Freeman MB, Vander Woude JC, et al: Comparison between the transabdominal and retroperitoneal approach for reconstruction of the infrarenal abdominal aorta. *J Vasc Surg* 5:19–27, 1987.
7. Johnson JN, McLoughlin GA, Walse PN, et al: Comparison of extraperitoneal and transperitoneal methods of aortoiliac reconstruction: 20 year experience. *J Cardiovasc Surg* 27:561–564, 1986.
8. Gregory RT, Wheeler JR, Snyder SO, et al: Retroperitoneal approach to aortic surgery. *J Cardiovasc Surg* 30:185–189, 1989.
9. Leather RP, Shah DM, Kaufman JL, et al: Comparative analysis of retroperitoneal and transperitoneal aortic replacement for aneurysm. *Surg Gynecol Obstet* 268:387–393, 1989.
10. Cambria RP, Brewster DC, Abbott WM, et al: Transperitoneal versus retroperitoneal approach for aortic reconstruction: A randomized prospective study. *J Vasc Surg* 11:314–325, 1990.
11. Hudson JC, Wurm WH, O'Donnell TF Jr, et al: Hemodynamics and prostacyclin release in the early phases of aortic surgery: Comparison of transabdominal and retroperitoneal approaches. *J Vasc Surg* 7:190–198, 1988.
12. Darling RC III, Shah DM, Chang BB, et al: Current status of the use of retroperitoneal approach for reconstructions of the aorta and its branches. *Ann Surg* 224:501–508, 1996.
13. Darling RC III, Shah DM, Chang BB, et al: Retroperitoneal approach for bilateral renal and visceral artery revascularization. *Am J Surg* 168:148–151, 1994.

14. Darling RC III, Kreienberg PB, Shah DM, et al: Aortic reconstruction and concomitant renal artery revascularization using the retroperitoneal approach: Techniques and results. *Semin Vasc Surg 9:231–235, 1996.*

15. Saifi J, Shah DM, Chang BB, et al: Left retroperitoneal exposure for distal mesenteric artery repair. *J Cardiovasc Surg* 31:629–633, 1990.

16. Chang BB, Paty PSK, Shah DM, et al: The right retroperitoneal approach for abdominal aortic surgery. *Am J Surg* 158:156–158, 1989.

17. Chang BB, Shah DM, Paty PSK, et al: Can the retroperitoneal approach be used for ruptured abdominal aortic aneurysms? *J Vasc Surg* 11:326–330, 1990.

18. Leather RP, Darling RC III, Chang BB, et al: Retroperitoneal in-line aortic bypass for treatment of infected infrarenal aortic grafts. *Surg Gynecol Obstet* 175:491– 494, 1992.

19. Shah DM, Chang BB, Paty PSK, et al: Treatment of abdominal aortic aneurysm by exclusion and bypass: An analysis of outcome. *J Vasc Surg* 13:15–22, 1991.

CHAPTER 12

Extrapleural Pneumonectomy for Malignant Mesothelioma

David J. Sugarbaker, M.D.
Chief, Division of Thoracic Surgery, Brigham and Women's Hospital, Harvard Medical School, Boston, Massachusetts

William G. Richards, Ph.D.
Research Associate, Division of Thoracic Surgery, Brigham and Women's Hospital, Harvard Medical School, Boston, Massachusetts

Jose P. Garcia, M.D.
Cardiothoracic Resident, Division of Thoracic Surgery, Brigham and Women's Hospital, Harvard Medical School, Boston, Massachusetts

M alignant pleural mesothelioma of the thorax is a disease that has been associated with asbestos exposure.[1] Asbestos fibers of the amphibole subgroup are particularly pathogenic.[2] Although asbestos exposure also increases the risk of lung carcinoma among cigarette smokers, tobacco use does not contribute to the etiology of malignant mesothelioma.[3]

The incidence of mesothelioma in the United States rose by 50% during the 1980s,[1] a reflection of the common industrial use of asbestos between 1940 and 1970.[4] In 1996 in the United States, 2,200 to 3,000 new diagnoses are expected.[4–6] A relatively long latency period justifies the prediction that regulation of industrial asbestos use in the 1960s will not be reflected in a decreased incidence until the 21st century.

Malignant pleural mesothelioma usually affects men between the ages of 50 and 70. Approximately 60% of the patients have chest pain or dyspnea, and significant pleural effusion will develop in most patients during their course. Other common initial symptoms include cough, fever, and weight loss. Patients seen with advanced disease will exhibit wasting, ascites, or chest wall deformity.

The diagnosis of malignant mesothelioma can be difficult to establish. Only 75% to 80% of the patients will report exposure to asbestos. The chest radiograph commonly shows pleural effusion, with or without pleural calcifications. Computed tomography of the chest is useful in determining the extent of disease, especially whether disease exists beyond the thoracic cavity. Recently, MRI has been used to assess mediastinal and transdiaphragmatic invasion in patients who are being considered for extrapleural pneumonectomy.[7] In this subgroup of patients, echocardiography has been found useful in assessing pericardial involvement and ventricular function. Pulmonary function tests are used to screen those patients who will need a ventilation-perfusion scan before being considered for extrapleural pneumonectomy. The diagnosis of malignant mesothelioma can sometimes be established by thoracentesis. The pleural fluid obtained is often yellow, as opposed to the bloody appearance of fluid associated with adenocarcinoma. Although cytologic examination of the fluid specimen is sometimes helpful, pleural biopsy is more commonly required for adequate tissue diagnosis.

Typically the tumor begins as small, discrete nodules on the visceral and parietal pleura that grow together and form a rind encompassing the lung. As the rind thickens, lung function may be mechanically affected, although the parenchyma is not usually involved with tumor.

Microscopically, these tumors are described as exhibiting epithelial, sarcomatoid, or mixed histology. Immunoperoxidase staining is used to differentiate between mesothelioma and adenocarcinoma of the lung.[8] Histologic subtyping of malignant mesothelioma is useful for prognosis. Patients with epithelial tumors have the best prognosis, whereas patients with pure sarcomatoid tumors, although rare, have the poorest survival.[9, 10] Overall, the median survival for diffuse malignant pleural mesothelioma is 4 to 12 months if left untreated.[11–14] These tumors are rarely associated with distant metastasis, instead being characterized by aggressive local extension. Most of the patients will succumb to cardiac or pulmonary involvement. In addition, bowel obstruction develops in approximately 30% as a result of tumor growth into the abdomen.[15]

Appropriate treatment of this disease can range from conservative to aggressive, depending on the stage of disease at time of diagnosis and on the overall health of the patient. No single-modality therapy has proved effective in improving the prognosis of malignant mesothelioma, although palliation of symptoms can be achieved by several approaches. Patients with advanced disease who are not candidates for surgical intervention may have symptomatic relief by drainage of pleural effusions followed by pleurodesis. Some studies have documented a tumor response to single-agent or combination chemotherapy,[16] although none to date has been shown to affect survival. Radiotherapy also confers a moderate palliative benefit in some patients.[17–20] Surgical resection using pleurectomy[21] or extrapleural pneumonectomy[22] can provide significant palliation, although with associated morbidity and mortality and no proven long-term benefit. Recently, the operative mortality associated with extrapleural pneumonectomy has declined.[21, 23, 24]

TRIMODALITY THERAPY

Several multimodality approaches have been reported with more promising results. In one series, cytoreductive pleurectomy with adjuvant chemotherapy and radiotherapy was associated with a 17-month median survival.[25] The theoretical basis for the trimodality approach described here[24, 26] is that a complete or nearly complete resection can be achieved by extrapleural pneumonectomy in selected patients with acceptable operative morbidity and mortality, thereby optimizing the setting for adjuvant therapies. High-dose radiotherapy can then be given after extrapleural pneumonectomy without the risk of radiation pneumonitis, and the effectiveness of chemotherapy is improved by minimizing residual disease.

PATIENT SELECTION

Patients without medical contraindications who had normal cardiac, hepatic, and renal function were candidates for trimodality therapy. Those who appeared to be completely resectable radiographically had an extrapleural pneumonectomy with adjuvant CAP (cyclophosphamide, Adriamycin [doxorubicin], and Platino [cisplatin]) chemotherapy and radiotherapy. Patients with compromised cardiac function (ejection fraction less than 45%), P_{CO_2} greater than 45 mm Hg, room-air P_{O_2} less than 65 mm Hg, or a predicted postoperative forced expiratory volume in 1 second less than 1 L were excluded.

EXTRAPLEURAL PNEUMONECTOMY

Right-Sided Procedure

The patient is ventilated with a double-lumen tube to allow for ventilation of the contralateral lung. For a right-sided extrapleural pneumonectomy, an extended right thoracotomy incision is made along the course of the sixth rib (Fig 1)[27] extending from midway between the posterior scapular ridge and the spine, and carried to the costochondral junction. The latissimus dorsi and serratus anterior muscles are divided. Previous biopsy sites are excised to prevent local recurrence. The sixth rib is resected for better exposure and for definition of the extrapleural plane. After identifying the extrapleural plane, blunt and sharp dissection proceeds superiorly

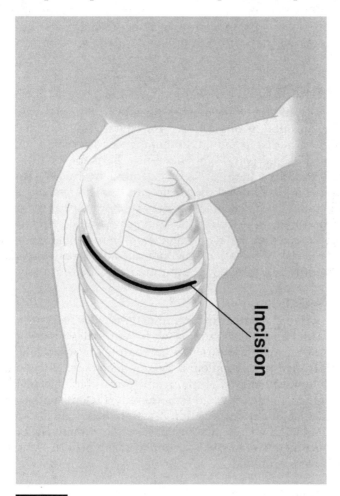

FIGURE 1.

The extended right thoracotomy incision. (Courtesy of Garcia JP, Richards WG, Sugarbaker DJ: Surgical treatment of malignant mesothelioma, in Kaiser KR, Kron IL, Spray TL (eds): *Mastery of Cardiothoracic Surgery.* Philadelphia, Lippincott-Raven, 1997, in press.)

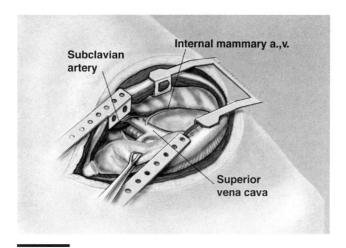

FIGURE 2.

Internal mammary artery and vein originating from the subclavian artery and superior vena cava, respectively. (Courtesy of Garcia JP, Richards WG, Sugarbaker DJ: Surgical treatment of malignant mesothelioma, in Kaiser KR, Kron IL, Spray TL (eds): *Mastery of Cardiothoracic Surgery.* Philadelphia, Lippincott-Raven, 1997, in press.)

toward the apex and is carried along the anterolateral aspect and inferiorly toward the diaphragm.

The lung is then mobilized and chest retractors are placed anteriorly and posteriorly to provide greater exposure of the posterior anatomy before proceeding with dissection around the azygous vein. The dissection then proceeds toward the cupola of the lung, with particular attention paid to the subclavian vessels to avoid injuring them. The internal mammary artery and vein can often pass through the extrapleural plane superomedially and can sometimes resemble adhesions. It is important to identify these vessels during this phase of the dissection to avoid avulsing them from the subclavian artery and superior vena cava (Fig 2).[27]

Dissection is continued from the lung apex to the azygous vein, continuing extrapleurally until the right upper lobe and main-stem bronchus are identified. The superior vena cava is then carefully dissected from the parietal pleural structures with sharp technique (Fig 3).[27]

A nasogastric tube is inserted to facilitate identification and palpation of the esophagus and help prevent its injury. A radial incision is made on the diaphragm posterolaterally and then carried anteromedially toward the pericardium, carefully dissecting to keep the pleural envelope intact. In some cases it is necessary

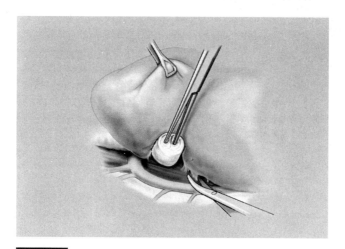

FIGURE 3.

Right lung dissected medially away from the azygous vein. (Courtesy of Garcia JP, Richards WG, Sugarbaker DJ: Surgical treatment of malignant mesothelioma, in Kaiser KR, Kron IL, Spray TL (eds): *Mastery of Cardiothoracic Surgery.* Philadelphia, Lippincott-Raven, 1997, in press.)

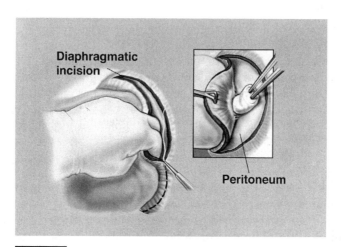

FIGURE 4.

Dissection of the pleural envelope off the diaphragm. (Courtesy of Garcia JP, Richards WG, Sugarbaker DJ: Surgical treatment of malignant mesothelioma, in Kaiser KR, Kron IL, Spray TL (eds): *Mastery of Cardiothoracic Surgery.* Philadelphia, Lippincott-Raven, 1997, in press.)

to remove the pleural envelope off the diaphragm before dividing it. To preserve the underlying peritoneum, blunt dissection with a sponge stick is used to remove the peritoneum off the diaphragm (Fig 4).[27] After the diaphragm has been divided anteromedially, the pericardium is divided along the inferior vena cava and esophageal hiatus. After entering the pericardium and identifying the inferior vena cava through the diaphragm, dissection proceeds just lateral to the inferior vena cava and esophagus to complete resection of the diaphragm (Fig 5).[27]

The pericardium is opened medially to the phrenic nerve and pulmonary vessels (see Fig 5). Careful dissection is necessary to avoid violating the parietal pleural envelope in this plane. The vena cava and superior pulmonary vein are then dissected off the main pulmonary artery, and the right pulmonary artery and superior pulmonary vein are divided intrapericardially with an endovascular stapler (Fig 6).[27] The pericardium is completely resected by dividing it posterior to the hilum. The lung is retracted to permit continued dissection posterior to the pericardium and lateral to the esophagus. A subcarinal lymph node dissection is routinely performed.

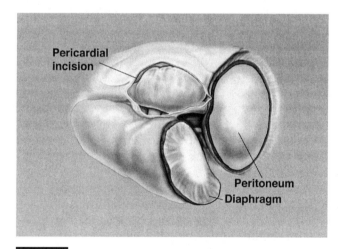

FIGURE 5.

The pericardium is opened anteromedially to the phrenic nerve and hilar vessels. (Courtesy of Garcia JP, Richards WG, Sugarbaker DJ: Surgical treatment of malignant mesothelioma, in Kaiser KR, Kron IL, Spray TL (eds): *Mastery of Cardiothoracic Surgery.* Philadelphia, Lippincott-Raven, 1997, in press.)

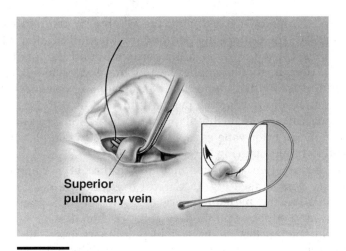

FIGURE 6.

The superior pulmonary vein is dissected within the pericardium. **Inset,** illustration of a safe technique for dissection of the hilar vessels using a pliable, plastic, self-dilating guidance catheter. One jaw of the endoscopic stapler will fit into the end of this catheter, thus allowing safe placement of the stapler. (Courtesy of Garcia JP, Richards WG, Sugarbaker DJ: Surgical treatment of malignant mesothelioma, in Kaiser KR, Kron IL, Spray TL (eds): *Mastery of Cardiothoracic Surgery.* Philadelphia, Lippincott-Raven, 1997, in press.)

The right main-stem bronchus is transected at the carina with a heavy-gauge stapler (Fig 7),[27] and the bronchial stump is covered with a pericardial fat pad. The pericardium is always reconstructed when performing a right extrapleural pneumonectomy to prevent cardiac herniation, which is a potentially fatal complication. Prolene suture is used to close the pericardium with a prosthetic patch (Fig 8),[27] and the patch is fenestrated in an effort to prevent cardiac tamponade (Fig 9).[27]

For reconstruction of the diaphragm, we currently use an impermeable patch to help prevent peritoneal fluid from accumulating too rapidly in the chest cavity and causing mediastinal shift or tamponade during the early postoperative period. A prosthetic impermeable patch is secured in place with multiple interrupted Prolene sutures (see Fig 9).

Specimens from multiple resection margins are examined microscopically in the pathology suite. Before wound closure, any remaining gross disease is outlined with clips to guide subsequent radiotherapy. Without the lung to tamponade chest wall bleeding sites, particular care is necessary to achieve complete hemostasis.

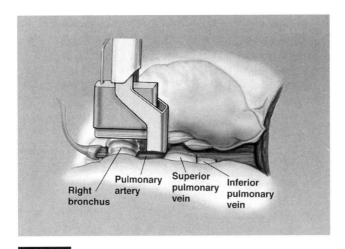

FIGURE 7.

The right main-stem bronchus is transected with a heavy-gauge stapler near the carina after the pulmonary artery and veins have been divided. (Courtesy of Garcia JP, Richards WG, Sugarbaker DJ: Surgical treatment of malignant mesothelioma, in Kaiser KR, Kron IL, Spray TL (eds): *Mastery of Cardiothoracic Surgery.* Philadelphia, Lippincott-Raven, 1997, in press.)

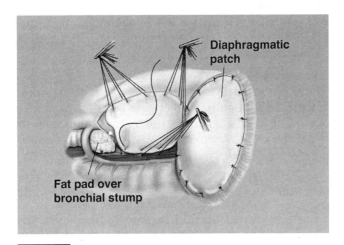

FIGURE 8.

The pericardium and diaphragm are reconstructed and a fat pad placed over the bronchial stump. (Courtesy of Garcia JP, Richards WG, Sugarbaker DJ: Surgical treatment of malignant mesothelioma, in Kaiser KR, Kron IL, Spray TL (eds): *Mastery of Cardiothoracic Surgery.* Philadelphia, Lippincott-Raven, 1997, in press.)

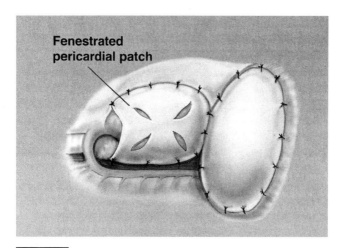

FIGURE 9.

Fenestrations and a pericardial patch are made to prevent tamponade. (Courtesy of Garcia JP, Richards WG, Sugarbaker DJ: Surgical treatment of malignant mesothelioma, in Kaiser KR, Kron IL, Spray TL (eds): *Mastery of Cardiothoracic Surgery.* Philadelphia, Lippincott-Raven, 1997, in press.)

The wound is closed in multiple layers to ensure a watertight closure, with a red rubber catheter left in the chest to allow for removal of air postoperatively (1,000 cc in men and 750 cc in women) and placement of the mediastinum in the midline.

Left-Sided Procedure

The left-sided procedure is similar to that on the right side, although there are subtle differences between the two approaches. During dissection of the medial aspect, particular note must be taken to enter the correct retroaortic plane to avoid avulsion of the intercostal vessels. The extent of tumor involvement of the aorta should be assessed at this time to determine resectability. After circumferential dissection of the specimen from the chest wall, the diaphragm is divided radially. On the left side, absence of the caval and esophageal hiatus makes the diaphragmatic dissection less technically demanding to perform, although care must be taken when dissecting around the aortic hiatus.

The pericardium is entered inferiorly and the incision carried superiorly to identify the pulmonary vasculature. We dissect the extrapleural pulmonary artery as it passes through the pericardium and enters the left chest. The left pulmonary artery is divided extrapericardially and extrapleurally. The veins are transected intrapericardially and the resection is completed posteriorly (Fig 10).[27]

The longer main-stem bronchus on the left side necessitates additional dissection to achieve a short bronchial stump, which is covered with a pericardial fat pad as for a right-sided procedure. Although it is not usually necessary to reconstruct the pericardium because of the small risk of cardiac herniation, the diaphragm must be reconstructed as described for a right-sided procedure. Finally, with the red rubber catheter, less air is removed from the left side (500 cc in women; 750 cc in men) than from the right; it is left in place for 48 hours.

POSTOPERATIVE MANAGEMENT

Postoperative management of patients undergoing extrapleural pneumonectomy focuses on pain control to facilitate early mobilization and intravascular fluid management. Thoracic epidural anesthesia during the first 3 to 5 postoperative days has been effective in achieving early ambulation. Pneumatic stockings are used for deep vein thrombosis prophylaxis until the patient is ambulating daily.

When stable, patients are transferred to a thoracic step-down unit with continuous monitoring via central lines and pulse oximetry. A 1-L/24hr fluid restriction is imposed for the first 3 to 5 postoperative days to prevent hypoxemia secondary to fluid retention

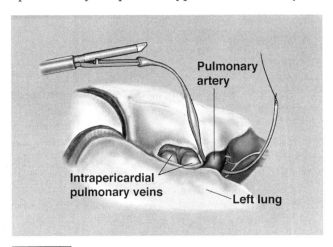

FIGURE 10.

The left pulmonary artery is divided as it leaves the pericardium and enters the left chest. (Courtesy of Garcia JP, Richards WG, Sugarbaker DJ: Surgical treatment of malignant mesothelioma, in Kaiser KR, Kron IL, Spray TL (eds): *Mastery of Cardiothoracic Surgery.* Philadelphia, Lippincott-Raven, 1997, in press.)

and contralateral lung capillary leak. Diuresis and chest physiotherapy are used to maintain appropriate oxygenation. Bronchoscopy is performed when indicated for pulmonary toilet. Daily chest radiographs are obtained for evaluation of mediastinal shift or fluid overload. They also allow for detection of early infiltrates, which are treated with broad-spectrum antibiotics until cultures are obtained. Patients are kept under aspiration precautions, and the nasogastric tube is not removed until the second postoperative day. The diet is advanced slowly after postoperative day 3.

ADJUVANT THERAPY

Patients used to receive chemotherapy (doxorubicin, 50 to 60 mg/m^2, and cyclophosphamide, 600 mg/m^2, for 4 to 6 cycles before 1985, n = 9; after 1985, 70 mg/m^2 cisplatin was added to the regimen) 4 to 6 weeks after surgery, followed by external-beam radiotherapy to the entire ipsilateral hemithorax and mediastinum to 30 Gy. At this time, patients receive taxol 200 mg/m^2 by continuous IV infusion (3 hr) and carboplatin AUC (area under the curve) 6 for 2 cycles 3 weeks apart. After radiation with concurrent, weekly taxol 60 mg/m^2, patients receive a repeat 2 cycles of taxol and carboplatin. When possible, a boost dose is delivered to areas of previous bulk disease to a total of 50 to 55 Gy.

RESULTS AND DISCUSSION

Among the first 120 consecutive patients undergoing extrapleural pneumonectomy at Brigham and Women's Hospital from 1980 to 1995, the overall median survival was 21 (1 to 96) months. Two- and 5-year survival rates were 45% and 22%, respectively (Fig 11).[26] Lack of lymph node involvement and epithelial histology were independent positive prognostic indicators. Thirty-nine of the 67 patients with epithelial tumors who had negative nodes demonstrated 74% 2-year and 39% 5-year survival rates, which were significantly longer than those of the 28 patients with epithelial tumors and positive nodes (52% 2-year and 10% 5-year survival rates; P = 0.002; Fig 12).[26]

Patients with microscopic transdiaphragmatic invasion (n = 14) had a poor prognosis regardless of cell type or node status (median survival, 11 months) (Fig 13).[26] Surprisingly, however, residual tumor, microscopically positive margins, or tumor involving (but not penetrating the full thickness of) the diaphragm or pericardium did not significantly affect survival. Additional factors found in this analysis to be unrelated to survival were age, gender,

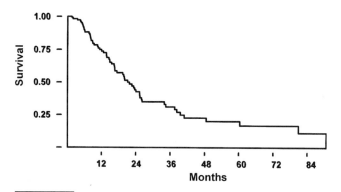

FIGURE 11.

Kaplan-Meier survival curve for all patients undergoing extrapleural pneumonectomy (N = 120; median survival, 20 months). (Courtesy of Sugarbaker DJ, Garcia JP, Richards WG, et al: Extrapleural pneumonectomy in
the multimodality therapy of malignant pleural mesothelioma: Results in
120 consecutive patients. *Ann Surg* 224:288–296, 1996.)

cigarette smoking, asbestos exposure, length of surgery, and side
affected by the tumor.

   Experience at our institution suggests that extrapleural pneumonectomy as a component of trimodality therapy for malignant
pleural mesothelioma can be safe and effective in carefully selected

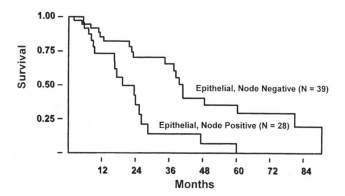

FIGURE 12.

Kaplan-Meier survival curve for patients with epithelial tumors and node-
negative vs. node-positive pathologic specimens. Patients with negative
nodes had a longer survival (*P* = 0.002). (Courtesy of Sugarbaker DJ, Garcia JP, Richards WG, et al: Extrapleural pneumonectomy in the multimodality therapy of malignant pleural mesothelioma: Results in 120 consecutive patients. *Ann Surg* 224:288–296, 1996.)

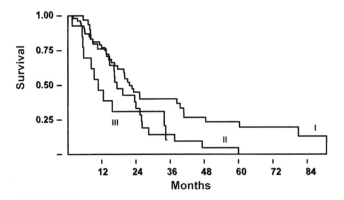

FIGURE 13.

Kaplan-Meier survival curve demonstrating a significant stratification of survival when all patients are classified as stage I, II, or III according to our proposed staging system. (Courtesy of Sugarbaker DJ, Garcia JP, Richards WG, et al: Extrapleural pneumonectomy in the multimodality therapy of malignant pleural mesothelioma: Results in 120 consecutive patients. *Ann Surg* 224:288–296, 1996.)

patients. The overall median survival associated with this trimodality strategy is superior to the historical results reported for single-modality therapy. Furthermore, the survival of patients treated with trimodality therapy is stratified with respect to nodal status, cell type, and transdiaphragmatic invasion, which validates a staging system that we previously proposed.[24]

Surgical resection alone was historically the sole treatment of mesothelioma. However, neither pleurectomy[21, 28–30] nor extrapleural pneumonectomy[22, 23, 31] alone increased the median survival. Extrapleural pneumonectomy was associated with operative mortality as high as 31%.[31] Most patients who underwent surgical resection later had invasion of the mediastinum or peritoneum and died of recurrent disease.

Chemotherapy alone is also ineffective in the treatment of malignant mesothelioma. Response rates are often difficult to determine because of the diffuse nature of most lesions and the common presence of pleural effusions, which make the extent of disease difficult to determine. In patients with measurable disease, chemotherapy has resulted in approximately 20% response rates, although no increase in survival has been demonstrated. Single-agent chemotherapy has been associated with median survival intervals from 4 to 12 months in a number of reported series (e.g., Adriamycin,[32] cyclophosphamide,[33] cisplatin,[34] doxorubicin,[32, 33] and mitomycin C).[35] For a comprehensive review, see elsewhere[16]). Although doublet combinations (doxorubicin-cyclophosphamide and doxorubicin-cisplatin) have some activity in mesothelioma, response rates have not been significantly greater than those of single-agent therapy, approximately 26%.[1, 36]

In some series, mesothelioma responds to high-dose radiotherapy as a single-treatment modality, but the median survival is not affected (for review, see elsewhere[17]). The risk of radiation-induced injury to underlying pulmonary parenchyma limits the dose that can be delivered to sites of pleural disease, and even suboptimal doses may result in significant morbidity.

The rationale for using adjuvant chemotherapy and radiotherapy after extrapleural pneumonectomy is founded on the assumption that this combination optimizes conditions for the effectiveness of each component modality. For example, in lung cancer, response rates to chemotherapy are improved as tumor burden and stage are reduced.[37] In esophageal cancer[38] and lung cancer,[39] chemotherapy and irradiation have been shown to augment the efficacy of surgery. The finding that platinum-based regimens are particularly active in epithelial tumors is consistent with the increased survival associated with epithelial histology and suggests that alternative chemotherapy might be used for sarcomatous tumors in future trials.

The current analysis of our experience confirms our previous findings in a subset (N = 52) of the same cohort of patients[24] in which epithelial histology and negative node status were independent prognostic factors predicting improved survival. In the current analysis, the 42 patients who were node-negative and had epithelial tumors demonstrated a 39% 5-year survival rate. Interestingly, positive resection margins do not predict reduced survival despite the overwhelming tendency for mesothelioma to recur locally.

In predicting survival, two systems that have been proposed for staging malignant pleural mesothelioma are of limited utility because stratification of survival has not been possible with previous treatment strategies. A staging system for any given malignancy is useful only to the degree that it stratifies survival, defines the success of standard treatment, and directs therapy. Because mesothelioma has been ineffectively treated with standard modes of therapy, it is not surprising that no accurate and predictive staging system has thus far been developed.

Butchart et al. proposed the most commonly used staging system in 1976.[31] Based on experience with 29 patients treated by pleural pneumonectomy, this staging system divides patients into stage I, including those patients with disease confined to the capsule of the pleural envelope, lung, pericardium, and diaphragm; stage II, those patients with tumors invading the chest wall or mediastinal structures with or without thoracic lymph node involvement; stage III, including patients with disease extending into the peritoneum with extrathoracic lymph node involvement; and stage IV, those rare patients with blood-borne metastases.[31] Unfortunately, this staging system does not reliably stratify survival probability by stage.

A second proposed staging system is based on the international TNM staging variables, although no correlation to survival has been made.[40] It is difficult to estimate preresectional T status because the extent of disease in mesothelioma is not typically discernible by radiographic techniques and can only be accurately assessed in the setting of a complete gross resection (extrapleural pneumonectomy). Nodal designations in non–small-cell lung cancer are based on lymphatic flow away from the tumor and therefore represent disease progression. In mesothelioma, the designation of N1, N2, or N3 status is not possible because there is no consistent progression of lymphatic drainage away from the primary tumor through identifiable nodal stations. The scarcity of blood-borne metastatic disease in patients with mesothelioma renders M status irrelevant for the majority of patients.[41]

We proposed a staging system based on survival stratification in an earlier analysis of a subset of the present cohort.[24] Stage I includes disease that can be resected by pleurectomy or extrapleural pneumonectomy. Stage II comprises patients with lymph node involvement detectable on MRI, at mediastinoscopy, or at thoracotomy. Stage III (Butchart stages II and III) includes patients with unresectable disease because of tumor extension into the mediastinum or across the diaphragm. Stage IV patients are those with extrathoracic metastatic disease.

The validity of this staging system is supported by analysis of 120 patients because survival was significantly stratified according to stage (Fig 13). It may be possible to select appropriate patients for aggressive therapy on the basis of resectability, histology, and node status. For example, MRI scanning to assess transdiaphragmatic and mediastinal invasion,[7] combined with noninvasive or minimally invasive methods for detecting lymph node metastases, including positron emission tomographic scanning, laparoscopy, thoracoscopy, and mediastinoscopy, could form the basis for more accurate preresectional staging. Our experience shows that aggressive trimodality therapy can extend survival in patients with node-negative epithelial tumors. Future clinical trials based on stage and cell type–specific adjuvant therapies may be useful in further validating this staging system.

REFERENCES

1. Antman KH, Pass HI, DeLaney T, et al: Benign and malignant mesothelioma, in DeVita VT Jr, Hellman S, Rosenberg SA (eds): *Cancer: Principles and Practice of Oncology,* ed 4. Philadelphia, JB Lippincott, 1993, pp 1489–1508.
2. Wagner JC, Sleggs EA, Marchand P: Diffuse pleural mesothelioma and asbestos exposure in the North Western Cape Province. *Br J Ind Med* 17:260–271, 1960.
3. Muscat JE, Wynder EL: Cigarette smoking, asbestos exposure, and malignant mesothelioma. *Cancer Res* 51:2263–2267, 1991.
4. Enterline PE, Henderson VL: Geographic patterns of pleural mesothelioma deaths in the United States, 1968–81. *J Natl Cancer Inst* 79:31–37, 1987.
5. Connelly RR, Spirtas R, Myers MH, et al: Demographic patterns for mesothelioma in the United States. *J Natl Cancer Inst* 78:1053–1060, 1987.
6. Walker AM, Loughlin JE, Freidlander ER, et al: Projections of asbestos-related disease 1980–2009. *J Occup Med* 25:409–425, 1983.
7. Patz EF Jr, Shaffer K, Piwnica-Worms DR, et al: Malignant pleural mesothelioma: Value of CT and MR imaging in predicting resectability. *AJR Am J Roentgenol* 159:961–966, 1992.
8. Corson JM: Pathology of mesothelioma, in Antman K, Aisner J (eds): *Asbestos-Related Malignancy.* Orlando, Fla, Grune & Stratton, 1986, p 179.
9. Antman K, Shemin R, Ryan L, et al: Malignant mesothelioma: Prognostic variables in a registry of 180 patients, the Dana-Farber Cancer Institute and Brigham and Women's Hospital experience over two decades, 1965–1985. *J Clin Oncol* 6:147–153, 1988.
10. Sugarbaker DJ, Heher EC, Lee TH, et al: Extrapleural pneumonectomy, chemotherapy, and radiotherapy in the treatment of diffuse malignant pleural mesothelioma. *J Thorac Cardiovasc Surg* 102:10–14, 1991.
11. Antman K, Pass HI, Recht A: Benign and malignant mesothelioma, in DeVita VT Jr, Hellman S, Rosenberg SA (eds): *Cancer: Principles and Practice of Oncology,* ed 3. Philadelphia, JB Lippincott, 1989, pp 1399–1414.
12. Chahinian AP, Ambinder RM, Mandel EM, et al: Evaluation of 63 patients with diffuse malignant mesothelioma. *Proc Am Soc Clin Oncol* 21:360A, 1980.
13. Law MR, Hodson ME, Turner-Warwick M: Malignant mesothelioma of the pleura: Clinical aspects and symptomatic treatment. *Eur J Respir Dis* 65:162–168, 1984.

14. Ruffie P, Feld R, Minkin S, et al: Diffuse malignant mesothelioma of the pleura in Ontario and Quebec: A retrospective study of 332 patients. *J Clin Oncol* 7:1157–1168, 1989.
15. Antman KH, Blum RH, Greenberger JS, et al: Multimodality therapy for malignant mesothelioma based on a study of natural history. *Am J Med* 68:356–362, 1980.
16. Sugarbaker DJ, Jaklitsch MT, Soutter AD, et al: Multimodality therapy of malignant mesothelioma, in Roth JA, Ruckdeschel JC, Weisenburger TH (eds): *Thoracic Oncology,* ed 2. Philadelphia, WB Saunders, 1996, pp 538–555.
17. Falkson G, Alberts AS, Falkson HC: Malignant pleural mesothelioma treatment: The current state of the art. *Cancer Treat Rev* 15:231–242, 1988.
18. Gordon W Jr, Antman KH, Greenberger JS, et al: Radiation therapy in the management of patients with mesothelioma. *Int J Radiat Oncol Biol Phys* 8:19–25, 1982.
19. Eschwege F, Schlienger M: [Radiotherapy of malignant pleural mesotheliomas. Apropos of 14 cases irradiated at high doses]. *J Radiol Electrol Med Nucl* 54:255–259, 1973.
20. Law MR, Gregor A, Hodson ME, et al: Malignant mesothelioma of the pleura: A study of 52 treated and 64 untreated patients. *Thorax* 39:255–259, 1984.
21. Allen KB, Faber LP, Warren WH: Malignant pleural mesothelioma: Extrapleural pneumonectomy and pleurectomy. *Chest Surg Clin North Am* 4:113–126, 1994.
22. Worn H: Moglichkeiten und Ergebnisse der chirurgischen Behandlung des malignen Pleuramesotheliomas. *Thoraxchir Vask Chir* 22:391–393, 1974.
23. Rusch VW, Piantadosi S, Holmes EC: The role of extrapleural pneumonectomy in malignant pleural mesothelioma. A Lung Cancer Study Group trial. *J Thorac Cardiovasc Surg* 102:1–9, 1991.
24. Sugarbaker DJ, Strauss GM, Lynch TJ, et al: Node status has prognostic significance in the multimodality therapy of diffuse, malignant mesothelioma. *J Clin Oncol* 11:1172–1178, 1993.
25. Rusch VW: Pleurectomy/decortication and adjuvant therapy for malignant mesothelioma. *Chest* 103:382S–384S, 1993.
26. Sugarbaker DJ, Garcia JP, Richards WG, et al: Extrapleural pneumonectomy in the multimodality therapy of malignant pleural mesothelioma: Results in 120 consecutive patients. *Ann Surg* 224:288–296, 1996.
27. Garcia JP, Richards WG, Sugarbaker DJ: Surgical treatment of malignant mesothelioma, in Kaiser LR, Kron IL, Spray TL (eds): *Mastery of Cardiothoracic Surgery.* Philadelphia, Lippincott-Raven, 230–236, 1997.
28. Mychalczak BR, Nori D, Armstrong JG, et al: Results of treatment of malignant pleural mesothelioma with surgery, brachytherapy, and external beam irradiation. *Endocurie Hypertherm Oncol* 5:245, 1989.

29. McCormack PM, Nagasaki F, Hilaris BS, et al: Surgical treatment of pleural mesothelioma. *J Thorac Cardiovasc Surg* 84:834–842, 1982.
30. Rusch VW: Trials in malignant mesothelioma. LCSG 851 and 882. *Chest* 106:359S–362S, 1994.
31. Butchart EG, Ashcroft T, Barnsley WC, et al: Pleuropneumonectomy in the management of diffuse malignant mesothelioma of the pleura. Experience with 29 patients. *Thorax* 31:15–24, 1976.
32. Harvey VJ, Slevin ML, Ponder BA, et al: Chemotherapy of diffuse malignant mesothelioma: Phase II trials of single agent 5-fluorouracil and Adriamycin. *Cancer* 54:961–964, 1984.
33. Gerner RE, Moore GE: Chemotherapy of malignant mesothelioma. *Oncology* 30:152–155, 1974.
34. Daboys G, Delajartre M, Le Mevel B: Treatment of diffuse pleural malignant mesothelioma by cisdichlorodiamine platinum in nine patients. *Cancer Chemother Pharmacol* 5:209–210, 1981.
35. Kelsen D, Bajorin D, Mintzer D: Phase II trial of mitomycin C in malignant mesothelioma. *Proc Am Soc Clin Oncol* 4:146A, 1985.
36. Chahinian AP, Antman K, Goutsou M, et al: Randomized phase II trial of cisplatin with mitomycin or doxorubicin for malignant mesothelioma by the Cancer and Leukemia Group B. *J Clin Oncol* 11:1559–1565, 1993.
37. Faber LP, Bonomi PD: Combined preoperative chemoradiation therapy. *Chest Surg Clin North Am* 1:43–59, 1991.
38. Forastiere AA, Orringer MB, Perez Tamayo C, et al: Concurrent chemotherapy and radiation therapy followed by transhiatal esophagectomy for local-regional cancer of the esophagus. *J Clin Oncol* 8:119–127, 1990.
39. Dillman RO, Seagren SL, Propert KJ, et al: A randomized trial of induction chemotherapy plus high-dose radiation versus radiation alone in stage III non–small-cell lung cancer. *N Engl J Med* 323:940–945, 1990.
40. Rusch VW, Venkatraman E: The importance of surgical staging in the treatment of malignant pleural mesothelioma. *J Thorac Cardiovasc Surg* 111:815–826, 1996.
41. Nauta RJ, Osteen RT, Antman KH, et al: Clinical staging and the tendency of malignant pleural mesotheliomas to remain localized. *Ann Thorac Surg* 34:66–70, 1982.

CHAPTER 13

Reoperation for Missed Parathyroid Adenoma

Jeffrey A. Norton, M.D.
Professor of Surgery, University of California, San Francisco

P rimary hyperparathyroidism (HPT) is a common clinical condition. The estimated incidence is 27.7 per 100,000 population in the United States, Great Britain, and Sweden.[1] In the majority of patients, HPT is caused by a solitary adenoma or a benign
tumor of one of the parathyroid glands (85%).[2, 3] From a surgical
point of view, HPT secondary to a parathyroid adenoma is ideal
because a relatively safe straightforward operation will result in
complete amelioration of the condition in approximately 90% of
the patients. However, if the initial procedure is unsuccessful, the
reoperation for a missed adenoma can be treacherous, difficult, and
more expensive[4] and turn an ideal procedure into a nightmare.

The estimated number of new cases of primary HPT in the
United States per year is 100,000.[1] The prevalence of the disease
(number of the total population affected) is between 1 per 100 and
1 per 1,000 population. Assuming that all patients with primary
HPT undergo surgery, that the success rate of initial operations for
primary HPT is 90%, and that 85% of the patients with primary HPT
have an adenoma as the cause, then 8,500 patients each year in the
United States will suffer a missed parathyroid adenoma and will
need to undergo a reoperation to remove it. Because reoperations for
primary HPT are more difficult than the initial operations, the success rate and complication rate of these operations have been significantly different from those of the initial operations,[3, 5–13] that is,
lower success rates and higher complication rates. However, significant advances have occurred over recent years that appear to have
improved the outcome for patients undergoing these difficult reoperations.[14–20] This chapter reviews these advances and describes a
uniform approach to these patients and the complexities of reoperations for missed parathyroid adenoma.

Advances in Surgery®, vol. 31
© 1998, Mosby–Year Book, Inc.

SIGNS AND SYMPTOMS

Because reoperations for missed parathyroid adenoma are much more difficult than the initial operations, most experts do not recommend repeat surgery unless the patient has significant symptoms and signs related to the primary HPT.[14, 21] These symptoms include bone pain, kidney stones, and symptoms suggestive of the involvement of other organ systems such as the gastrointestinal tract and muscle joints, as well as neuropsychiatric symptoms.

The classic bone disease of severe primary HPT is osteitis fibrosa cystica. This disease causes severe bone pain, and pathologic fractures may occur. Serum levels of bony alkaline phosphatase are elevated. Overt bone resorption associated with HPT can be detected on plain radiographs of the hands, skull, and clavicles. Subperiosteal bone resorption is seen most commonly on the radial side of the distal middle phalanges. The skull may have a salt-and-pepper or moth-eaten appearance on plain radiographs. The cortex of the lateral third of the clavicle is thin, so it appears tapered on plain roentgenograms. Brown tumors, or bone cysts, can be seen in the long bones or the pelvis. Patients with these findings of bone resorption have severe HPT. The number of these patients is decreasing because surgery generally corrects the disease before such severe signs develop. However, patients who have had unsuccessful initial operations and have missed parathyroid adenomas have evidence of more severe bone disease.[3, 12, 13, 21]

Bone density is now measured to more accurately quantitate the effects of excessive parathyroid hormone (PTH) on bone.[1] Bone density is generally measured at three sites to evaluate the mass of both cortical and cancellous bone: radius (cortical), vertebrae (cancellous), and hip (both). Heightened bone resorption and demineralization are secondary to the catabolic effects of excessive PTH on cortical bone. In patients with primary HPT, the density of cortical bone is primarily decreased such that the maximal decrease in bone density will be seen in the radius, the vertebrae will not have a decrease in density, and the hip will have a moderate decrease. Current data from patients undergoing initial operations for HPT indicate that only 2% have decreased bone density. However, experience with reoperations suggests that between 30% and 50% of the patients have a significant decrease in bone density.[1, 3, 12, 13, 21]

Nephrolithiasis is another manifestation of primary HPT. The incidence of kidney stones is between 15% and 20% of all patients with primary HPT. The incidence in individuals undergoing reoperation is 55%.[1, 3, 12, 13, 21] Besides nephrolithiasis, the kidneys may also be affected by the deposition of calcium phosphate crystals throughout the renal parenchyma, called nephrocalcinosis. Nephrocalcinosis may result in the development of frank kidney stones or a reduction in creatinine clearance. The presence of either nephrocalcinosis or nephrolithiasis is an indication for reoperation for primary HPT.

Primary HPT is also associated with weakness and easy fatiguability. It is not clear how excessive concentrations of calcium and PTH produce these symptoms. It is especially evident in proximal muscle groups, and patients may experience difficulty climbing stairs or getting up from a chair. Some patients describe a general feeling of tiredness and lack of energy. Muscle weakness is present in approximately 2% of the patients with HPT at the time of initial surgery and in 22% of the patients at reoperation.[1, 3, 12, 13, 21] The symptom itself is an indication for reoperation, especially if the patient has significant proximal muscle group weakness or the fatigue is lifestyle limiting such that the patient cannot function in the present state.

Primary HPT may also affect the gastrointestinal tract, and symptoms of peptic ulcer disease and pancreatitis have been linked to HPT. It is now clear that a major association between HPT and peptic ulcer disease occurs in patients with multiple endocrine neoplasia type 1; such patients may have concomitant primary HPT and Zollinger-Ellison syndrome (ZES).[22, 23] Certainly, the major clinical manifestation of the ZES is severe peptic ulcer disease, and it has been convincingly demonstrated that surgery to correct the primary HPT markedly ameliorates the ZES.[22] The exact relationship between non-ZES peptic ulcer disease and primary HPT is not clear. Similarly, the exact relationship between primary HPT and pancreatitis remains to be elucidated. However, approximately 17% of the patients undergoing reoperations for missed adenoma will have some upper gastrointestinal symptoms such as pain or dyspepsia that will resolve with successful surgery.[1, 3, 12, 13, 21]

Gout or pseudogout may be associated with primary HPT.[1] Older patients with chondrocalcinosis of the knees and bones in whom primary HPT develops may be at risk for the development of gout. Hypertension may also be associated with primary HPT.[24] This sign may be more population based than individual based because hypertensive patients with HPT may not have an improvement in blood pressure control after resection of a parathyroid adenoma.[25] The neuropsychiatric symptoms of HPT are controversial. Affective disorders, depression, anxiety, cognitive difficulties, and memory loss may all be associated with HPT in some instances.

Interestingly, reversal of some of these symptoms has been described after correction of HPT.[26, 27] Some investigators have documented improvement in cognitive test results after resection of a parathyroid adenoma.[27] However, others contend that it is still unclear as to what neuropsychiatric symptoms are related to HPT because these symptoms may be multifactorial.[28]

In patients who are to undergo a reoperation for a missed adenoma, it is critical to be certain that significant symptoms are being caused by the HPT such that it is deemed necessary to proceed with another more risky operation. Recently, we described our experience with 222 consecutive patients who underwent reoperation for missed parathyroid adenoma (Table 1).[14] Only 32 (14%) were thought to be asymptomatic, and the most common symptoms were either pain from kidney stones (48%) or bone pain with decreased bone density (41%). This should be contrasted to patients undergoing initial operations for HPT, 80% of whom are asymptomatic and only 20% and 2% of whom have either kidney stones or bone pain, respectively.[29] Therefore it is clear that most surgeons select patients for parathyroid reoperation with more stringency than they do for initial operations.

TABLE 1.
Incidence of Symptoms
of Primary Hyperparathyroidism
in 222 Patients Who Underwent
Reoperations for Missed
Adenoma

Symptom	Number (%)
Kidney stones	106 (48)
Bone pain	91 (41)
Fatigue	61 (28)
Neuropsychiatric	46 (21)
Gastrointestinal	43 (19)
Weakness	32 (14)
None	32 (14)

(Courtesy of Jaskowiak N, Norton JA, Alexander HR, et al: A prospective trial evaluating a standard approach to reoperation for missed parathyroid adenoma. *Ann Surg,* in press.)

REVIEW OF PREVIOUS OPERATIONS

Every surgeon who has written about reoperations for primary HPT describes the importance of careful review of the results of each of the previous operations.[14–20] The surgeon who plans the reoperation should obtain the operative notes and the pathology report from the initial operation and any subsequent operations. The pathology slides should also be reviewed by a pathologist capable of accurately assessing the presence of either normal or abnormal parathyroid tissue. Records including preoperative and postoperative serum levels of calcium should be reviewed to discern whether the patient has *persistent* or *recurrent* primary HPT. Careful questioning of the patient should be performed to determine whether postoperative hypocalcemia has developed. For example, did the previous surgeon prescribe supplemental calcium or vitamin D? Did the patient have any tingling or other symptoms of tetany that were relieved by supplemental calcium? Most successful operations for HPT will result in symptoms of tingling and the use of supplemental calcium and/or vitamin D.

Primary HPT occurring after the surgery to correct it is divided into either *persistent* disease or *recurrent* disease. Persistent disease is defined as persistent hypercalcemia, which means that the initial operation failed to normalize the serum level of calcium. Recurrent disease means that either hypocalcemia or normalization of the serum level of calcium was present for a time period of at least 6 months and then subsequently hypercalcemia recurred. Persistent disease usually means that the surgeon failed to remove a parathyroid adenoma or failed to recognize multiglandular disease (hyperplasia) and did not remove sufficient parathyroid tissue. Recurrent disease suggests that all pathologic tissue was removed at the initial operation; however, it either regrew because a remnant of pathologic tissue subsequently enlarged or a parathyroid adenoma was incompletely resected and subsequently regrew.[30] Parathyroid tumors may recur locally if they are incompletely excised or they are carcinoma.[30] The operative note may contain clues to incomplete excision of an adenoma. Such clues include excessive bleeding during resection and propinquity to the recurrent laryngeal nerve. These may cause the surgeon to inadvertently leave a small amount of parathyroid adenoma.

When reading operative notes from unsuccessful surgical procedures, discrepancies are usually present and lead to uncertainty about what actually occurred during the original procedure. For example, it may be that the right and left side of the neck are confused or it may be that what was referred to as the superior gland is really an inferior gland. One important rule is to never believe the previous surgeon without biopsy confirmation of the presence of parathyroid tissue. For example, if the surgeon states that the left superior parathyroid gland was identified and appeared normal, this statement is disregarded unless the pathology review corroborates it. For the diagnosis of an adenoma, it is essential to identify one abnormal gland and one normal gland. Occasionally the adenoma will contain a suppressed normal gland that can be identified histologically. A normal parathyroid gland measures approximately 3 $\times$ 4 mm and weighs between 30 and 50 mg. In the case of a missing adenoma, the initial operative note and pathology result will, it is hoped, identify by biopsy at least one normal parathyroid gland. If a normal gland has been sampled for biopsy during the initial operation, the reoperation focuses solely on finding and removing an abnormal gland. The surgeon performing a reoperation does not need to identify other normal parathyroid glands under these circumstances. If an abnormal parathyroid gland was removed at the initial operation and the pathology report corroborates it, the diagnosis is most likely parathyroid hyperplasia and the reoperating surgeon must account for and remove four parathyroid glands during all the operative procedures combined together. If the rare instance of a locally recurrent parathyroid adenoma is diagnosed, the patient has recurrent disease in the same location as the original surgery.[30] In these instances when the etiology is unclear (adenoma or hyperplasia), it may be useful to measure either PTH[31] or urinary cyclic adenosine monophosphate (cAMP)[18] levels during the operation as an on-line marker to determine when all the abnormal parathyroid tissue has been removed. Each study has been demonstrated to be useful in this regard.

DIAGNOSIS

The measurement of hypercalcemia is an essential component of the diagnosis of primary HPT, as is a concomitant measurement of elevated serum levels of PTH. The diagnosis is dependent on elevated levels of both calcium and PTH. A serum level of calcium greater than 12 mg/dL (severe hypercalcemia) is considered a clear indication for reoperation. There are many different immunologic assays for PTH, including the C-terminal, N-terminal, midmolecule, and intact PTH molecule. Use of the intact PTH assay has virtually eliminated false positive results inasmuch as the great majority of PTH-related protein molecules do not cross-react with the intact assay. A serum intact PTH level greater than 100 pg/mL (an indication of more severe disease) is also an indication for parathyroid re-exploration.

A 24-hour urine test for calcium and creatinine should also be performed before a reoperation for HPT. Familial hypocalciuric hypercalcemia (FHH) must be excluded before a reoperation because this diagnosis will lead to an unsuccessful result. Familial hypocalciuric hypercalcemia is identified primarily by very low urinary excretion of calcium and only minimally elevated levels of intact PTH, whereas patients with HPT usually have markedly elevated PTH levels and either normal or elevated urinary excretion of calcium. Patients with FHH have urinary calcium clearance/creatinine clearance values less than 0.01. Patients with FHH will also have high to normal serum levels of magnesium.[32]

The diagnosis of persistent or recurrent primary HPT can be made in all patients by measuring these parameters. It is critical that the correct diagnosis be obtained and the patient known to be symptomatic before performing localization studies.

LOCALIZATION STUDIES

Before initial operations for primary HPT, no localization studies are recommended and the operation is very safe and cost-effective.[4] However, unsuccessful initial operations lead to considerable cost that is primarily due to the localization procedures needed to identify the missed parathyroid adenoma. The major nuclear medicine study that has accurately guided a reoperation for a missed parathyroid adenoma is the sestamibi scan (Fig 1).[14, 15] The sestamibi scan has a success rate of approximately 67% to 80% and it has few false positive results (Table 2). The sestamibi scan is able to image adenomas in both the neck and chest with equal clarity. Single photon emission CT is used with sestamibi to determine whether the adenoma is within the anterior of the neck, posterior of the neck, or the chest. Ultrasound, another imaging study frequently used for parathyroid adenomas, is noninvasive and inexpensive. Abnormal parathyroid glands appear sonolucent when compared with the more echo-dense thyroid (Fig 2). Ultrasound cannot image mediastinal parathyroid adenomas because of the sternum. We perform both sestamibi scanning and US in each patient because US can provide spatial resolution for very precise localization of the adenoma and can be used in the operating room to guide operative identification and removal of the adenoma. Ul-

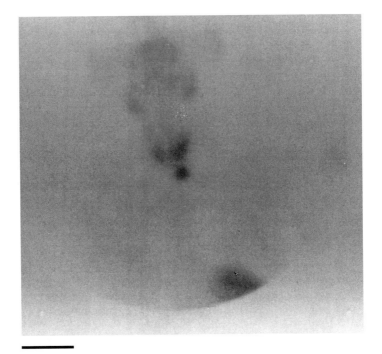

FIGURE 1.

Sestamibi scan of missed parathyroid adenoma. The image identifies a left
inferior parathyroid adenoma *(darkest circular spot)* just inferior to the
thyroid gland. Submandibular glands are also seen.

trasound by itself has approximately a 48% true positive rate, and
it has some false positive results (21%).[14] When US is combined
with sestamibi scans, we have recently seen a true positive rate of
nearly 90% and few false positive results.[33] Therefore, in most patients with missed adenomas, we have performed only US and a
sestamibi scan. If the studies identify an adenoma, we proceed with
surgery (Fig 3). If they do not, we proceed with either CT or selective arteriography. If US identifies an adenoma but it is uncertain
that it is an adenoma, US-guided fine-needle aspiration (FNA) can
be performed. The aspirate is diluted in saline and PTH is measured.[34] Detection of PTH in the aspirate is pathognomonic for a
parathyroid adenoma.

Computed tomography and MRI are equivalent. Both provide
cross-sectional imaging and both are useful for imaging mediastinal
parathyroid adenomas (Fig 4) and adenomas within the tracheoesophageal groove. Magnetic resonance imaging does not use any ra-

TABLE 2.
Localization Study Results in 222 Patients Who Underwent
Reoperations for Missed Parathyroid Adenoma

	n	True Positive, %	False Positive, %
Sestamibi	39	67	0
US	225	48	21
CT	218	52	16
MRI	155	48	14
Angiography	150	59	9
Venous sampling	98	76	4

(Courtesy of Jaskowiak N, Norton JA, Alexander HR, et al: A prospective trial evaluating a standard approach to reoperation for missed parathyroid adenoma. *Ann Surg* 224:308–320, 1996.)

diation, and parathyroid adenomas appear very bright on the T2 and stir sequence. However, it is much more expensive than CT, and in numerous studies it has similar sensitivity to CT,[14, 16] approximately 50% (Table 2). Furthermore, CT-guided FNA for PTH can also be performed.[16] Therefore, we no longer recommend MRI to image parathyroid adenomas. If the sestamibi scan initially suggests that the abnormal parathyroid gland is in the mediastinum, CT is indicated in an attempt to image the exact location of the density identified on the sestamibi scan (Fig 4).

If all the imaging studies are negative, arteriograms may be used to image a parathyroid adenoma. Parathyroid adenoma appears as a blush on selective angiograms (Fig 5). These studies have few false positive results (9%), but the sensitivity is only 59%.[14, 17] If a parathyroid angiogram is performed, selective injections of the internal mammary arteries are indicated to exclude a mediastinal parathyroid adenoma. Parathyroid adenomas have been identified within the aortopulmonary window.[35] We have purposefully treated 27 patients with mediastinal parathyroid adenomas by angiographic ablation. This had been done in a serendipitous fashion at the time of the selective angiogram. Long-term complete resolution of the HPT was achieved in 17 (63%) patients.[36] This procedure was performed with only minimal pain and no complications. In the 10 patients who had recurrences after ablation, each was able to have the adenoma removed surgically for cure without complication. Thus an-

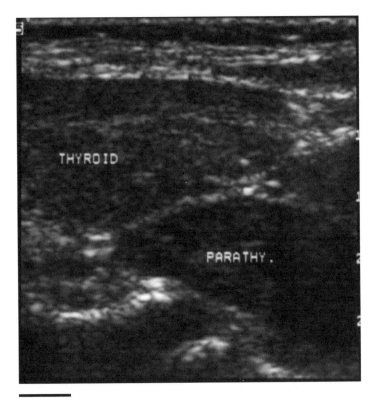

FIGURE 2.
Ultrasound of missed parathyroid adenoma: sagittal US of the left side of the neck in the same patient shown in Figure 1. Ultrasound shows a sonolucent parathyroid adenoma *(parathy)* measuring 3 × 2 cm that is inferior and posterior to the left lobe of the thyroid *(thyroid)*. The parathyroid adenoma is clearly separable from the thyroid and has fewer internal echoes.

giography can identify some patients with mediastinal adenomas who are able to have the tumor ablated without surgical techniques for cure.

Finally, we have performed selective venous sampling for concentrations of PTH in 86 patients who had equivocal localization studies and needed reoperations for HPT.[37] The study depends on the observation that the concentration of PTH in the vein that selectively drains the parathyroid adenoma will be markedly higher than the concentrations in other veins (Fig 6). Parathyroid hormone venous sampling identified a significant gradient in 76 of 86 patients (88%).[37] Any gradient in a thymic vein suggests that the para-

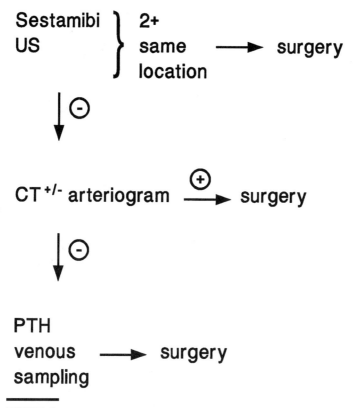

FIGURE 3.
Imaging strategy to localize missed parathyroid adenomas. *Abbreviation: PTH,* parathyroid hormone.

thyroid adenoma is within the thymus, usually within the mediastinum. The sensitivity of PTH sampling was 88% and the specificity was 86%. In reoperations for missed adenoma, venous sampling had true positive results in 76% with a false positive rate of only 4% (Table 2).[14] Venous sampling appears to be the study of choice for guiding reoperations in uncommon (approximately 10%) patients in whom all other imaging studies fail to identify the parathyroid adenoma (Fig 6). It will provide regional localization in most of these patients and suggest a region on which to focus the dissection. Often, if the adenoma is not visualized at the time of surgery, it may be necessary to remove part of the thyroid or the thymus based on the location of the gradient (Fig 6). In these instances, the parathyroid adenoma may be found within the resected specimen.

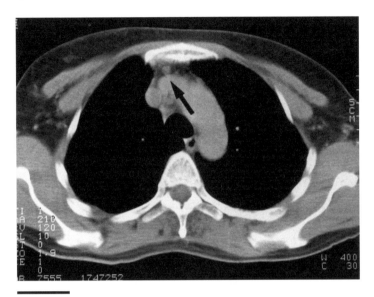

FIGURE 4.

Computed tomography of a mediastinal parathyroid adenoma showing a parathyroid adenoma *(arrow)* within the thymus in the anterior superior mediastinum.

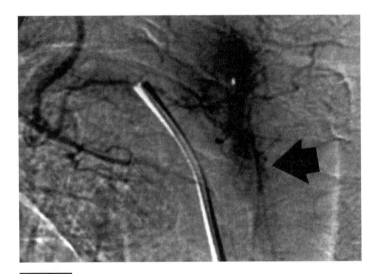

FIGURE 5.

Selective angiogram of a right inferior parathyroid adenoma. A catheter is in the right inferior thyroid artery. Digital subtraction techniques are used to identify the blush of a right inferior parathyroid adenoma *(arrow)* inferior and posterior to the right lobe of the thyroid.

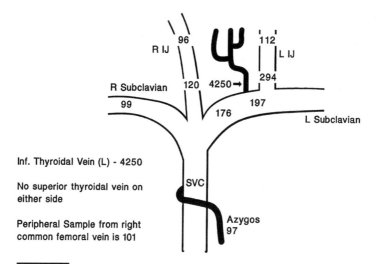

FIGURE 6.

Diagram of the results of selective venous sampling for parathyroid hormone concentrations in a patient with missed parathyroid adenoma. Peripheral levels of parathyroid hormone are 97 pg/mL. Levels in the left inferior thyroid vein are markedly elevated, 4,250 pg/mL, which suggests that the missed adenoma is in the left side of the neck associated with the left lobe of the thyroid. All other imaging studies were negative, and at surgery no parathyroid adenoma could be found. A left thyroid lobectomy was performed based solely on the results of the venous sampling. Postoperatively, the patient's serum level of calcium dropped and an intrathyroidal parathyroid adenoma was identified within the thyroid lobe.

In review, currently we rely primarily on US and sestamibi scanning as the initial localization studies in patients with previously missed parathyroid adenomas. We find that when the studies are examined and reviewed together, the sensitivity is approximately 90%.[33] If the sestamibi scan identifies an adenoma within the mediastinum that is not able to be seen by US, we order a CT scan. If both the sestamibi study and US are negative, we select CT and angiography, which are positive in approximately 50% of the patients in this situation. If these studies are negative, we obtain selective venous sampling for PTH, which provides some useful information in approximately 76% to 88% of the patients (see Fig 3). Therefore, most patients will have the adenoma imaged by cost-effective US and sestamibi scans, and the majority of the remainder will have important useful localization information obtained by using the aforementioned strategy.

SURGERY

NECK RE-EXPLORATION

The surgical strategy for reoperations for a missed parathyroid adenoma is markedly different from that for initial operations. During initial operations, the surgeon attempts to identify all four parathyroid glands and should perform a biopsy on at least one normal gland and remove any abnormal gland(s).[38] In fact, during initial explorations for HPT, we try to perform biopsies on four glands and remove the abnormal ones.

It is important to know and understand the anatomical relationships of the neck structures critical for successful parathyroid surgery.[2, 39] In each initial operation, the surgeon should be able to accurately identify four structures on both sides of the neck: inferior thyroid artery, recurrent laryngeal nerve, and superior and inferior parathyroid gland. The superior parathyroid gland is named for its relationship to the inferior thyroid artery: it is always superior to it. The inferior parathyroid gland is also named for its relationship to the inferior thyroid artery: it is inferior to it. Importantly, both these glands also have a relationship to the recurrent laryngeal nerve. The superior gland is posterolateral to the nerve, whereas the inferior gland is anteromedial to it. The superior gland is tucked underneath the superior pole of the thyroid and is usually visible only after incising the investing cervical fascia. When the superior parathyroid gland massively enlarges as a parathyroid adenoma, it frequently descends along the esophagus into the posterior superior mediastinum. Many surgeons have called these glands ectopic, but when the anatomy is completely dissected out, the usual anatomical relationships prevail such that this location is not ectopic. The inferior gland is often associated with the thymus and can be found either within the thymic tissue or within the thyrothymic ligament.[2, 40] Furthermore, the inferior gland is more often ectopic and variable in location.

The reoperation is a more focused procedure that is dependent on the results of the initial operation and the localization studies.[3, 10, 21, 41] If during the initial operation the surgeon found and performed a biopsy on one normal gland and the patient has persistent HPT, a diagnosis of missed parathyroid adenoma is assumed and the procedure is designed to dissect in the exact area based on the results of preoperative localization studies. Intraoperative US (IOUS) can also be used to further facilitate the dissection.[19] The major difficulty is dense scar tissue from the initial procedure that obliterates tissue planes and greatly impedes the ability to dissect the usual structures necessary for success. It is important for the operating surgeon to review the images from the localization procedures because they will allow a planned focused dissection. This type of focused dissection is necessary to avoid complications. Of course, the surgeon needs to understand the usual anatomy to avoid the recurrent laryngeal nerve. Parathyroid glands intimately associated with the recurrent laryngeal nerve are frequently missed or incompletely removed during the initial procedure because the surgeon may have been afraid to critically dissect near the nerve.[30]

Initial operations are performed by dividing the fascia between the strap muscles in the midline. Reoperations are performed by an alternate route along the medial border of the sternocleidomastoid muscle.[10, 21, 42, 43] This allows rapid identification of the jugular vein and the common carotid artery. Parathyroid glands are generally medial to these structures (except the rare gland within the carotid sheath), and the carotid sheath can be retracted laterally to allow excellent exposure of the posterior compartment of the neck. The strap muscles are generally divided in the inferior aspect of the neck along the insertion on the clavicular head and are then separated from the anterior surface of the thyroid. At this point, IOUS can be performed with a high-resolution small-parts transducer, either 7.5 or 10 MHz.[19] This is done early in the procedure before dissection of the central block of tissue that contains the parathyroid adenoma. Frequently, IOUS identifies the parathyroid adenoma, which appears sonolucent when compared with the more echodense thyroid tissue (see Fig 2). Furthermore, US can be used to differentiate a parathyroid adenoma from an enlarged lymph node by blood flow measurement. Parathyroid adenomas have much greater blood flow than do lymph nodes. Intraoperative US identifies approximately 75% to 80% of parathyroid adenomas, including adenomas within the lobe of the thyroid.[19, 21, 44] It can facilitate excision of these intrathyroidal adenomas without performing a complete thyroid lobectomy. If IOUS fails to detect the abnormal gland, complete dissection of that side of the neck is necessary to exclude the possibility that the imaging study was falsely negative. Care should be taken to identify with certainly the recurrent laryngeal nerve because even if IOUS is negative, it is sometimes necessary to remove the ipsilateral thyroid lobe. The surgeon should always dissect along the esophagus into the posterior superior mediastinum because upper adenomas will migrate along the esophagus and this is the most common site of missed adenomas (Fig 7). The dissection should proceed superior to the hyoid bone inasmuch as unde-

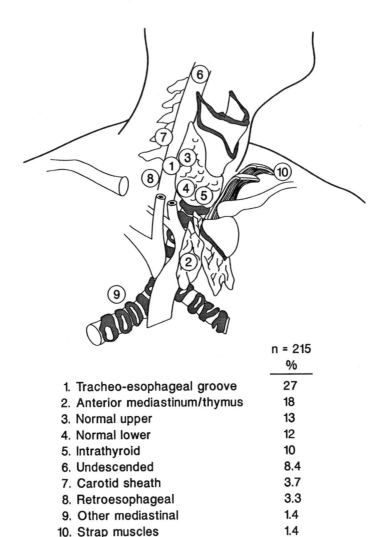

	n = 215
	%
1. Tracheo-esophageal groove	27
2. Anterior mediastinum/thymus	18
3. Normal upper	13
4. Normal lower	12
5. Intrathyroid	10
6. Undescended	8.4
7. Carotid sheath	3.7
8. Retroesophageal	3.3
9. Other mediastinal	1.4
10. Strap muscles	1.4

FIGURE 7.

Location of 222 previously missed parathyroid adenomas found during re-operations for primary hyperparathyroidism. (Courtesy of Joskowiak N, Norton JA, Alexander HR, et al: A prospective trial evaluating a standard approach to reoperation for missed parathyroid adenoma. *Ann Surg,* 224:308–320, 1996.)

scended parathyroid adenomas can occur near the carotid bifurcation.[45–47] These glands may have the appearance of a lymph
node, but in actuality there may be a parathyroid adenoma in the
center completely surrounded by thymic tissue. This is the
so-called parathymus or parathymic parathyroid adenoma, which
results from failure of the thymus and the parathyroid to descend
normally during embryologic development. If selective venous
sampling identifies a significant gradient of PTH draining from
one lobe of the thyroid and IOUS fails to identify an intrathyroidal parathyroid adenoma, we would still remove that thyroid lobe
(see Fig 6). In these conditions, we have had intrathyroidal
parathyroid adenomas found on final pathology and the surgery
has been successful. A marked parathyroid hormone gradient is a
significant clue to the region of the adenoma. Occasionally there
will be unusual venous drainage and aberrant anatomy secondary
to the initial surgery. However, if there is a dramatic increment in
PTH concentration in comparison to the peripheral hormone
concentration, the adenoma is generally being drained by that
vein, and if the adenoma is not identified at surgery, as much as
possible from the area is removed.

MEDIASTINAL EXPLORATION

Mediastinal exploration is often indicated during reoperative parathyroid surgery.[20, 48] The inferior parathyroid glands develop and
migrate with the thymus and can be found within the anterior mediastinum. Three techniques are used for mediastinal exploration:
closed exploration and thymectomy with a special retractor that
elevates the sternum,[49] endoscopic exploration of the anterior mediastinum with minimally invasive techniques, and standard median sternotomy.[20] A complete thymectomy should be done no
matter what the approach. Closed exploration and endoscopic exploration have the advantage of less pain and shorter recovery. The
median sternotomy has the advantage of better exposure and the
ability to explore other areas within the mediastinum in which an
ectopic parathyroid gland may occur, that is, along the aortic arch,
along the superior vena cava, and in the aortopulmonary window
(see Fig 7).[35] We prefer the standard median sternotomy because it
allows excellent exposure of the root of the neck and the anterior
mediastinum. It also facilitates identification of difficult adenomas
in the lower part of the neck that may be behind the head of the
clavicles or near the origin of the carotid. We have used IOUS
within the mediastinum to identify parathyroid adenomas within
the thymus and along the arch. Furthermore, median sternotomy

is not as painful as many believe if the sternum is properly wired at the conclusion of the procedure.

ECTOPIC LOCATIONS

It is important to remember that most missed parathyroid adenomas during reoperations for HPT are found within the neck in normal anatomical positions (Fig 7). This implies that the initial surgeon may not have understood the anatomy and was not able to explore the neck properly. Previously, some surgeons have stated that localization procedures are not necessary for the majority of patients who need reoperations because these adenomas can be found by individuals who are aware of the parathyroid anatomy.[50] However, parathyroid adenomas can occur in ectopic locations, so surgeons performing reoperations must know all the possibilities (see Fig 7).

Many studies have demonstrated that the most common site for a missed parathyroid adenoma is along the esophagus in the posterior superior mediastinum.[10, 14, 21] This has been described as an ectopic location, but it really represents the position of a markedly enlarged superior gland that descends posterior to the recurrent laryngeal nerve into the mediastinum. Importantly, because of its location deep in the posterior of the neck, it is often missed on preoperative US but is usually well visualized on CT as a density in the tracheoesophageal groove. It is the cause of the hyperparathyroidism necessitating 27% of all reoperations. The next most common site for ectopic parathyroid adenoma is within the thymus in the anterior mediastinum (see Fig 4). Eighteen percent of resected adenomas from our recent series were in this location,[14] and we had previously demonstrated that 17 other patients with these adenomas were managed by angiographic ablation.[36] Wang et al. have previously reported that the most common location of supernumerary parathyroid glands is within the mediastinal thymus,[40] so it makes sense that ectopic adenomas occur there.[51] In fact, some of these adenomas have been removed only because the surgeon performed a complete thymectomy; that is, they were only subsequently discovered postoperatively on pathologic analysis.[20]

The next most common location for a missed adenoma is within the thyroid.[14, 44] Ten percent were found there. These glands can usually be identified intraoperatively with the use of US, which can also be used to remove the intrathyroidal adenoma without removing the entire lobe. However, in several instances in which IOUS has been negative, we have removed the thyroid lobe based primarily on preoperative venous sampling (see Fig 6). An intrathyroidal parathyroid adenoma was identified only on pathologic analysis of the removed thyroid lobe. Therefore, a negative US scan of the thyroid does not exclude the possibility of an intrathyroidal parathyroid adenoma despite the fact that most of these glands are visible on US.

An undescended parathyroid adenoma was first described by Edis et al.[46] We have previously reported our results with it and have cited it as a common cause of missed adenomas.[45] As originally described, this adenoma was completely surrounded by thymus tissue and thus the term *parathymus*.[46] Despite the term parathymus, we have seen some undescended parathyroid adenomas that were not associated with thymic tissue.[47] They occur high in the neck at the level of the hyoid bone or at the carotid bifurcation. This was the site of missed adenomas in 8% of our patients. It is important to instruct radiologists about this possibility because CT and US must image high in the neck to the angle of the jaw to identify it. It is usually medial to the carotid artery at the bifurcation. If an undescended parathyroid adenoma is imaged preoperatively, an alternate route is recommended with an incision high in the neck to remove it without encountering the previous surgery site and scar tissue.[45, 47] This approach greatly simplifies operative management.

Despite the fact that carotid sheath parathyroid adenomas have been described and occur in approximately 4% of missed adenomas, this site is not a common location for a missed parathyroid adenoma. Most adenomas of the parathyroid glands are medial to the carotid artery, so a mass identified lateral to the jugular vein is usually a lymph node. We have identified one parathyroid adenoma that originated in the fibers of the vagus nerve within the carotid sheath. Certainly, retroesophageal locations have been identified (3%), and it is important to dissect along the esophagus into the posterior mediastinum. Rarely, we have found local seeding of parathyroid adenoma that has evolved as a consequence of the initial operation.[30] The surgeon may have cut into the capsule of the adenoma and spilled tumor cells that subsequently grew in the tissue of the neck. A most unusual location that has recently been identified is within the floor of the mouth. Finally, unusual locations within the mediastinum have been reported and include locations along the aortic arch, along the superior vena cava, posterior to the innominate vein, and in the aortopulmonary window.[35] It is critical to review the preoperative imaging studies with all these ectopic locations in mind so that unsuccessful surgery will not be the outcome of a search for a missed adenoma.

PARATHYROID CRYOPRESERVATION

Abnormal parathyroid tissue removed during reoperations for HPT should be cryopreserved. Patients undergoing reoperations for missed adenoma have a higher incidence of hypoparathyroidism.[3, 5–13] Cryopreservation is performed by keeping the tissue in iced saline solution on the operating table and slicing it into 2 × 1-mm fragments. The fragments are transferred to RPMI 1640 tissue culture solution containing autologous serum and dimethyl sulfoxide and then frozen in a programmable freezer. Programmable freezers decrease the temperature by 1°C per minute until a temperature of −40°C is reached. Then the tissue is stored in liquid nitrogen. If evidence of permanent hypoparathyroidism develops postoperatively (the patient still needs vitamin D and calcium 6 months postoperatively), the tissue is removed from the freezer and grafted into a nondominant forearm (approximately 20 fragments).

RESULTS

Two hundred twenty-two reoperations for missed adenoma were performed on 222 patients with either persistent or recurrent primary hyperparathyroidism.[14] The outcome was successful as judged by resolution of the hypercalcemia in 209 patients (94%) (Table 3). We subsequently performed 6 additional reoperations on

TABLE 3.
Results and Complications of Reoperations for Missed Adenoma in 222 Patients

Adenoma found at initial reoperation	209 (94%)
Adenoma found at second reoperation	6 (100%)
Overall success	215 (97%)
Mean operative time (range), min	172 (25–550)
Recurrent laryngeal nerve injury	3 (1.3%)
Blood transfusion	3 (1.3%)
Hypoparathyroidism	12 (5.3%)
Parathyroid autograft	12 (5.3%)
Normal autograft function	8/12 (75%)
Permanent hypoparathyroidism	4 (1.5%)
Death	0 (0%)

(Courtesy of Jaskowiak N, Norton JA, Alexander HR, et al: A prospective trial evaluating a standard approach to reoperation for missed parathyroid adenoma. *Ann Surg* 224:308–320, 1996.)

6 patients who initially underwent unsuccessful reoperations; each had resolution of the hypercalcemia for an overall success rate of 97%. Furthermore, by using the localization strategy described (see Fig 3), the average time of the reoperation was 2.8 hours. The operative success rate compares favorably with that of other series in that previous success rates were between 78% and 91% with a mean rate of 82%.[5–10] The 1.3% recurrent laryngeal nerve injury rate was a dramatic decrease from our initial report of nearly a 5% injury rate.[52] The right recurrent laryngeal nerve was injured much more commonly than the left nerve because it takes a more oblique course and is occasionally nonrecurrent whereas the left is more medial and protected within the tracheoesophageal groove. One permanent tracheostomy was necessary secondary to bilateral recurrent laryngeal nerve injury. Although 25% of our patients required oral vitamin D replacement before discharge, only 5% had postoperative permanent hypoparathyroidism. These patients were subsequently managed by delayed cryopreserved transplantation of autologous adenomatous tissue into the nondominant forearm. The graft procedure was performed in 12 patients, and 8 had resolution of the hypoparathyroidism. The cryopreserved autografts worked normally in these 8 patients and worked subnormally in 4. The overall incidence of hypoparathyroidism was 2%. No cryopreserved autograft caused hypercalcemia despite the fact that it has previously been reported that transplantation of fresh adenomatous tissue can cause recurrent hyperparathyroidism.[53] One life-threatening transection of the carotid artery was repaired without sequelae, only 3 patients required blood transfusion, and there was one myocardial infarction and no deaths (see Table 3).

SUMMARY

These results in difficult patients with previously missed parathyroid adenomas demonstrate that a prospective strategy to treat these patients surgically can be used with a high degree of success. This strategy required collaboration among endocrinologists, radiologists, and surgeons. Prospectively, only patients with symptomatic persistent or recurrent primary hyperparathyroidism were included. Operative reports and pathology results from the initial operation and all previous operations were reviewed in detail. Patients with FHH or hypercalcemia from other causes were excluded. State-of-the-art radiologic localization procedures were used to localize the abnormal parathyroid gland. Most patients had only noninvasive procedures, such as the sestamibi scan, but some whose results were equivocal underwent invasive localization, including selective angiography and venous sampling. All patients underwent surgery even if the localization procedures were negative. The operative approach and strategy were dependent on the previous operative result and results of the imaging studies. Operative techniques like IOUS and urinary cAMP determination helped facilitate a more rapid successful outcome. However, in some patients, operative success was only achieved by complete dissection and removal of all tissue that might harbor the adenoma such as a lobe of the thyroid or the thymus. Abnormal parathyroid tissue was cryopreserved for possible subsequent autotransplantation in the event of hypoparathyroidism. The reoperative success rate for missed adenoma was 97%, the highest ever reported with a very acceptable complication rate and no deaths. Postoperative hypoparathyroidism, which was really a complication of the initial previous operations during which normal parathyroid tissue was removed, was treated by autotransplantation of cryopreserved tissue in 12 patients, and 8 functioned perfectly. With attention to details and possible pitfalls, reoperations for missed parathyroid adenomas can be performed safely and effectively.

REFERENCES

1. Bilezikian JP, Silverberg SJ, Gartenberg F, et al: Clinical presentation of primary hyperparathyroidism, in Bilezikian JP, Levine MA, Marcus R (eds): *The Parathyroids.* New York, Raven Press, 1994, pp 457–469.
2. Thompson NW, Eckhauser F, Harness J: Anatomy of primary hyperparathyroidism. *Surgery* 92:814, 1982.
3. Thompson NW, Vinik AI: The technique of initial parathyroid exploration and reoperative parathyroidectomy, in Thompson NW, Vinik AI (eds): *Endocrine Surgery Update.* New York, Grune & Stratton, 1983, p 368.
4. Doherty GM, Weber B, Norton J: Cost of unsuccessful surgery for primary hyperparathyroidism. *Surgery* 116:954–958, 1994.
5. Grant CS, van Heerden JA, Charboneau JW, et al: Clinical management of persistent and/or recurrent primary hyperparathyroidism. *World J Surg* 10:555–565, 1986.
6. Billings PJ, Milroy EJG: Reoperative parathyroid surgery. *Br J Surg* 70:542–546, 1983.
7. Granberg P-O, Johansson G, Lindvall N, et al: Reoperation for primary hyperparathyroidism. *Am J Surg* 143:296–300, 1982.
8. Palmer JA, Rosen IB: Reoperative surgery for hyperparathyroidism. *Am J Surg* 144:406–410, 1982.
9. Prinz RA, Gamvros OI, Allison DJ, et al: Reoperations for hyperparathyroidism. *Surg Gynecol Obstet* 152:760–764, 1981.

10. Wang C: Parathyroid re-exploration. A clinical and pathological study of 112 cases. *Ann Surg* 186:140–145, 1977.
11. Clark OH, Way LW, Hunt TK: Recurrent hyperparathyroidism. *Ann Surg* 184:391–402, 1976.
12. Brennan MF, Marx SJ, Doppman J, et al: Results of reoperation for persistent and recurrent hyperparathyroidism. *Ann Surg* 194:671, 1981.
13. Brennan MF, Norton JA: Reoperation for persistent and recurrent hyperparathyroidism. *Ann Surg* 201:40–44, 1985.
14. Jaskowiak N, Norton JA, Alexander HR, et al: A prospective trial evaluating a standard approach to reoperation for missed parathyroid adenoma. *Ann Surg* 224:308–320, 1996.
15. Weber CJ, Vansant J, Alazraki N, et al: Value of technetium 99m sestamibi iodine 123 imaging in reoperative parathyroid surgery. *Surgery* 114:1011–1018, 1993.
16. Miller DL, Doppman JL, Shawker TH, et al: Localization of parathyroid adenomas in patients who have undergone surgery Part I. Noninvasive imaging methods. *Radiology* 162:133–137, 1987.
17. Miller DL, Doppman JL, Krudy AG, et al: Localization of parathyroid adenomas in patients who have undergone surgery Part II. Invasive procedures. *Radiology* 162:138–141, 1987.
18. Norton JA, Brennan MF, Saxe AW, et al: Intraoperative urinary cyclic adenosine monophosphate as a guide to successful reoperative parathyroidectomy. *Ann Surg* 200:389–395, 1984.
19. Norton JA, Shawker TH, Jones BL, et al: Intraoperative ultrasound and reoperative parathyroid surgery: An initial evaluation. *World J Surg* 10:631–639, 1986.
20. Norton JA, Schneider PD, Brennan MF: Median sternotomy in reoperations for primary hyperparathyroidism. *World J Surg* 9:807–813, 1985.
21. Carty SE, Norton JA: Management of patients with persistent or recurrent primary hyperparathyroidism. *World J Surg* 15:716–723, 1991.
22. Norton JA, Cornelius MJ, Doppman JL, et al: Effect of parathyroidectomy in patients with hyperparathyroidism, Zollinger-Ellison syndrome, and multiple endocrine neoplasia type 1: A prospective study. *Surgery* 102:958–966, 1987.
23. McCarthy DM, Peikin SR, Lopatin RN: Hyperparathyroidism—A reversible cause of cimetidine-resistant gastric hypersecretion. *BMJ* 1:765, 1979.
24. Heath H, Hodgson SF, Kennedy MA: Primary hyperparathyroidism: Incidence, morbidity and potential economic impact in a community. *N Engl J Med* 302:189–193, 1980.
25. Sancho JJ, Rouco J, Riera-Vidal R, et al: Long-term effect of parathyroidectomy for primary hyperparathyroidism on arterial hypertension. *World J Surg* 16:732–735, 1992.
26. Joborn C, Hetta J, Johanson H, et al: Psychiatric morbidity in primary hyperparathyroidism. *World J Surg* 12:476, 1988.

27. Alarcon RD, Franceschini JA: Hyperparathyroidism and paranoid psychosis case report and review of the literature. *Br J Psychiatry* 145:477–486, 1984.

28. Brown GG, Preisman RC, Kleerekoper MD: Neurobehavioral symptoms in mild primary hyperparathyroidism; related to hypercalcemia but not improved by parathyroidectomy. *Henry Ford Hosp Med J* 35:211–215, 1987.

29. Silverberg SJ, Shane E, Jacobs TP: Nephrolithiasis and bone involvement in primary hyperparathyroidism. *Am J Med* 89:327–334, 1990.

30. Fraker DL, Travis WD, Merendino JJJ, et al: Locally recurrent parathyroid neoplasms as a cause for recurrent and persistent primary hyperparathyroidism. *Ann Surg* 213:58–65, 1991.

31. Irvin GL, Dembrow VD, Prudhomme DL: Clinical usefulness of an intraoperative "quick parathyroid hormone" assay. *Surgery* 114:1019–1023, 1993.

32. Heath DA: Familial hypocalciuric hypercalcemia, in Bilezikian JP, Levine MA, Marcus R (eds): *The Parathyroids*. New York, Raven Press, 1994, pp 699–710.

33. Yim J, Doherty GM, Norton JA: Reoperations for symptomatic hyperparathyroidism in the era of sestamibi. Unpublished data, 1996.

34. Doppman JO, Krudy AG, Marx SJ, et al: Aspiration of enlarged parathyroid glands for parathyroid hormone assay. *Radiology* 148:31–35, 1983.

35. Doppman JL, Skarulis MC, Chene CC, et al: Parathyroid adenomas in the aortopulmonary window. *Radiology* 201:456–462, 1996.

36. Doherty GM, Doppman JL, Miller DL, et al: Results of a multidisciplinary strategy for management of mediastinal parathyroid adenoma as a cause of persistent primary hyperparathyroidism. *Ann Surg* 215:101–106, 1992.

37. Sugg SL, Fraker DL, Alexander HR, et al: Prospective evaluation of selective venous sampling for parathyroid hormone concentration in patients undergoing reoperations for primary hyperparathyroidism. *Surgery* 114:1004–1010, 1993.

38. Norton JA, Brennan MF, Wells SA Jr: Surgical management of hyperparathyroidism, in Bilezikian JP, Levine MA, Marcus R (eds): *The Parathyroids*. New York, Raven Press, 1994, pp 531–551.

39. Wang CA: The anatomic basis of parathyroid surgery. *Ann Surg* 183:271, 1975.

40. Wang CA, Mahaffey JE, Axelrod L, et al: Hyperfunctioning supernumerary parathyroid glands. *Surg Gynecol Obsetet* 148:711, 1979.

41. Lange JR, Norton JA: Surgery for persistent or recurrent primary hyperparathyroidism. *Curr Pract Surg* 4:56–62, 1992.

42. Saxe AW, Brennan MF: Strategy and technique of reoperative parathyroid surgery. *Surgery* 89:417, 1981.

43. Cheung PSY, Borgstrom A, Thompson NW: Strategy in reoperative surgery for hyperparathyroidism. *Arch Surg* 124:676–680, 1989.

44. Wang CA: Hyperfunctioning intrathyroid glands: A potential cause of failure in parathyroid surgery. *J R Soc Med* 74:49, 1981.
45. Fraker DL, Doppman JL, Shawker TH, et al: Undescended parathyroid adenoma: An important etiology for failed operations for primary hyperparathyroidism. *World J Surg* 14:342–348, 1990.
46. Edis AJ, Purnell DC, van Heerden JA: The undescended parathymus: An occasional cause of failed neck exploration of hyperparathyroidism. *Ann Surg* 190:64–68, 1979.
47. Billingsley KG, Fraker DL, Doppman JL, et al: Localization and operative management of undescended parathyroid adenomas in patients with persistent primary hyperparathyroidism. *Surgery* 116:982–990, 1994.
48. Clark OH: Mediastinal parathyroid tumors. *Arch Surg* 123:1096–1100, 1988.
49. Wells SA Jr, Cooper JD: Closed mediastinal exploration in patients with persistent hyperparathyroidism. *Ann Surg* 214:555–561, 1991.
50. Edis AJ, Sheedy PF II, Beahrs OH, et al: Results of reoperation for hyperparathyroidism, with evaluation of preoperative localization studies. *Surgery* 84:384–393, 1978.
51. Wang C, Gaz RD, Moncure AC: Mediastinal parathyroid exploration: A clinical and pathologic study of 47 cases. *World J Surg* 10:687–695, 1986.
52. Patow CA, Norton JA, Brennan MF: Vocal cord paralysis and reoperative parathyroidectomy. *Ann Surg* 203:282–285, 1986.
53. Brennan MF, Brown EM, Marx SJ, et al: Recurrent hyperparathyroidism from an autotransplanted parathyroid adenoma. *N Engl J Med* 299:1057–1059, 1978.

CHAPTER 14

Surgical Infections in Immunocompromised Patients—Prevention and Treatment

Shimon Kusne, M.D.
Associate Professor of Medicine and Surgery, Division of Transplantation Medicine, Thomas E. Starzl Transplantation Institute, Division of Infectious Diseases, University of Pittsburgh, Pittsburgh, Pennsylvania

Ron Shapiro, M.D.
Associate Professor of Surgery, Director, Renal Transplantation, Thomas E. Starzl Transplantation Institute, University of Pittsburgh, Pittsburgh, Pennsylanvia

A dvances in both organ transplantation and the treatment of cancer, and the specter of the AIDS epidemic have led to an increase in the number of immunocompromised patients. Surgeons who perform transplant procedures commonly have to deal with infectious complications as part of the postoperative course. With the improved survival of patients with cancer or AIDS, surgical intervention is becoming increasingly common, and it is important to be able to recognize infectious complications.

This chapter discusses the common infections seen in immunocompromised patients, as well as prevention and treatment strategies. Transplant recipients are discussed in detail, and the unique problems related to cancer and neutropenia, AIDS, splenectomized patients, and burn patients are also described. Infections associated with emergency laparotomies are discussed separately because an acute abdomen may often be a manifestation of gastrointestinal infection in an immunocompromised patient.

INFECTIOUS COMPLICATIONS IN TRANSPLANT RECIPIENTS

EPIDEMIOLOGIC AND RISK FACTORS

Signs and symptoms of infection can be very subtle in immuno-suppressed transplant recipients. The absence of fever does not rule out an infectious complication. Therefore, physicians must use their clinical judgment and experience when a transplant recipient is being assessed.

Three main risk factors for infectious complications in transplant recipients are recognized:

1. The operation itself
2. Nosocomial factors and remote exposure to infectious agents
3. Immunosuppression

1. Infections that occur soon after the surgical procedure are almost always related to the operation itself. Often the site of infection is the area in which the transplant operation occurred. Urosepsis may be associated with ureteral obstruction or urinary extravasation after kidney transplantation. Bacteremia after liver transplantation may originate from cholangitis secondary to biliary stricture, hepatic artery thrombosis, or infected intra-abdominal fluid collections. In addition, a survey of infectious complications after liver transplantation done in our institution[1] found a direct correlation between the length of the operative time and the frequency of infectious episodes (Fig 1).

2. Exposure to infectious agents may occur before, during, or after transplantation. Infection can be transmitted from the donor organ to the recipient. Many cases of transmission of bacterial, viral, fungal, and protozoal infections have been documented.[2] A wound infection or peritonitis may develop secondary to spillage of material from the gastrointestinal tract during anastomosis between the bile duct and the intestine during liver transplantation or secondary to urinary leakage at time of kidney transplantation. Exposure to a fungus may occur in the postoperative period or remotely before surgery. *Aspergillus* spores may be inhaled and cause invasive aspergillosis. *Histoplasma capsulatum* may have been acquired many years before transplantation and then show signs of reactivation after transplantation. Most cases of tuberculosis (TB) after transplantation occur in patients who have had exposure to TB in the remote past.

3. Immunosuppression is the most important risk factor for opportunistic infections. Unfortunately, there is no way of determining in a precise way the extent to which a given transplant

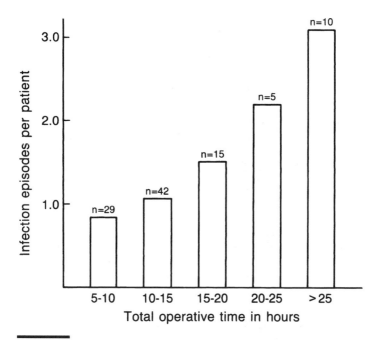

FIGURE 1.

Frequency of severe infections in relation to total operative time (hours) per patient in 101 consecutive liver transplant recipients. (Adapted from Kusne S, Summer JS, Singh N, et al: Infections after liver transplantation. *Medicine [Baltimore]* 67[2]:132–143, 1988.)

recipient is immunosuppressed. Various immunosuppressive regimens differ in terms of their effect on the immune system and their association with infectious complications. Cadaveric kidney transplant recipients are more prone to infectious complications than living related transplant patients are because of increased requirements for immunosuppression. The use of antilymphocyte agents, such as antithymocyte globulin or OKT3, is associated with increased rates of *Pneumocystis carinii* pneumonia (PCP), disseminated cytomegalovirus (CMV), and posttransplant lymphoproliferative disorder (PTLD). Nonviral infection rates in patients receiving tacrolimus have been lower than those in patients receiving cyclosporine-based immunosuppression, probably as a result of lower steroid requirements and less use of antilymphocyte preparations.

The timing of infections in relation to transplantation can be very useful. Rubin divided the postoperative period after kidney transplantation into three intervals[3]: the first month, when infections are mostly related to technical and mechanical problems; from 1 to 6 months, when two thirds of the febrile illnesses are caused by CMV; and after the sixth month, when the pattern of infection is usually similar to that seen in the general population. Similarly, in our survey of infectious complications after liver transplantation,[1] most bacterial and fungal infection episodes occurred within the first 2 months after surgery, and CMV infection usually occurred in the second month after transplantation (Fig 2).

BACTERIAL INFECTIONS

Urinary tract infection and urosepsis are the most common infectious complications after kidney transplantation. In one study of the portal of entry of bacteremia in recipients of different transplanted organs, 41% of the bacteremias originated from the urinary tract in kidney transplant recipients, whereas the most frequent source in liver transplant recipients was biliary/abdominal.[4] The most important bacterial infections after liver transplantation include infected fluid collections, peritonitis, cholangitis, and liver abscess.[1] The pathogens are usually enteric organisms and include enterococci, enteric gram-negatives, and rarely, anaerobes. Technical surgical complications and nosocomial factors are probably the most important etiologic factors. For example, vesicoureteral reflux after kidney transplantation can be associated with urosepsis.[5] Enteric drainage in pancreas transplantation has been associated with a higher rate of wound infection[6] than has bladder drainage, although this has been much less of a problem in more recent series.[7]

Listeria monocytogenes

Listeria monocytogenes can be cultured from animals and plants and can be carried in the human intestine. In a survey of fecal carriage, 2.3% of the stool specimens from renal transplant recipients, home hemodialysis patients, or patients seeing a general practitioner because of diarrhea yielded Listeria.[8] Most of the reported cases of listeriosis are in kidney transplant recipients. In one series of 102 kidney transplant patients with listeriosis, 50% had meningitis.[9] The infection may be difficult to eradicate and may recur.[10] About a third of the patients may have bacteremia and no identifiable source.[9] The treatment of listeriosis usually requires IV penicillin or ampicillin, and gentamicin is added for synergy. Trimethoprim-sulfamethoxazole (TMP-SMX) is an option in patients with penicillin allergy.

Mycobacterium

Mycobacterial disease should be considered in any case of fever of unclear etiology after transplantation. Most cases of TB in trans-

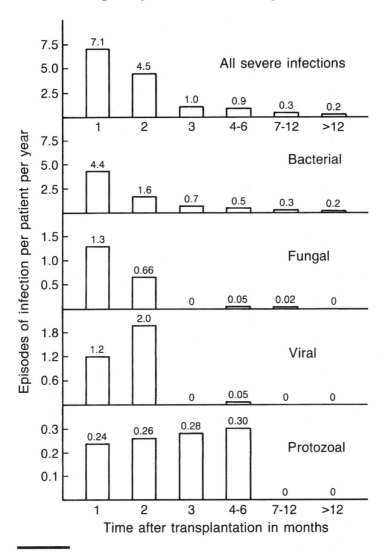

FIGURE 2.
Incidence of episodes of severe infections per patient per year and time of occurrence after transplantation in 101 consecutive liver transplant recipients. (Adapted from Kusne S, Summer JS, Singh N, et al: Infections after liver transplantation. *Medicine [Baltimore]* 67[2]:132–143, 1988.)

plant recipients are due to reactivation of old tuberculous lesions, although primary TB infections have been reported. In one epidemic of *Mycobacterium tuberculosis,* epidemiologic and DNA analysis showed transmission of TB from the source case to five renal transplant recipients.[11] The median incubation time for the development of TB was 7.5 weeks.[11] In another recent report, the infection was transmitted through a lung donor 12 weeks after transplantation.[12]

Tuberculosis cases have increased in the United States, as well as cases of multidrug-resistant TB.[13] During 1990–1991, the Centers for Disease Control investigated a few such outbreaks. All *M. tuberculosis* isolates were resistant to isoniazid, and some were also resistant to other anti-TB drugs. After exposure to multidrug-resistant TB, isoniazid obviously cannot be given. Prophylactic drugs to be considered in such exposure are pyrazinamide together with ethambutol or pyrazinamide with fluoroquinolones.[13] Candidates with chronic liver or renal disease may be anergic, and very often skin tests cannot be reliably used to assess exposure to TB.

Legionella

In one recent series, pneumonia developed in 15% of the patients after liver transplantation, and 27% of the bacterial pneumonias were secondary to *Legionella*.[14] Nosocomial sources can be determined by molecular techniques. The source of legionellosis is usually the water supply. In one series the source of *Legionella pneumophila* in three heart-lung recipients was an ice machine.[15] In a recent epidemic in Brazil in a renal transplant unit, periodic hyperchlorination and flushing of the hospital pipes with hot water were not effective in ending the outbreak.[16] Only after the installation of small independent electric showers and disconnection from the general contaminated system did the transplant unit eliminate *Legionella* from its water.[16]

Treatment of *Legionella* pneumonia has traditionally been with erythromycin, but the quinolones have also proved to be effective and have the advantage of not interacting with the immunosuppressive agents cyclosporine or tacrolimus.

Nocardia

A filamentous branching aerobic bacterium, *Nocardia* is soil borne and can affect transplant recipients. Long-term steroids, lymphoma, and renal and cardiac transplantation are risk factors. In one report, nocardiosis developed in seven patients from the same kidney transplant unit, and cultures of the air and dust grew *Nocardia asteroides*.[17] Two other cases occurred after maintenance work in a transplant unit, which suggests that inhalation of dust could be a source of infection.[18] Treatment of *Nocardia* has usually relied on sulfonamides, but combination therapy (e.g., cefotaxime, imipenem, and amikacin) has also been used to obtain synergy.

As a general rule, antibiotic treatment should target the specific bacterial pathogen. At times, when acute infection occurs, empirical antibiotic coverage is needed because the etiology of the sepsis is not yet known. The choice of antibiotics should be based on the type of infection. For example, line-related sepsis is an indication for gram-positive coverage. Abdominal sepsis after liver transplantation is most likely caused by an enteric organism. At the same time that antibiotic therapy is started, it is important to remove or change foreign bodies and resolve any mechanical problems. For example, stent in the urinary or biliary tract may be the cause of urosepsis or cholangitis.

Bacterial prophylaxis is given in the immediate perioperative period to prevent wound and urinary tract infections. Ninety percent of wound infections occur within the first 21 days after surgery,[19] and obesity has been associated with an increased rate of wound infection.[19, 20] Selective bowel decontamination has been used in some liver transplant centers as a routine prophylactic strategy.[21] Nonabsorbable antibiotics are given orally to selectively reduce aerobic gut flora, but not anaerobic gut flora. The benefits of this method of prophylaxis are still controversial because no reduced mortality or reduction in length of stay in the ICU has been observed.[22] The prophylactic regimens used currently in our institution for adult liver transplant recipients are listed in Table 1.

VIRAL INFECTIONS

Cytomegalovirus

Cytomegalovirus is the most frequent cause of infectious complications after kidney and liver transplantation. The reported incidence of CMV infection has remained constant over time, between 50% and 90%. The following patients are at highest risk for the development of CMV after transplantation[23]:

1. Seronegative individuals receiving an organ from a seropositive donor
2. Seronegative individuals receiving a significant volume of seropositive blood
3. Seropositive individuals receiving antilymphocyte preparations

Seropositive patients may reactivate their own virus or get a superinfection with a new virus strain from the donor. Seronegative patients who receive organs from CMV-seronegative donors are usually at low risk of acquiring CMV. As a general rule, symptom-

TABLE 1.
Prophylaxis in Liver Transplant Recipients at the University
of Pittsburgh

Infection	Prophylaxis
Bacterial	
Perioperative	Cefotaxime and ampicillin IV, 3 g/day for 72 hr
Viral	
CMV	Preemptive therapy is used by monitoring weekly pp65 CMV antigenemia; seronegative recipients are given a course of ganciclovir when the antigenemia level becomes positive; seropositive recipients are treated when the antigenemia level is 10 positive cells per 200,000 leukocytes or greater; ganciclovir is continued until the antigenemia level is zero
HSV	Acyclovir, 200 mg po bid or tid or 400 mg po bid, is adequate for prevention. In patients with recurrent oral or genital HSV, oral suppressive treatment may be used for 1 yr
Fungal	
Candida	Nystatin suspension, po or through a nasogastric tube, 2–4 million U/day in 4 divided doses for the duration of the admission or for 3 mo; clotrimazole troches, 10 mg qid po, is also adequate; fluconazole, 50–100 mg/day po, is also effective but interferes with CyA or FK 506 metabolism Amphotericin solution is used for wound irrigation, usually 50 mg diluted in 1 L of D_5W
Protozoal	
PCP	Trimethoprim/sulfamethoxazole, 80 mg/400 mg po once a day (the dose is reduced to every other day when creatinine is 2.5 mg/dL or greater) for the first 6–12 mo and then 3 times a week or diaminodiphenylsulfone (dapsone), 100 mg/day or 3 times a week, or aerosolized pentamidine, 300 mg diluted in sterile water and given by inhalation every 4 weeks
Toxoplasma gondii	Routinely not given after liver transplantation, but in special circumstances, pyrimethamine, 25 mg/day po, may be given for 6 wk

Abbreviations: CMV, cytomegalovirus; *HSV,* herpes simplex virus; *CyA,* cyclosporine; D_5W, 5% dextrose in water; *PCP, Pneumocystis carinii* pneumonia.

atic infection will more commonly develop in seronegative patients who receive an organ from a seropositive donor than in seropositive patients, who have protecting antibodies. The differentiation between symptomatic infection (disease) and asymptomatic infection is important because most of the patients will have viral "shedding," i.e., the virus can be cultured from many body fluids. Symptomatic infection may manifest itself as either a febrile illness or as an invasive process affecting one or more specific organs, e.g., hepatitis, colitis, pneumonitis.

Prophylaxis with several agents has been attempted, with variable results. Successful prophylaxis using high-dose oral acyclovir was originally reported by Balfour et al. in kidney transplant recipients.[24] This was a randomized, placebo-controlled, double-blind trial that used 800 to 3,200 mg/day of acyclovir adjusted for renal function.[24] Another prospective, randomized trial showed the usefulness of specific anti-CMV hyperimmune globulin in seronegative recipients of kidneys from seropositive donors.[25] By contrast, in similarly mismatched liver transplant recipients, no striking benefit of prophylaxis was seen with either ganciclovir[26] or anti-CMV hyperimmune globulin.[27] However, a recent trial of oral ganciclovir in liver transplant recipients showed a reduction in CMV disease in the seropositive donor/seronegative recipient subgroup.[28]

An alternative approach has looked at preemptive therapy,[29] i.e., using antiviral therapy in patients in whom subclinical infection develops to prevent CMV disease. Cytomegalovirus antigenemia (pp65) can be used as a marker in preemptive therapy. The pp65 antigen is a 65-kd lower matrix phosphoprotein that can be detected in polymorphonuclear cells by immunoperoxidase[30] or immunofluorescence techniques.[31] High antigenemia levels correlate with CMV disease, and low levels are correlated with asymptomatic disease.[32] Seronegative recipients are treated with a course of ganciclovir as soon as the antigenemia becomes positive, whereas seropositive patients are treated only if they reach a threshold level. The optimal level for initiation of preemptive therapy in seropositive patients is not yet clear. Some authors use 100 positive cells per 200,000 polymorphonuclear cells,[33] but the threshold may be lower. With preemptive therapy, we have seen an 8% incidence of symptomatic CMV infection after liver transplantation.[34] This method is also effective in mismatched CMV patients,[35] but frequent monitoring is required. Other methods that can be used for monitoring of patients for preemptive therapy include quantitative polymerase chain reaction (PCR) in urine,[36] blood,[37, 38] or serum.[39]

Intravenous ganciclovir, 5 mg/kg twice daily (with adjustment for renal function), is the treatment of choice for patients with symptomatic disease. Occasionally, foscarnet is required in cases of ganciclovir resistance, but it is nephrotoxic.

Epstein-Barr Virus

Epstein-Barr virus (EBV) belongs to the herpes family. It infects B lymphocytes primarily, where it causes blast transformation, and can be transmitted by saliva or blood. The virus has been associated with infectious mononucleosis, Burkitt's lymphoma, nasopharyngeal carcinoma, and hairy leukoplakia. Epstein-Barr virus infection can be found in up to 40% to 70% of transplant recipients and may cause PTLD. The incidence of PTLD is about 3% and is higher in children than in adults. OKT3 and CMV mismatch are also risk factors and can act independently and synergistically.[40] Posttransplant lymphoproliferative disorder may involve any organ, but areas rich in lymphoid tissue are more commonly involved. The syndrome of PTLD involving the gut is of particular interest to surgeons because it may be characterized by local invasion, necrosis, and perforation and lead to a surgical emergency.

The treatment of PTLD is to decrease drastically or stop the immunosuppression. Antiviral agents such as acyclovir and ganciclovir inhibit EBV in the laboratory and have been used together with reduction of immunosuppression. Preemptive therapy in high-risk patients may have a role in the treatment of this infection. Monitoring of EBV by quantitative PCR techniques,[41, 42] or by detection of EBV antigens[43] with immunocytochemical techniques may be a useful strategy. New potential treatments include EBV-specific cytotoxic T-lymphocytes in bone marrow transplant patients,[44] use of LAK cells,[45] and use of an anti–B-cell monoclonal antibody.[46]

Herpes Simplex and Herpes Zoster Virus

Herpes simplex virus (HSV) is a common infection in transplant recipients. Infection with HSV usually represents reactivation of a latent virus. Although it is generally limited to mucocutaneous areas, hepatitis or even disseminated HSV infection may occur after transplantation.[47] Acyclovir, 200 mg orally twice daily, is useful prophylactically; infection normally requires IV acyclovir, 5 to 10 mg/kg three times daily. Herpes zoster infection (varicella-zoster virus [VZV]), which usually causes skin lesions that follow a dermatomal distribution, is a manifestation of the reactivation of old VZV infection.

Varicella, which is a primary VZV infection, can be a serious problem in pediatric or adult recipients who have not had varicella before transplantation. Exposure to an individual with varicella is treated with varicella zoster immune globulin, 125 to 625 U IM, if the exposure has occurred within the last 96 hours. Varicella infection is treated with IV acyclovir, 10 mg/kg three times daily for 10 to 14 days. Although both HSV and VZV are usually associated with mild illness, even in transplant patients, they can both lead to fulminant hepatic necrosis and death in a small percentage of cases.[47, 48]

Other antiviral compounds that have similar antiviral activity but better bioavailability than acyclovir, such as the acyclovir analogues (valacyclovir and famciclovir), have been released for use.[49] Prospective trials are needed to assess the efficacy of these antivirals in immunosuppressed hosts.

Adenovirus

Infection with adenovirus may occur in transplant recipients, usually in children. There have been several reports of adenovirus-associated hepatitis.[50–52] Adults may rarely be affected. Therefore, this virus should be considered a potential cause of hepatitis, mostly in the pediatric population. In a review of the literature in 1990, 15 of 16 (94%) cases occurred in immunosuppressed patients.[53] There is no treatment, but some new antivirals such as HPMPC (cidofovir), which is approved for CMV retinitis, have antiviral activity.

Parvovirus B19

Parvovirus B19 is the smallest single-stranded DNA virus that infects vertebrates. It spreads by the respiratory route and is the cause of erythema infectiosum. In transplant recipients and patients with chronic hemolytic anemia, it can cause anemia because the virus affects red blood cell progenitors. Parvovirus B19 has been reported in kidney, liver, heart, and bone marrow transplant recipients.[54] Improvement may occur with a reduction in immunosuppression and the use of IV immunoglobulin.[54]

Herpesvirus-6

Herpesvirus-6 has been cultured from transplant patients, but the relationship to symptomatic disease is still controversial. Of 65 kidney transplant recipients who were monitored prospectively by viral culture and serologic testing, viremia developed in 14%,[55] and reactivation of the virus occurred in 54%. All recipients and their donors were seropositive.[55] In a recent report by Singh et al.,[56] encephalopathy, maculopapular rash, fever, and thrombocytopenia developed in a liver transplant recipient.[56] Herpesvirus-6 DNA was detected in his peripheral blood, and his bone marrow was positive by immunohistochemical staining.[56] The virus is sensitive to both ganciclovir and foscarnet.

Hepatitis C Virus

The rate of hepatitis C virus (HCV) infection has been increasing after transplantation. The rate of transmission of the virus from positive donors to negative recipients is very high, and most centers will only transplant HCV-positive organs into HCV-positive recipients. In a survey of centers performing heart and lung transplant operations, 22% would still accept positive donors, 44% would accept them only for positive recipients, and 27% would not accept them under any circumstance.[57, 58] Hepatitis C virus–positive kidney transplant recipients have a 5-fold increased risk of posttransplant liver disease, a 3.3-fold increased risk of death, and a 9.9-fold increased risk of death secondary to sepsis when compared with HCV-negative recipients.[59] On the other hand, when HCV-positive recipients received a kidney from either an HCV-positive or HCV-negative donor, there was no difference in patient or graft survival, with a follow-up of 3.5 years.[60, 61]

There is still no effective treatment for HCV infection. The use of interferon alfa-2b is effective in controlling disease activity, but it is associated with a high relapse rate.[62] Interferon is also associated with a high incidence of rejection.[63]

Hepatitis B Virus

The rate of hepatitis B infection after transplantation has been decreasing, probably because of careful testing of blood products for hepatitis B. Although some transplant centers perform liver transplantation for end-stage liver disease secondary to hepatitis B, no center is performing transplants in patients with positive hepatitis B DNA because of a 100% recurrence rate in the new organ. Passive immunization with hepatitis B immune globulin in high doses is used to prevent recurrence of hepatitis in the transplanted liver. Transmission of the virus can also occur through the donor organ. A recent report[64] of transmission of hepatitis B through organs that were positive for antibody to the hepatitis B core antigen but IgM-negative is worrisome and suggests that some of these donors may be able to transmit the virus.

The original observation that both ganciclovir and foscarnet have some activity in the inhibition of hepatitis B virus unfortunately has not held up in clinical practice.[65, 66]

FUNGAL INFECTIONS

Liver transplant recipients have a higher incidence of fungal infection (up to 40%) than do other transplant recipients. These infections usually occur in patients who have surgical complications and/or a long ICU stay and who receive multiple courses of antibiotic therapy. Fungal infections are associated with a high mortality rate. The most frequent fungal infections after transplantation include candidiasis and aspergillosis. In our survey of invasive fungal infections in liver transplant recipients, we had an overall incidence of 16% (14 patients with candidiasis and 4 patients with aspergillosis).[67] In another series of 186 consecutive liver transplant procedures, the incidence of invasive fungal infections was very similar, 16.5%.[68] Risk factors found in this series to be associated with invasive fungal infection were the amount of fresh frozen plasma given and the development of acute renal failure requiring hemofiltration.[68]

Candida

The most common fungal infection after transplantation is candidiasis. *Candida* usually colonizes mucosa and may cause a superficial mucositis such as esophagitis or cystitis. *Candida* is a known colonizer of the bowel and, in liver transplant recipients, may cause abdominal infections, possibly related to spillage from the gut.[69] Between December 1985 and December 1992, candidemia developed in 1.4% of 2,621 liver transplant recipients, with an overall mortality of 81%. The risk factors that were identified for the development of candidemia in this population were exposure to multiple antibiotics and hyperglycemia necessitating insulin treatment.[70]

The drug of choice for the treatment of *Candida* infection remains amphotericin B, although its nephrotoxicity is a limiting factor. Fluconazole is a good alternative, but some strains of *Candida* are relatively resistant, such as *Candida krusei* and *Candida glabrata*.[71] Prophylaxis for *Candida* mucositis is usually given to transplant recipients for the first 3 to 4 months and consists of oral mycostatin suspension, 5 mL four times daily. Clotrimazole troches are a useful alternative.[72] Fluconazole prophylaxis has also been shown to reduce the incidence of superficial and invasive fungal infections after bone marrow transplantation,[73] but it interferes with the metabolism of cyclosporine and tacrolimus. Low-dose IV amphotericin B (0.1 mg/kg/day) prophylaxis has also been effective in the prevention of invasive fungal infections after bone marrow transplantation.[74] Early diagnosis of invasive candidiasis by monitoring serum metabolites of *Candida* such as D-arabinitol may be an important diagnostic tool in the future.[75]

Aspergillus

Aspergillus is the second most frequent fungal infection in transplant patients. The fungus is acquired by inhalation and may colonize the airways first and then cause invasive disease. Clusters of cases of invasive aspergillosis in transplant units have occurred in association with construction and maintenance work, which have led to dispersion of the conidia in the environment. The fungus is angioinvasive, tends to disseminate to the CNS, and can cause infarcts and cavitations in the lung. Risk factors in bone marrow transplantation are neutropenia and steroid use.[76] Solid organ transplant recipients are not usually neutropenic. Between 1981 and 1990, we had a 1.5% incidence of invasive aspergillosis in our liver transplant population, with a mortality rate close to 100%.[77]

The drug of choice for aspergillosis remains amphotericin B, which has to be administered at a relatively high dose (1.0 to 1.5 mg/kg/day), a dose associated with significant nephrotoxicity. The introduction of a liposomal formulation is promising because such preparations are less toxic to the kidney and may have similar efficacy.[78] Itraconazole, an oral triazole, is effective against *Aspergillus,* although its absorption via the nasogastric tube is marginal and an IV formulation is not available. In addition to medical treatment, surgery may also have a role in selected cases, e.g., resection of solitary lung nodules.[79] Early diagnosis is crucial in obtaining a favorable outcome because the disease carries a very high mortality when diagnosed late. Antigen detection of *Aspergillus* galactomannan by enzyme-linked immunosorbent assay and PCR may be useful in the future.[80]

Cryptococcus neoformans

Infection usually occurs months or years after transplantation. *Cryptococcus* is the most frequent cause of meningitis in transplant recipients. In a recent review of our own cases of cryptococcal meningitis, we identified ten patients after liver transplantation, for an incidence of 0.25%.[81] In this series, meningismus was present in only three patients, and the initial symptoms were more commonly headache, fever, and mental status changes.[81] Because the signs and symptoms may be subtle, a delay in diagnosis is not uncommon. Treatment is usually with a course of amphotericin B together with flucytosine, supplemented by oral fluconazole.

PROTOZOAL INFECTIONS

Pneumocystis carinii

With the introduction of routine TMP-SMX prophylaxis, the incidence of PCP has decreased dramatically in all centers. Before this prophylaxis, the reported incidence of PCP was around 10%. In 1981, PCP developed in 14 of 156 (8.9%) kidney recipients.[82] Since prophylaxis was instituted, PCP has occurred only in patients who do not receive prophylaxis.[82] In our program, single-strength oral TMP-SMX (80 mg trimethoprim plus 400 mg sulfamethoxazole) is administered daily for the first 6 to 12 months and then three times per week indefinitely. Other drugs used for prophylaxis include aerosolized pentamidine, 300 mg diluted in 6 mL of sterile water given monthly, and oral dapsone at a dose of 100 mg daily or three times per week.

Possible transmission of PCP from AIDS patients has recently been reported. In one such report, seven patients in a renal transplant unit contracted PCP in 1991; they were not receiving prophylaxis.[83]

Although not directly supported by the literature, it has been our impression that TMP-SMX prophylaxis not only prevents PCP but may also prevent *Legionella, Listeria, Nocardia,* and *Toxoplasma.*

Toxoplasma gondii

Although a febrile illness or lymphadenopathy usually develops in normal individuals after infection with *T. gondii,* visceral disease with pneumonitis, meningoencephalitis, or myocarditis may develop in immunocompromised hosts. The risk of the development of toxoplasmosis is relatively low after kidney or liver transplantation and may be related to the routine use of TMP-SMX prophylaxis. However, in heart transplant recipients, transmission of *Toxoplasma* is known to occur when an organ from a positive donor is transplanted into a seronegative recipient. In some centers, prophylaxis with oral pyrimethamine, 25 mg/day for 6 weeks, is used to prevent toxoplasmosis in high-risk heart transplant recipients. Otherwise, routine prophylaxis for *T. gondii* is not indicated. Finally, PCR might have a role in the early diagnosis of toxoplasmosis.[84]

PARASITES

Strongyloides stercoralis

Strongyloides stercoralis is a nematode that can infect patients with impaired T-lymphocyte function. In a review of the English literature in 1990, 33 kidney transplant patients had contracted this infestation after traveling or residing in endemic areas.[85] The nematode can be quiescent for years and then develop into an active infection after transplantation.[85] The two main manifestations are gastrointestinal, with abdominal pain, diarrhea, nausea, and vomiting, or pulmonary, with progressive lung infiltrates. Treatment is with thiabendazole. Unexplained eosinophilia and a history of travel or residence in an endemic area will help establish the diagnosis.[85]

Others

With the gradual increase in transplantation in developing countries, one would expect an increase in the occurrence of tropical diseases among transplant recipients.[86] Two examples have been reported recently: two patients from Taiwan contracted malaria after receiving a living unrelated kidney in India,[86] and a patient in Hong Kong contracted the liver fluke *Clonorchis sinensis* from a donor liver.[87] These two examples illustrate the importance of taking a good travel and residence history.

PATIENTS WITH CANCER OR NEUTROPENIA

RISK OF INFECTION

Patients with neutropenia have an increased risk of infection. The risk starts when the white blood cell count is below $1,000/mm^3$ neutrophils and increases when the count is lower than $500/mm^3$ neutrophils. The highest risk is with counts of less than $100/mm^3$ cells. There are different risk categories depending on the duration of neutropenia. In patients with solid tumors who are receiving chemotherapy, the neutropenia usually lasts only about 7 days and rarely longer than 14 days. Neutropenia lasting more than 14 days can develop in leukemia patients and bone marrow transplant patients. With long-lasting neutropenia, not only is the risk of bacterial sepsis higher, but also the risk of invasive fungal infection is increased. Most of the infections in neutropenic patients originate from the gastrointestinal tract and the skin. The risk is significantly higher with chemotherapeutic agents that cause mucositis of the gastrointestinal mucosa and with various catheters and invasive devices. Another source of infection is the environment. Plants and fresh fruits may be the source of gram-negative infection. In one series of *Xanthomonas maltophilia* infections, the source identified was two water faucets in an ICU.[88]

Bacterial

Most of the pathogenic bacteria in this population have traditionally been gram-negative rods (e.g., *Klebsiella, Escherichia coli,* and *Pseudomonas*). More recently, infections with gram-positive bacteria such as coagulase-negative *Staphylococcus* and α-hemolytic streptococci have become more frequent.[89] These infections may be caused by the increased use of central lines and other invasive instruments, mucositis secondary to chemotherapy, and the increased use of quinolones, which have mostly anti–gram-negative activity.[89]

An entity that may require surgery is typhlitis, which occurs in cases of severe neutropenia and is associated with a high mortality. Typhlitis is characterized by bacterial invasion, with mucosal and submucosal necrosis of the colon, particularly the cecum. Treatment is usually medical, but surgery may be indicated in cases of imminent perforation.[90, 91]

Fungal
The most common invasive fungal pathogens are *Candida* and *Aspergillus.* In general, the diagnosis is more difficult to make than with bacterial infection because it is more difficult to culture these organisms. Fungal infections are associated with a high mortality. In cases of invasive candidiasis, blood cultures are positive less than half the time. The outcome of invasive fungal infection depends on recovery of the neutrophil count, and treatment with antifungal agents in the absence of marrow recovery is doomed to failure. Although both *Candida* and *Aspergillus* may be colonizers or contaminants, in neutropenic hosts, a positive culture (one positive *Candida* blood culture or one positive *Aspergillus* culture from respiratory secretions) may be a manifestation of invasive disease and should be investigated and treated promptly.

The use of central vein and other intravascular catheters has been associated with a higher rate of gram-positive infections in recent years. Subcutaneous ports offer a viable alternative to right atrial catheters and are associated with a lower risk of infection.[92] They consist of a subcutaneously implanted reservoir attached to a central venous catheter.[92] Ports have no extracutaneous component and require no patient maintenance, as opposed to central lines, which required detailed care to prevent infection. These advantages may help explain the reduced infection rate.[92] In the case of catheter or reservoir infection, many authors believe that in most cases, treatment with antibiotics without removal of the catheter is possible. However, a tunnel infection or port pocket infection is an indication for device removal, as are septic emboli, refractory hypotension, and persistent culture positivity.[92] Some authors also believe that in cancer patients, fungemia is an indication for catheter removal.[93]

TREATMENT AND PREVENTION
Many centers have abandoned the practice of reverse isolation in neutropenic patients. Although it is true that the infection rate is

decreased by this practice, especially with prolonged neutropenia, patient survival does not differ significantly from that of nonisolated patients.[94] In addition, the overall improved management of infections has made reverse isolation less important.[94]

Infection in neutropenic patients can have catastrophic consequences if not diagnosed and treated promptly, and empirical treatment is crucial. Early regimens included a combination of aminoglycosides and a β-lactam.[89] This regimen was associated with renal, auditory, and vestibular toxicity. Other regimens that have been evaluated included two β-lactams, a single broad-spectrum third- or fourth-generation cephalosporin, a quinolone, or a carbapenem (e.g., imipenem).[89] A number of trials have shown that combination treatment is associated with outcomes similar to those with a single agent such as ceftazidime.[89] The use of a quinolone (e.g., ciprofloxacin or norfloxacin) as a single agent was associated with failure secondary to gram-positive organisms.[89, 95] At present, the consensus is that ceftazidime or imipenem as a single agent is as effective as a combination regimen for the initial treatment of febrile neutropenic patients,[89] although single-agent therapy may not be sufficient in patients with long-lasting neutropenia (>15 days).[96]

Various antibacterial and antifungal prophylactic agents are used in neutropenic patients. The use of TMP-SMX prophylaxis was not associated with a reduced incidence of bacterial infections in neutropenic cancer patients,[94] although it was useful in preventing PCP. Use of the triazoles for fungal prophylaxis (e.g., fluconazole) has been associated with the emergence of resistant organisms such as *C. krusei* and *C. glabrata*. Selective gut decontamination using the principle of "colonization resistance" was initially greeted with great enthusiasm. The idea is that by preserving the anaerobic flora with the use of nonabsorbable antibiotics, gram-negative pathogens would not colonize the gut. Unfortunately, the development of resistant organisms occurred. In one series, 37% of 35 episodes of *E. coli* bacteremia were resistant to quinolones (which had been used for prophylaxis).[97]

Finally, the use of cytokines to stimulate the marrow may have a role in the prevention and treatment of infectious complications in neutropenic hosts. In a randomized trial, autologous marrow transplantation patients given granulocyte-macrophage colony-stimulating factor (GM-CSF) had recovery of the neutrophil count to 500×10^6 per liter 7 days earlier than did patients who received placebo, had fewer infections, and required 3 fewer days of antibiotics, although the survival rate was not different.[98] The role of these agents as adjuvant treatment of invasive fungal infections is being evaluated. In a pilot study, four of eight patients given GM-CSF together with amphotericin B were cured[99]; however, capillary leak syndrome developed in 3 patients in association with an excessively high dose of GM-CSF.[99] The initial dose was 400 μg/m²/day given as a continuous infusion over a 24-hour period.[99]

SURGICAL PATIENTS WITH ACQUIRED IMMUNODEFICIENCY SYNDROME

COMMON INFECTIONS AND ADVANCES IN ANTIRETROVIRAL THERAPY

Because of the nature of their disease, patients with AIDS, in contrast to other immunocompromised patients, become more immunosuppressed with time. Transplant patients are more susceptible to infection relatively soon after transplantation, when the level of immunosuppression is high. Cancer patients tend to get infected in association with chemotherapy-induced neutropenia. In AIDS patients, the absolute CD4 lymphocyte count has been considered to be the best test to assess the likelihood of infection developing. Over time, the CD4 count falls and the risk of opportunistic infection increases. Table 2 shows regimens used for prophylaxis and CD4 counts in patients with AIDS. Different types of opportunistic infections are more common, depending on the CD4 count. *Candida* esophagitis and thrush are more common in patients with higher CD4 counts and occur relatively early, whereas CMV infection, toxoplasmosis, and *Mycobacterium avium-intracellulare* infection occur late in the course of the disease. Because the CD4 count progressively falls, patients who recover from an acute infectious complication will need lifelong maintenance therapy. When prophylaxis is prescribed for patients with AIDS, the CD4 count is an important value to take into consideration. The lower it is, the greater number of different opportunistic pathogens that need to be considered for prophylaxis.

Significant progress has been made in the quantitative diagnosis of HIV over the past few years. Concentrations of HIV-1 virus RNA have been quantified by different PCR techniques, and viral load has been correlated with various stages of disease activity.[100] Plasma viral load was found to be a good predictor of the progression of HIV infection to AIDS and death and was a better predictor than the CD4 cell count.[101] Along with the advances made in quantification of the virus, new antivirals in the form of nucleoside analogues and protease inhibitors have been released for clinical use.

TABLE 2.
Prophylactic Regimens and CD4 Counts in Patients with Acquired
Immunodeficiency Syndrome

CD4 Count (/μL)	Infection	Prophylaxis
200–500	Thrush, *Candida* esophagitis	Fluconazole, 50–100 mg/day po
200–500	Tuberculosis	If the patient is PPD+ or anergic with risk factors for TB: INH, 300 mg/day po/vitamin B_6, 50 mg/day po, for 1 yr. In cases of suspected INH resistance, use po rifampin, 600 mg/day, together with pyrazinamide, 20–30 mg/kg/day po
<200	*Pneumocystis carinii* pneumonia	TMP-SMX, 1 DS tablet daily, or Dapsone, 100 mg/day po, or Aerosolized pentamidine, 300 mg/mo
<200	*Cryptococcus* meningitis	Fluconazole, 200 mg/day po after the first episode of infection or possibly before infection occurs
<100	Toxoplasmosis	Seropositive patients: TMP-SMX, 1 DS tablet daily. Pyrimethamine together with dapsone may be effective
<100	MAI infection	Rifabutin, 300 mg/day po
<50	Cytomegalovirus	Ganciclovir, po?

Abbreviations: PPD, purified protein derivative; Tb, tuberculosis; INH, isoniazid; TMP-SMX, trimethoprim-sulfamethoxazole; DS, double strength; MAI, Mycobacterium avium-intracellulare complex.

The effect of various combinations of antivirals on viral load has been evaluated, and some of these antiviral drug combinations are very potent in inhibiting the virus. As a corollary, startling clinical improvements have been observed in many patients.[102] However, more follow-up will be required to assess the long-term efficacy of these new combinations.

INFECTIONS ASSOCIATED WITH EMERGENCY ABDOMINAL SURGERY

Surgeons are frequently called to assess AIDS patients with abdominal pain. Some of these patients require emergency laparotomy and are occasionally discovered to have a surgical complication of an infection and/or neoplasm. In about 50% of these patients, AIDS-related opportunistic infections had not been diagnosed before surgery. The following are most commonly associated with such events.

Cytomegalovirus

Cytomegalovirus may cause perforation of ulcers in the bowel.[103, 104] A review of 13 cases in the literature disclosed a 54% mortality within 1 month of surgery and an overall mortality of 87%.[103] The triad of pneumoperitoneum, AIDS, and a history of CMV infection may suggest this complication.[103] These patients frequently have only minimal abdominal tenderness, no fever, and a normal white blood cell count. The perforation usually occurs between the distalmost portion of the ileum and the splenic flexure.[103] Eight perforations occurred in the colon, six in the ileum, and one in the appendix.[103] Sigmoidoscopy may miss these findings because of the location of the lesions.[103]

Cryptosporidium

A protozoan parasite of the gastrointestinal tract, *Cryptosporidium* frequently causes debilitating diarrhea in AIDS patients.[105] It may cause cholecystitis or cholangitis in patients with AIDS. In 7 years, 13 patients with AIDS had cholangitis associated with *Cryptosporidium* in one institution.[105] All had right upper quadrant pain, fever, nausea, vomiting, and diarrhea.[105] *Cryptosporidium* was found in the intestine in all patients and in the biliary tract in 9 patients.[105] Papillitis may cause stenosis, which can lead to dilatation of the common bile duct and pancreatic duct.[105] Cytomegalovirus may produce a clinical and radiologic picture similar to that of *Cryptosporidium.*

Lymphoma/Sarcoma

Various non-Hodgkin's and Hodgkin's lymphomas may be associated with bowel perforation.[106] Kaposi's sarcoma may be a cause of bleeding from or obstruction and perforation of the small bowel, colon, and rectum.[106]

BURN PATIENTS

FACTORS CONTRIBUTING TO INFECTION

The most important causes of morbidity and mortality in burn patients are infections.[107] About 50% of the deaths in burn units are from infection.[108] Contributing factors include the elimination of skin as a barrier; the formation of exudate and eschar, which serve as a culture medium for bacteria; decreased complement and immunoglobulin levels; diminished cell-mediated immunity; and reduced neutrophil chemotaxis.[108] In severe burns, immunoglobulin levels reach their nadir on the second to third day.[109] Depletion of IgG, an important opsonizing antibody, correlates with septic complications.[110] In addition, patients with burns involving more than 20% of the total body surface area have depressed chemotaxis, which may also contribute to sepsis.[107]

WOUND INFECTION

Wound infection is obviously the most important infectious complication after burn injury. The predominant pathogens causing wound infections in burn patients are gram-negative bacteria.[108] The syndrome of burn wound sepsis occurs when bacteria invade the subcutaneous layer and disseminate to the general circulation.[111] The external appearance of the wound may be deceptive because local symptoms at the wound site may be minimal.[111] Fungi such as *Aspergillus, Candida, Mucor,* and *Geotrichum* may also colonize and invade the burn wound and may disseminate distantly.[111] Extensive excision and even amputation may be necessary.[111]

TREATMENT AND PREVENTION

Mortality has declined in burn centers from 24% in 1974 to 7% in 1979–1984.[112] Most authors believe that the improvement is related mainly to better care of these patients.[112] Aggressive and prompt excision of the burn eschar and immediate closure of the wound with grafts, together with better metabolic and nutritional support, have been important factors.[112] The use of routine systemic antibiotic prophylaxis is controversial because of the occurrence of resistance and fungal superinfection.[108] Organisms obtained through surveillance culture may not always be the real pathogen, but this may help in the selection of initial antibiotic coverage.[108] Topical agents reduce the rate of both colonization and invasive wound infection,[108, 112] but they do not reduce mortality in very large burns (70% of the body surface area).[111] Quantitative biopsy culture allows monitoring of bacterial colonization of the wound.[111] Invasion of bacteria usually occurs when the colony count reaches 10^5 organisms per gram of tissue.[111] Reverse isolation does not seem to prevent fatal burn wound sepsis.[111]

POSTSPLENECTOMY PATIENTS

Patients who undergo splenectomy are prone to infectious complications. These risks are not only for patients whose spleens have been surgically removed but also for people who have functional asplenia, such as patients with sickle cell anemia or chronic lymphocytic leukemia, bone marrow recipients with graft-vs.-host disease, and patients with chronic liver disease and portal hypertension.[113, 114]

The infections in these patients are with encapsulated organisms, mainly *Pneumococcus, Meningococcus,* and *Haemophilus influenzae.* Other entities also reported to cause infection in splenectomized patients include *Gonococcus, Pseudomonas,* babesiosis, and malaria. An unusual association has been described with DF-2 *(Capnocytophaga canimorsus)* in infections after dog bites.[114] Of all these organisms, *Pneumococcus* sepsis is associated with the highest mortality.[113]

Although most infections occur within 2 years of splenectomy, patients are still at risk up to 30 years later. Therefore, although children are at higher risk for infection after splenectomy, adults may die of fulminant sepsis many years after splenectomy.[114, 115] As an example, of 226 family members with hereditary spherocytosis, 4 died of infection.[115] The calculated risk of fatal infection in this group was 0.73 per 1,000 years.[115]

Sepsis after splenectomy occurs more commonly in patients with lymphoma or a hematologic abnormality than in patients who undergo splenectomy for trauma. The lower rate of infection in trauma patients may be related to immunologic reasons but could also be secondary to functioning accessory spleens found in some trauma patients.[114]

TREATMENT AND PREVENTION

Postsplenectomy infection may range from pneumonia to fulminant sepsis.[116] Fatal sepsis has been reported even 30 years after splenectomy.[116] In many cases, even the most aggressive therapeutic measures, including prompt institution of IV antibiotics and intensive care monitoring, fail to prevent mortality.[117] The overwhelming postsplenectomy syndrome is associated with massive bacterial invasion, and the patient goes into shock and dies within 24 to 72 hours. At times, no source of infection can be identified.[116] In a splenectomized patient, any fever or systemic symptoms are enough to warrant admission to the hospital for observation, cultures, and empirical antibiotics.[114]

Vaccination against encapsulated organisms, which include *Pneumococcus, H. influenzae,* and *Meningococcus,* is recommended in splenectomized patients.[113, 116] Although there are clear guidelines regarding pneumococcal vaccine in adults, the indications for the other two are not absolute. Because of the important role of the spleen in antibody response, pneumococcal vaccine is recommended at least 2 weeks before splenectomy.[113] Vaccination should be delayed for 6 months after immunosuppression, chemotherapy, and radiation treatment,[113] and revaccination should be given every 5 to 10 years.[113] The vaccine for *H. influenzae* type b is given to children.[113] Meningococcal vaccine is not recommended routinely but may be indicated in a patient who travels a great deal.[113] With regard to oral antibiotic prophylaxis, the data are derived from children with sickle cell anemia. Prophylaxis with oral penicillin has been effective.[113] Oral amoxicillin or erythromycin can also be used.[113] The indications for long-term oral antibiotics in adults are more controversial.

INFECTION CONTROL CONSIDERATIONS

Nosocomial infections have become a serious problem and have led to considerable morbidity, prolonged hospitalization, and increased mortality.[118] Infection control measures have thus assumed critical importance in the prevention of infections, particularly in immunocompromised patients. Outbreaks of multidrug-resistant TB have occurred in hospitals among HIV patients, sometimes because physicians have failed to recognize atypical manifestations and have not placed patients in respiratory isolation quickly enough. There has been an increase in resistant organisms causing infections in every hospital (more, perhaps, in teaching hospitals because of the patient population they tend to attract). In part, this increase is due to the indiscriminate use of antibiotics, which selects out resistant organisms. Outbreaks of multiple drug–resistant *Klebsiella* have been reported after the use of ceftazidime.[119] Critical care units have been colonized with very resistant gram-negative bacteria such as *X. maltophilia* and *Pseudomonas cepacia*, which can cause nosocomial infections.[120] *Candida* colonization has been found to be a predictor of *Candida* infection in critically ill surgical patients.[121] The increased use of fluconazole prophylaxis after bone marrow transplantation has been associated with an increased rate of infection with *C. krusei* and *C. glabrata*.[122, 123] There is no better example of nosocomial spread of resistant organisms than that of vancomycin-resistant *Enterococcus faecium* (VREF), in this case an organism with no effective antibiotic treatment. Many outbreaks of VREF have occurred recently, mostly in immunocompromised individuals.[124, 125] Risk factors for the development of VREF bacteremia include the severity of illness, underlying disease, and the administration of vancomycin.[126]

Relatively simple infection control guidelines, such as routine hand washing,[127] institution of prompt respiratory isolation,[128] and the conscientious use of anti-infectious agents, will have an important impact on reducing nosocomial infections.

SUMMARY

The care of immunocompromised patients is a challenge to all physicians. The variety of opportunistic infections that can develop in these patients underscores the importance of the immune response. The key to success in the prevention and management of infections in these patients lies in knowing what kind of infections to expect and instituting empirical treatment even before a specific diagnosis is made. With the advent of better preventive strategies, the use of prophylactic and preemptive therapies, and the introduction of new immunomodulators, successful outcomes in these interesting and challenging patients may be more easy to achieve in the future.

REFERENCES

1. Kusne S, Dummer JS, Singh N, et al: Infections after liver transplantation. *Medicine (Baltimore)* 67:132–143, 1988.
2. Gottesdiener KM: Transplanted infections: Donor-to-host transmission with the allograft. *Ann Intern Med* 110:1001– 1016, 1989.
3. Rubin RH: Infectious disease complications of renal transplantation. *Kidney Int* 44:221–236, 1993.
4. Wagener MM, Yu VL: Bacteremia in transplant recipients: A prospective study of demographics, etiologic agents, risk factors, and outcomes. *Am J Infect Control* 20:239–247, 1992.
5. Mastrosimone S, Pignata G, Maresca MC, et al: Clinical significance of vesicoureteral reflux after kidney transplantation. *Clin Nephrol* 40:38–45, 1993.
6. Everett JE, Wahoff DC, Statz C, et al: Characterization and impact of wound infection after pancreas transplantation. *Arch Surg* 129:1310–1317, 1994.
7. Corry RJ, Egidi MF, Shapiro R, et al: Pancreas transplantation with enteric drainage under tacrolimus induction therapy. *Transplant Proc* 29(1–2):642, 1997.
8. MacGowan AP, Marshall RJ, MacKay IM, et al: *Listeria* faecal carriage by renal transplant recipients, haemodialysis patients and patients in general practice: Its relation to season, drug therapy, foreign travel, animal exposure and diet. *Epidemiol Infect* 106:157–166, 1991.
9. Stamm AM, Dismukes WE, Simmons BP, et al: Listeriosis in renal transplant recipients: Report of an outbreak and review of 102 cases. *Rev Infect Dis* 4:665–682, 1982.

10. Chang J, Powles R, Mehta J, et al: Listeriosis in bone marrow transplant recipients: Incidence, clinical features, and treatment. *Clin Infect Dis* 21:1289–1290, 1995.

11. Jereb JA, Burwen DR, Dooley SW, et al: Nosocomial outbreak of tuberculosis in a renal transplant unit: Application of a new technique for restrictions fragment length polymorphism analysis of *Mycobacterium tuberculosis* isolates. *J Infect Dis* 168:1219–1924, 1993.

12. Miller RA, Lanza LA, Kline JN, et al: *Mycobacterium tuberculosis* in lung transplant recipients. *Am J Respir Crit Care Med* 152:374–376, 1995.

13. Management of persons exposed to multidrug-resistant tuberculosis. *MMWR* 41:(RR-11):61–69, 1992.

14. Singh N, Gayowski T, Wagener M, et al: Pulmonary infections in liver transplant recipients receiving tacrolimus. *Transplantation* 61:396–401, 1996.

15. Bangsborg JM, Uldum S, Jensen JS, et al: Nosocomial legionellosis in three heart-lung transplant patients: Case reports and environmental observations. *Eur J Clin Microbiol Infect Dis* 14:99–104, 1995.

16. Levin ASS, Gobara S, Scarpitta CM, et al: Electric showers as a control measure for *Legionella* spp. in a renal transplant unit in Sao Paulo, Brazil. *J Hosp Infect* 30:133–137, 1995.

17. Stevens DA, Peir AC, Beaman BL, et al: Laboratory evaluation of an outbreak of nocardiosis in immunocompromised hosts. *Am J Med* 71:928–934, 1981.

18. Bauwens M, Hauet T, Crevel J, et al: Nocardiosis in recipients of renal transplants: Two case reports. *Transplant Proc* 27:2430, 1995.

19. Weigelt JA, Dryer D, Haley RW: The necessity and efficiency of wound surveillance after discharge. *Arch Surg* 127:77–82, 1992.

20. Forse RA, Karam B, MacLean LD, et al: Antibiotic prophylaxis for surgery in morbidly obese patients. *Surgery* 106:750–757, 1989.

21. Wiesner RH, Hermans PE, Rakela J, et al: Selective bowel decontamination to decrease gram-negative aerobic bacterial and *Candida* colonization and prevent infection after orthotopic liver transplantation. *Transplantation* 45:570–574, 1988.

22. Ledingham IM, Alcock SR, Eastaway FT, et al: Triple regimen of selective decontamination of the digestive tract, systemic cefotaxime, and microbiological surveillance for prevention of acquired infection in intensive care. *Lancet* 1:787–790, 1988.

23. Snydman DR: Cytomegalovirus prophylaxis strategies in high-risk transplantation. *Transplant Proc* 26:20S–22S, 1994.

24. Balfour HH Jr, Chace BA, Stapleton JT, et al: A randomized, placebo-controlled trial of oral acyclovir for the prevention of cytomegalovirus disease in recipients of renal allografts. *N Engl J Med* 320:1381–1387, 1989.

25. Snydman DR, Werner BG, Heinze-Lacey B, et al: Use of cytomegalovirus immune globulin to prevent cytomegalovirus disease in renal transplant recipients. *N Engl J Med* 317:1049–1054, 1987.

26. Martin M, Manez R, Linden P, et al: A prospective randomized trial comparing sequential ganciclovir–high dose acyclovir to high dose acyclovir for prevention of cytomegalovirus disease in adult liver transplant recipients. *Transplantation* 58:779–785, 1994.

27. Snydman DR, Werner BG, Dougherty NN, et al: Cytomegalovirus immune globulin prophylaxis in liver transplantation. *Ann Intern Med* 119:984–991, 1993.

28. Pescovitz M, Gane E, Saliba F, et al: Efficacy and safety of oral ganciclovir in the prevention of cytomegalovirus (CMV) disease in liver transplant recipients (abstract). Presented at the 36th Meeting of the Interscience Conference on Antimicrobial Agents and Chemotherapy, New Orleans, 1996.

29. Rubin RH: Preemptive therapy in immunocompromised hosts. *N Engl J Med* 324:1057–1059, 1991.

30. The TH, Van Der Ploeg M, Van Den Berg AP, et al: Direct detection of cytomegalovirus in peripheral blood leukocytes—a review of the antigenemia assay and polymerase chain reaction. *Transplantation* 54:193–198, 1992.

31. Gerna G, Zipeto D, Percivalle E, et al: Human cytomegalovirus infection of the major leukocyte subpopulations and evidence for initial viral replication in polymorphonuclear leukocytes from viremic patients. *J Infect Dis* 166:1236–1244, 1992.

32. Grossi P, Minoli L, Percivalle E, et al: Clinical and virological monitoring of human cytomegalovirus infection in 294 heart transplant recipients. *Transplantation* 59:847–851, 1995.

33. Lautenschlager I, Hockerstedt K, Salmela K: Quantitative CMV-antigenemia test in the diagnosis of CMV infection and in the monitoring of response to antiviral treatment in liver transplant recipients. *Transplant Proc* 26:1719–1720, 1994.

34. Kusne S, Grossi P, Irish W, et al: Incidence of cytomegalovirus (CMV) disease after introduction of routine use of PP65-antigenemia (Ant) for preemptive therapy in adult liver transplant recipients (abstract). Presented at the 36th Meeting of the Interscience Conference on Antimicrobial Agents and Chemotherapy, New Orleans, 1996.

35. Grossi P, Kusne S, Rinaldo C, et al: Guidance of ganciclovir therapy with pp65 antigenemia in cytomegalovirus-free recipients of livers from seropositive donors. *Transplantation* 61:1659–1660, 1996.

36. Fox JC, Kidd IM, Griffiths PD, et al: Longitudinal analysis of cytomegalovirus load in renal transplant recipients using a quantitative polymerase chain reaction: Correlation with disease. *J Gen Virol* 76:309–319, 1995.

37. Drouet E, Colimon R, Michelson S, et al: Monitoring levels of human cytomegalovirus DNA in blood after liver transplantation. *J Clin Microbiol* 33:389–394, 1995.

38. Manez R, Kusne S, Rinaldo C, et al: Time to detection of cytomegalovirus (CMV) DNA in blood leukocytes is a predictor for the develop-

ment of CMV disease in CMV-seronegative recipients of allografts from CMV-seropositive donors following liver transplantation. *J Infect Dis* 173:1072–1076, 1996.

39. Cunningham R, Harris A, Frankton A, et al: Detection of cytomegalovirus using PCR in serum from renal transplant recipients. *J Clin Pathol* 48:575–577, 1995.

40. Walker RC, Marshall WF, Strickler JG, et al: Pretransplantation assessment of the risk of lymphoproliferative disorder. *Clin Infect Dis* 20:1346–1353, 1995.

41. Riddler SA, Breinig MC, McKnight JLC: Increased levels of circulating Epstein-Barr virus (EBV)-infected lymphocytes and decreased EBV nuclear antigen antibody responses are associated with the development of posttransplant lymphoproliferative disease in solid-organ transplant recipients. *Blood* 84:972–984, 1994.

42. Rooney CM, Loftin SK, Holladay MS, et al: Early identification of Epstein-Barr virus–associated post-transplantation lymphoproliferative disease. *Br J Haematol* 89:98–103, 1995.

43. Hornef MW, Wagner HJ, Fricke L, et al: Immunocytochemical detection of Epstein-Barr virus antigens in peripheral B lymphocytes after renal transplantation. *Transplantation* 59:138–140, 1995.

44. Rooney CM, Smith CA, Ng CYC, et al: Use of gene-modified virus-specific T lymphocytes to control Epstein-Barr-virus– related lymphoproliferation. *Lancet* 345:9–13, 1995.

45. Nalesnik M, Rao A, Furukawa H, et al: Autologous lymphokine-activated killer cell therapy of Epstein-Barr virus-positive and -negative lymphoproliferative disorders arising in organ transplant recipients. *Transplantation* 63:1200–1205, 1997.

46. Fischer A, Blanche S, Le Bidois J, et al: Anti–B cell monoclonal antibodies in the treatment of severe B-cell lymphoproliferative syndrome following bone marrow and organ transplantation. *N Engl J Med* 324:1451–1456, 1991.

47. Kusne S, Schwartz M, Breinig MK, et al: Herpes simplex virus hepatitis after solid organ transplantation in adults. *J Infect Dis* 163:1001–1007, 1991.

48. Kusne S, Pappo O, Manez R, et al: Varicella-zoster virus hepatitis and a suggested management plan for prevention of VZV infection in adult liver transplant recipients. *Transplantation* 60:619–621, 1995.

49. Esterbrook P, Wood MJ: Successors to acyclovir. *J Antimicrob Chemother* 34:307–311, 1994.

50. Cames B, Rahier J, Burtomboy G, et al: Acute adenovirus hepatitis in liver transplant recipients. *J Pediatr* 120:33–37, 1992.

51. Koneru B, Jaffe R, Esquivel CO, et al: Adenoviral infections in pediatric liver transplant recipients. *JAMA* 258:489–492, 1987.

52. Michaels MG, Green M, Wald ER, et al: Adenovirus infection in pediatric liver transplant recipients. *J Infect Dis* 165:170–174, 1992.

53. Krilov LR, Rubin LG, Frogel M, et al: Disseminated adenovirus infec-

tion with hepatic necrosis in patients with human immunodeficiency virus infection and other immunodeficiency states. *Rev Infect Dis* 12:303–307, 1990.

54. Torok TJ: Parvovirus B19 and human disease. *Adv Intern Med* 37:431–455, 1992.

55. Yoshikawa T, Suga S, Asano Y, et al: A prospective study of human herpesvirus-6 infection in renal transplantation. *Transplantation* 54:879–883, 1992.

56. Singh N, Carrigan DR, Gayowski T, et al: Variant B human herpesvirus-6 associated febrile dermatosis with thrombocytopenia and encephalopathy in a liver transplant recipient. *Transplantation* 60:1355–1357, 1995.

57. Sanchez-Tapias JM, Rodes J: Dilemmas of organ transplantation from anti-HCV–positive donors. *Lancet* 345:469–470, 1995.

58. Milfred SK, Lake KD, Anderson DJ, et al: Practices of cardiothoracic transplant centers regarding hepatitis C–seropositive candidates and donors. *Transplantation* 57:568–572, 1994.

59. Pereira BJG, Wright TL, Schmid CH, et al: The impact of pretransplantation hepatitis C infection on the outcome of renal transplantation. *Transplantation* 60:799–805, 1995.

60. Pereira BJG, Wright TL, Schmid CH, et al: A controlled study of hepatitis C transmission by organ transplantation. *Lancet* 345:484–487, 1995.

61. Morales JM, Campistol JM, Castellano G, et al: Transplantation of kidneys from donors with hepatitis C antibody into recipients with pretransplantation anti-HCV. *Kidney Int* 47:236–240, 1995.

62. Rostaing L, Izopet J, Baron E, et al: Treatment of chronic hepatitis C with recombinant interferon alpha in kidney transplant recipients. *Transplantation* 59:1426–1431, 1995.

63. Kramer P, Ten Kate FWJ, Bijnen AB, et al: Recombinant leucocyte interferon A induces steroid-resistant acute vascular rejection episodes in renal transplant recipients. *Lancet* 1:989–990, 1984.

64. Wachs ME, Amend WJ, Ascher NL, et al: The risk of transmission of hepatitis B from HBsAg(-), HBcAb(+), HBIgM(-) organ donors. *Transplantation* 59:230–234, 1995.

65. Singh N, Gayowski T: Lack of sustained efficacy of combination ganciclovir and foscarnet for hepatitis B virus recurrence after liver transplantation. *Transplantation* 59:1629–1630, 1995.

66. Yoshida EM, Wolber RA, Mahmood WA, et al: Attempted resolution of acute recurrent hepatitis B in a transplanted liver allograft by the administration of ganciclovir. *Transplantation* 58:956–958, 1994.

67. Kusne S, Dummer JS, Singh N, et al: Fungal infections after liver transplantation. *Transplant Proc* 20:650S–651S, 1988.

68. Briegel J, Forst H, Spill B, et al: Risk factors for systemic fungal infections in liver transplant recipients. *Eur J Clin Microbiol Infect Dis* 14:375–382, 1995.

69. Kusne S, Tobin D, Pasculle AW, et al: *Candida* carriage in the alimentary tract of liver transplant candidates. *Transplantation* 57:398–402, 1994.
70. Nieto-Rodriguez JA, Kusne S, Manez R, et al: Factors associated with the development of candidemia and candidemia-related death among liver transplant recipients. *Ann Surg* 223:70–76, 1996.
71. Wingard JR: Importance of *Candida* species other than *C. albicans* as pathogens in oncology patients. *Clin Infect Dis* 20:115–125, 1995.
72. Gombert ME, duBouchet L, Aulicino TM, et al: A comparative trial of clotrimazole troches and oral nystatin suspension in recipients of renal transplants: Use in prophylaxis of oropharyngeal candidiasis. *JAMA* 258:2553–2555, 1987.
73. Goodman JL, Winston DJ, Greenfield RA, et al: A controlled trial of fluconazole to prevent fungal infections in patients undergoing bone marrow transplantation. *N Engl J Med* 326:845–851, 1992.
74. Riley DK, Pavia AT, Beatty PG, et al: The prophylactic use of low-dose amphotericin B in bone marrow transplant patients. *Am J Med* 97:509–514, 1994.
75. Walsh TJ, Merz WG, Lee JW, et al: Diagnosis and therapeutic monitoring of invasive candidiasis by rapid enzymatic detection of serum D-arabinitol. *Am J Med* 99:164–172, 1995.
76. DeBock R: Epidemiology of invasive fungal infections in bone marrow transplantation. *Bone Marrow Transplant* 14:1S–2S, 1994.
77. Kusne S, Torre-Cisneros J, Manez R, et al: Factors associated with invasive lung aspergillosis and the significance of positive *Aspergillus* culture after liver transplantation. *J Infect Dis* 166:1379–1383, 1992.
78. Oppenheim BA, Herbrecht R, Kusne S: The safety and efficacy of amphotericin B colloidal dispersion in the treatment of invasive mycoses. *Clin Infect Dis* 21:1145–1153, 1995.
79. Wang SS, Chu SH, Lee YC, et al: Successful treatment of invasive pulmonary aspergillosis in heart transplantation. *Transplant Proc* 26:2329–2332, 1994.
80. Verweij PE, Stynen D, Rijs AJMM, et al: Sandwich enzyme-linked immunosorbent assay compared with Pastorex latex agglutination test for diagnosing invasive aspergillosis in immunocompromised patients. *J Clin Microbiol* 33:1912– 1914, 1995.
81. Jabbour N, Reyes J, Kusne S, et al: Cryptococcal meningitis after liver transplantation. *Transplantation* 61:146–167, 1996.
82. Hardy AM, Wajszczuk CP, Hakala TR, et al: Infection in renal transplant recipients on cyclosporine: *Pneumocystis* pneumonia. *Transplant Proc* 25:2773S–2774S, 1983.
83. Hennequin C, Page B, Roux P, et al: Outbreak of *Pneumocystis carinii* pneumonia in a renal transplant unit. *Eur J Clin Microbiol Infect Dis* 14:122–126, 1995.
84. Bretagne S, Costa JM, Kuentz M, et al: Case report: Late toxoplasmosis evidenced by PCR in a marrow transplant recipient. *Bone Marrow Transplant* 15:809–811, 1995.

85. DeVault GA Jr, King JW, Rohr MS, et al: Opportunistic infections with *Strongyloides stercoralis* in renal transplantation. *Rev Infect Dis* 12:653–671, 1990.

86. Lee PC, Lee PY, Lei HY, et al: Malaria infection in kidney transplant recipients. *Transplant Proc* 26:2099–2100, 1994.

87. Ho JK, Lau WY, Leung N, et al: Liver infested with *Clonorchis sinensis* in orthotopic liver transplantation: A case report. *Transplant Proc* 26:2269–2271, 1994.

88. Khardori N, Elting L, Wong E, et al: Nosocomial infections due to *Xanthomonas maltophilia* in patients with cancer. *Rev Infect Dis* 12:997–1003, 1990.

89. Kibbler CC: Neutropenic infections: Strategies for empirical therapy. *J Antimicrob Chemother* 36107S–117S, 1995.

90. Varki AP, Armitage JO, Feagler JR: Typhlitis in acute leukemia: Successful treatment by early surgical intervention. *Cancer* 43:695–697, 1979.

91. Mulholland MW, Delaney JP: Neutropenic colitis and aplastic anemia. *Ann Surg* 197:84–90, 1983.

92. Groeger JS, Lucas AB, Thaler HT, et al: Infectious morbidity associated with long-term use of venous access devices in patients with cancer. *Ann Intern Med* 119:1168–1174, 1993.

93. Lecciones JA, Lee JW, Navarro EE, et al: Vascular catheter-n-associated fungemia in patients with cancer: Analysis of 155 episodes. *Clin Infect Dis* 14:875–883, 1992.

94. Pizzo PA: Considerations for the prevention of infectious complications in patients with cancer. *Rev Infect Dis* 11:1551S–1562S, 1989.

95. Kotilainen P, Nikoskelainen J, Huovinen P: Emergence of ciprofloxacin-resistant coagulase-negative staphylococcal skin flora in immunocompromised patients receiving ciprofloxacin. *J Infect Dis* 161:41–44, 1990.

96. Boogaerts MA: Anti-infective strategies in neutropenia. *J Antimicrob Chemother* 36:167S–178S, 1995.

97. Carratala J, Fernanzez-Sevilla A, Tubau F, et al: Emergence of quinolone-resistant *Escherichia coli* bacteremia in neutropenic patients with cancer who have received prophylactic norfloxacin. *Clin Infect Dis* 20:557–560, 1995.

98. Nemunaitis J, Rabinowe SN, Singer JW, et al: Recombinant granulocyte-macrophage colony-stimulating factor after autologous bone marrow transplantation for lymphoid cancer. *N Engl J Med* 324:1773–1778, 1991.

99. Bodey GP, Anaissie E, Gutterman J, et al: Role of granulocyte-macrophage colony-stimulating factor as adjuvant therapy for fungal infection in patients with cancer. *Clin Infect Dis* 17:705–707, 1993.

100. Feinberg MB: Changing the natural history of HIV disease. *Lancet* 348:239–246, 1996.

101. Mellors JW, Rinaldo CR Jr, Gupta P, et al: Prognosis in HIV-1 infection

predicted by the quantity of virus in plasma. *Science* 272:1167–1170, 1996.

102. Carpenter CCJ, Fischl MA, Hammer SM, et al: Antiretroviral therapy for HIV infection in 1996. *JAMA* 276:146–154, 1996.
103. Kram HB, Shoemaker WC: Intestinal perforation due to cytomegalovirus infection in patients with AIDS. *Dis Colon Rectum* 33:1037–1040, 1990.
104. Dieterich DT, Kim MH, McMeeding A, et al: Cytomegalovirus appendicitis in a patient with acquired immunodeficiency syndrome. *Am J Gastroenterol* 86:904–906, 1991.
105. Texidor HS, Godwin TA, Ramirez EA: Cryptosporidiosis of the biliary tract in AIDS. *Radiology* 180:51–56, 1991.
106. Ferguson CM: Surgical complications of human immunodeficiency virus infection. *Am Surg* 54:4–9, 1988.
107. Altman LC, Furukawa CT, Klebanoff SJ: Depressed mononuclear chemotaxis in thermally injured patients. *J Immunol* 119:199–203, 1977.
108. Warren S, Burke JF: Infection of burn wounds: Evaluation and management, in Remington JS, Swartz MN (eds): *Current Clinical Topics in Infectious Diseases,* vol 11, Cambridge, Mass, Blackwell Scientific, 1991, pp 206–217.
109. Arturson G, Johansson SGO, Hogman CF, et al: Changes in immunoglobulin levels in severely burned patients. *Lancet* 1:546–548, 1969.
110. Moran K, Munster AM: Alterations of the host defense mechanism in burned patients. *Surg Clin North Am* 67:47–56, 1987.
111. Luterman A, Dacso CC, Curreri PW: Infections in burn patients. *Am J Med* 81:45S–52S, 1986.
112. Tompkins RG, Burke JF, Schoenfeld DA, et al: Prompt eschar excision: A treatment system contributing to reduced burn mortality. *Ann Surg* 204:272–281, 1986.
113. Working Party of the British Committee for Standards in Haematology Clinical Haematology Task Force: Guidelines for the prevention and treatment of infection in patients with an absent or dysfunctional spleen. *BMJ* 312:430–434, 1996.
114. Brigden ML: Overwhelming postsplenectomy infection still a problem. *West J Med* 157:440–443, 1992.
115. Schilling RF: Estimating the risk for sepsis after splenectomy in hereditary spherocytosis. *Ann Intern Med* 122:187–188, 1995.
116. Shaw JHF, Print CG: Postsplenectomy sepsis. *Br J Surg* 76:1074–1081, 1989.
117. Cole JT, Flaum MA: Postsplenectomy infections. *South Med J* 85:1220–1224, 1992.
118. Dinkel RH, Lebok U: A survey of nosocomial infections and their influence on hospital mortality rates. *J Hosp Infect* 28:297–304, 1994.
119. Meyer KS, Urban C, Eagan JA, et al: Nosocomial outbreak of *Klebsiella* infection resistant to late-generation cephalosporins. *Ann Intern Med* 119:353–358, 1993.

120. Maningo E, Watanakunakorn C: *Xanthomonas maltophilia* and *Pseudomonas cepacia* in lower respiratory tracts of patients in critical care units. *J Infect* 31:89–92, 1995.

121. Pittet D, Monod M, Suter PM, et al: *Candida* colonization and subsequent infections in critically ill surgical patients. *Ann Surg* 220:751–758, 1994.

122. Wingard JR, Merz WG, Rinaldi MG, et al: Increase in *Candida krusei* infection among patients with bone marrow transplantation and neutropenia treated prophylactically with fluconazole. *N Engl J Med* 325:1274–1277, 1991.

123. Wingard JR, Merz WG, Rinaldi MG, et al: Association of *Torulopsis glabrata* infections with fluconazole prophylaxis in neutropenic bone marrow transplant patients. *Antimicrob Agents Chemother* 37:1847–1849.

124. Edmond MB, Ober JF, Weinbaum DL, et al: Vancomycin-resistant *Enterococcus faecium* bacteremia: Risk factors for infection. *Clin Infect Dis* 20:1126–1133, 1995.

125. Linden PK, Pasculle AW, Manez R, et al: Differences in outcomes for patients with bacteremia due to vancomycin-resistant *Enterococcus faecium* or vancomycin-susceptible *E. faecium*. *Clin Infect Dis* 22:663–670, 1996.

126. Shay DK, Maloney SA, Montecalvo M, et al: Epidemiology and mortality risk of vancomycin-resistant enterococcal bloodstream infections. *J Infect Dis* 172:993–1000, 1995.

127. Larson EL: APIC guidelines for handwashing and hand antisepsis in health care settings. *Am J Infect Control* 23:251–269, 1995.

128. McGowan JE Jr: Nosocomial tuberculosis: New progress in control and prevention. *Clin Infect Dis* 21:489–505, 1995.

CHAPTER 15

Laparoscopic Adrenalectomy

Scott R. Schell, M.D., Ph.D.
Chief Resident, Department of Surgery, School of Medicine, Johns Hopkins University, Baltimore, Maryland

Mark A. Talamini, M.D.
Associate Professor and Director of Minimally Invasive Surgery, Department of Surgery, School of Medicine, Johns Hopkins University, Baltimore, Maryland

Robert Udelsman, M.D.
Associate Professor and Director of Endocrine and Oncologic Surgery, Department of Surgery, School of Medicine, Johns Hopkins University, Baltimore, Maryland

M inimally invasive techniques have revolutionized the field of surgery. Successful application of laparoendoscopic techniques to cholecystectomy, Nissen fundoplication, and nephrectomy have demonstrable advantages over open techniques. Laparoscopic adrenalectomy is a new example of the successful application of minimally invasive techniques to an organ that is relatively inaccessible because of its location in the retroperitoneum.

The first laparoscopic adrenalectomy was performed by Gagner et al. in 1992.[1] They used an anterior transabdominal approach in patients with Cushing's syndrome and pheochromocytoma. Since then, this procedure has been performed with increasing frequency, and the world literature has grown to over 50 reports of the application and modification of this procedure to include nearly 500 patients. Subsequent reports have described expanded indications, alternative approaches to the adrenal gland, and refinements in laparoendoscopic technique.

Laparoscopic adrenalectomy has been used for virtually all nonmalignant neoplasms of the adrenal gland. In skilled hands, transfusion requirements and postoperative recovery times are significantly reduced. Furthermore, with decreases in patient length of stay and shorter time requirements for return to regular activity, laparoscopic adrenalectomy appears to have economic advantages over open adrenalectomy and will thus almost certainly become the preferred adrenalectomy technique.

This report reviews the reported series of laparoscopic adrenalectomy. In addition, the indications, perioperative evaluation, operative technique, and postoperative results are described.

INDICATIONS

The indications for laparoscopic adrenalectomy have expanded. Recent reviews suggest that the majority of adrenal masses are amenable to laparoscopic resection, with tumor size representing the single most significant limiting factor.[2–5] It has recently been estimated that at least 60% of surgically treatable adrenal lesions could be extirpated laparoscopically.[6]

Adrenal masses are either hormonally active or inactive. Virtually all hormonally active primary adrenal tumors should be resected, as listed in Table 1. Hormonally active adrenal tumors suitable for laparoscopic resection include aldosterone-producing adenomas (APAs), glucocorticoid-producing adenomas, androgen-producing adenomas, pheochromocytomas, highly selected cases of bilateral adrenal hyperplasia secondary to either Cushing's disease or the ectopic adrenocorticotropic (ACTH) syndrome, and bilateral macronodular adrenal hyperplasia.

TABLE 1.

Indications for Laparoscopic Adrenalectomy

Hormonally active
   Aldosterone-producing adenoma
   Glucocorticoid-producing adenoma
   Androgen-producing adenoma
   Pheochromocytoma
   Selected cases of bilateral adrenal hyperplasia caused by Cushing's
     disease or the ectopic ACTH syndrome
   Bilateral macronodular adrenal hyperplasia
Hormonally inactive
   Tumors larger than 4.5 cm
   Tumors larger than 3.0 cm that demonstrate growth on serial imaging
     studies

Abbreviation: ACTH, adrenocorticotropic hormone.

ALDOSTERONE-PRODUCING ADRENAL ADENOMA

Primary aldosteronism (Conn's syndrome) results from the over-production of aldosterone by an adenoma of the adrenal cortex (APA). Although the majority of these adenomas are small, endocrine evaluation and imaging techniques can usually localize these tumors, and their small size lends them ideally to laparoscopic resection. Several series have reported the use of laparoscopic adrenalectomy for removal of APAs with excellent results and few complications.[7–9] Approximately 30% of the Hopkins' series is composed of APAs, and our results compare favorably with these previous reports.

CUSHING'S SYNDROME

Patients with glucocorticoid-producing adenomas represent particular challenges for surgical resection. Cushingoid patients present greater technical difficulties because of their large deposition of retroperitoneal fat and poor tissue quality. These patients are also at increased risk for significant metabolic abnormalities and infection and display marked impairments in wound healing. Laparoscopic techniques in these patients, although challenging, have been successful in several series.[10–13] Avoidance of a large incision in laparoscopic adrenalectomy is a major advance in the management of cushingoid patients.[14] Ultrasound visualization and use of an argon-beam coagulator have also been helpful adjuncts in these patients.[10, 13] Thirty-five percent of our patients underwent successful laparoscopic adrenalectomy in the setting of advanced Cushing's syndrome.[14] None of our patients required blood transfusions or experienced problems with wound healing. A typical left-sided glucocorticoid-producing adrenal adenoma is demonstrated in Figure 1. This is an ideal indication for laparoscopic adrenalectomy.

Bilateral laparoscopic adrenalectomy has also been used in highly selected patients with Cushing's disease, which is caused by an ACTH-secreting pituitary adenoma. Although the preferred treatment of Cushing's disease is resection of the pituitary adenoma, a subset of patients fail neurosurgical intervention. Occasionally, adrenalectomy is required for these patients because of life-threatening complications of Cushing's syndrome. Bilateral adrenal hyperplasia results from Cushing's disease or the ectopic ACTH syndrome. Because these diseases requires removal of both adrenal glands, previous reports have recommended the posterior or retroperitoneal approach for laparoscopic resection.[4, 5, 11, 15, 16] The posterior approach requires the use of a dissecting balloon and

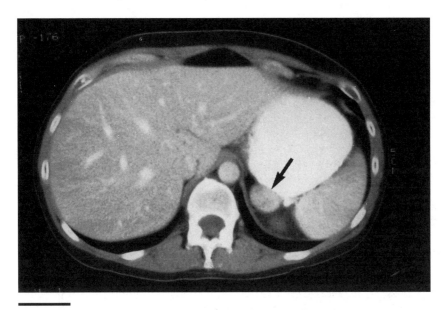

FIGURE 1.
Computed tomographic scan demonstrating a glucocorticoid-producing left-sided adrenal adenoma *(arrow).*

is technically more challenging because of limited visualization. We have successfully performed bilateral adrenalectomy with a transperitoneal flank approach in two patients with refractory Cushing's disease.

VIRILIZING ADRENAL ADENOMAS
Androgen-producing, or virilizing, adrenal adenomas occur rarely and are also amenable to laparoscopic resection.[15, 16]

PHEOCHROMOCYTOMAS
Laparoscopic adrenalectomy has been used to resect pheochromo-cytomas.[1, 4, 11, 15–25] Before endosurgical approaches to adrenal surgery, most authors expressed their preference for the open anterior abdominal technique, which allows careful exploration of both adrenals, as well as exploration for potential extra-adrenal pheo-chromocytomas. However, with improvements in CT and MRI imaging, as well as meta-iodobenzylguanidine localization scans, application of endosurgical techniques has expanded with excellent results.

BILATERAL MACRONODULAR ADRENAL HYPERPLASIA
Laparoscopic adrenalectomy also appears applicable for the treatment of bilateral macronodular adrenal hyperplasia. To date, there

have been no reports of laparoscopic resections for this condition; however, because both glands are involved, bilateral resection would be indicated.

INCIDENTALOMAS

Hormonally inactive, or nonfunctioning, adenomas of the adrenals discovered on abdominal imaging studies ("incidentalomas") represent ideal candidates for laparoscopic resection. However, we do not advocate resection of small, nonfunctional adrenal masses unless they are either larger than 4.5 cm in greatest diameter or larger than 3.0 cm and demonstrate growth on serial imaging studies. Because tumors greater than 4.5 cm in diameter are more likely to be malignant, evidence of local invasion or metastasis is a contraindication to laparoscopic resection.

CONTRAINDICATIONS

Contraindications to laparoscopic adrenalectomy are listed in Table 2. Adrenocortical carcinomas should be extirpated by an open en bloc resection. These cancers often extend into adjacent structures, including the kidney, perinephric tissues, retroperitoneal lymph nodes, liver, tail of the pancreas, splenic hilum, and diaphragm. The wide margins of resection required for these invasive carcinomas cannot be adequately achieved with endoscopic techniques.

Morbid obesity is a relative contraindication. These patients often require very high intra-abdominal pressures to maintain an adequate pneumoperitoneum. However, these patients are also at increased risk of complications when an open anterior, flank, or posterior approach is used. Therefore, in experienced hands even these patients can often undergo successful laparoscopic adrenalectomy.

TABLE 2.
Contraindications to Laparoscopic Adrenalectomy

Adrenal carcinoma
Morbid obesity
Bleeding disorder
Poorly controlled pheochromocytoma
Multiple previous abdominal procedures
Need for simultaneous intra-abdominal procedure not amenable to the
 laparoscopic approach

Uncorrected therapeutic or idiopathic anticoagulation is a relative contraindication to laparoscopic adrenalectomy.[3] Coagulation parameters should be fully investigated preoperatively and corrected if possible. Thrombocytopenia should also be investigated and treated before endoscopic surgery.

Pheochromocytomas were once considered an absolute indication for open anterior adrenalectomy to allow for early control of the main adrenal vein and to provide adequate exposure for bilateral adrenal and extra-adrenal exploration. However, because of increased sensitivity of preoperative imaging studies, the ability to obtain early control of the adrenal vein, and adequate blood pressure management, we and others believe that laparoscopic adrenalectomy is well suited for select patients with pheochromocytomas.[2, 4, 26] We have used this technique in asymptomatic patients whose tumors were discovered as a result of family screening in multiple endocrine neoplasia IIa kindreds, as well as in sporadic cases. In all cases we have used preoperative α-adrenergic receptor blockade with phenoxybenzamine.

Another relative contraindication to a laparoscopic approach occurs in patients who have undergone multiple previous intraabdominal procedures that may have resulted in extensive adhesion formation, particularly those who have undergone previous nephrectomy, splenectomy, or liver resection. In these patients, placement of a Veress needle for insufflation and placement of trochars should be undertaken with an open technique. Dissection of intraabdominal adhesions can often be achieved laparoscopically provided that adhesion formation is not excessively dense. These patients may also be better treated by using a posterior laparoscopic approach. Patients with concurrent intra-abdominal or retroperitoneal pathology who require open exploration and should not undergo laparoscopic adrenalectomy because the benefits of reduced morbidity and shorter length of stay from a laparoscopic approach are negated.

PREOPERATIVE EVALUATION

A detailed history and physical examination must be obtained in all patients. Careful attention should be paid to systemic symptoms, changes in blood pressure, and alterations in body habitus and skin to assess the potential function of the adrenal mass. Careful review of imaging studies should be undertaken to determine the size, location, and extension of the adrenal mass and to evaluate the contralateral adrenal as well as other sites of intraabdominal pathology.

In patients without clinical symptoms and signs of hormonal excess, we routinely screen for aldosteronomas, pheochromocytomas, and glucocorticoid-producing adrenal adenomas. If the patient is normotensive and not receiving any medication, our aldosteronoma evaluation is limited to the measurement of serum potassium. If the potassium level is normal, additional studies are not obtained. However, if the patient has findings suggestive of hyperaldosteronism, including hypokalemia and/or hypertension, additional studies, including an assessment of aldosterone levels and plasma renin activity, are indicated. It is extremely important to confirm that the patient has hyperaldosteronism, distinguish between an adrenal APA and idiopathic hyperaldosteronism, (a bilateral process treated pharmacologically,) and localize the aldosteronoma to the affected adrenal gland.

The mainstay screening assays for both pheochromocytomas and glucocorticoid-producing adrenal adenomas are 24-hour urinary collections. These include metanephrines, vanillylmandelic acid or fractionated catecholamines for pheochromocytomas, and 17-hydroxy steroids or urinary free cortisol for glucocorticoid-producing adenomas. These results, if positive, often lead to additional evaluations, particularly in patients with Cushing's syndrome, to ascertain that the patient has ACTH-independent hormone secretion. These include a dexamethasone suppression test, pituitary MRI, and in selected patients, inferior petrossal sinus sampling and a corticotropin releasing hormone stimulation test.

PREOPERATIVE PREPARATION

Patients with hormone-producing adrenal tumors may require preoperative treatment for several weeks before surgery. Particularly in the case of pheochromocytoma, phenozybenzamine or other α- and occasionally β-adrenergic receptor blocking agents may be used. Profoundly cushingoid patients, as well as patients with aldosteronomas, often have significant metabolic derangements that must be corrected preoperatively. In addition, adrenal insufficiency will develop in patients with ACTH-independent Cushing's syndrome once their primary adrenal tumor is resected, and such patients will therefore require postoperative glucocorticoid replacement therapy.

The majority of patients without significant co-morbid pathology can be admitted to the hospital on the morning of surgery. Patients with pheochromocytomas are admitted the evening before surgery and undergo IV volume expansion. Patients undergoing laparoscopic adrenalectomy require limited bowel preparation. In our practice, patients receive a Fleet's enema on the night before surgery and another enema the morning of surgery. Patients should be instructed to take nothing by mouth after midnight before surgery, but they are allowed to take their routine medications on the morning of surgery with a sip of water.

OPERATIVE TECHNIQUE

The preferred technique for laparoscopic adrenalectomy in the majority of centers is the transperitoneal lateral approach, described here in detail.

Patients undergo general endotracheal anesthesia, and a nasogastric tube and Foley catheter are inserted. In selected cases, notably those with pheochromocytomas, an arterial line and central venous access are established. The patient is placed in the lateral decubitus position with the affected adrenal gland placed in the upper position. An axillary roll is used and the extremities carefully padded to minimize the chance of neurologic injury. The patient's position is such that the kidney rest of the operating table is placed in the midpoint between the costal margin and the anterior superior iliac spine. The operating table is then placed in the flexed position so that the patient's flank is maximally exposed in the extended position, and the kidney rest is then elevated. Finally, the legs are slightly elevated to minimize venous pooling. Patient positioning is illustrated in Figure 2.

The operating table is then placed in the side-to-side position so that during the procedure the patient can be manipulated in a lateral position to take advantage of "gravitational exposure" obtained by allowing the spleen and liver to fall out of the operative field. The patient is then carefully taped to the operating room table (shoulders and hips) to maintain a stable position in anticipation of lateral rotation during the operative procedure. The abdomen is prepared and draped in a generous fashion so that if required, conversion to open adrenalectomy can easily be accomplished. In addition, the instruments required for open adrenalectomy should be present in the operating room.

Entrance to the abdominal cavity is established with a Veress needle, and insufflation of the abdominal cavity is obtained with carbon dioxide. Once a pneumoperitoneum of 4 to 5 L has been established, a disposable 10/12-mm port is inserted and a 30-degree side-viewing rigid telescope is used. We use two separate video screens so that surgeons on both sides of the table have ready ac-

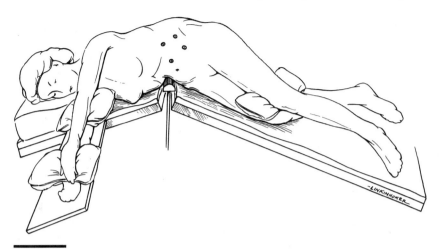

FIGURE 2.

Patient positioning and port location for laparoscopic left adrenalectomy. Positioning and port placement for laparoscopic right adrenalectomy are a mirror image of that for left adrenalectomy.

cess to the image. The abdominal cavity is inspected for evidence of adhesions or other pathology, and attention is then focused directly on the adrenal gland. For both right and left adrenalectomy, we generally use four separate ports, among them the video port. These are placed in a quadrilateral fashion as depicted in Figure 2, which demonstrates port placement for a left adrenalectomy. Port placement for a right adrenalectomy is a mirror image of the left. Throughout the procedure, the camera is moved between ports to aid in visualization. Instruments required for the procedure include cauterization scissors, a clamp-type instrument such as a Babcock or Maryland dissector, and an expanding retractor system such as a fan retractor. Additional special equipment required for laparoscopic adrenalectomy includes a pouch retrieval device (EndoPouch, Ethicon Corp.), as demonstrated in Figure 3,A and B.

The approach to the right adrenal gland is somewhat easier than the left. Occasionally mobilization of the right colon is required. We begin our right adrenalectomy by mobilizing the lateral attachments of the liver such that the liver can be rotated and eventually elevated. By continuing along the posterior and lateral attachments of the liver, one quickly approaches the vena cava. This is the exact position of the adrenal gland. Rarely is it necessary to perform a Kocher procedure inasmuch as the duodenum is normally rotated adequately to obtain posterior exposure to the ad-

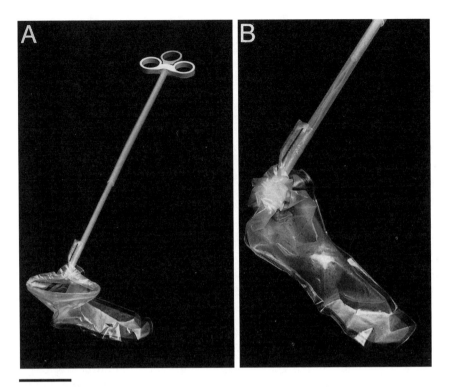

FIGURE 3.

A, endoscopic retrieval pouch device. This plastic closure device is extremely useful and markedly improves the ability to insert the specimen into the retrieval pouch and extirpate it from the abdominal cavity. **B,** pouch containing a specimen in the closed position.

renal gland. The vena cava is approached directly because virtually all right-sided adrenal glands have their venous drainage through a dominant vessel into the posterior aspect of the vena cava. The kidney is then retracted inferiorly, which allows additional dissection along the vena cava. In most cases, the adrenal vein is approached early in the dissection by using fan retractors on both the right kidney and the liver. However, in some cases it is easier to approach laterally by mobilizing the liver, opening Gerota's fascia, and then approaching the caval aspect of the dissection. Generally speaking, when operating for a pheochromocytoma, it is advantageous to obtain early control of the adrenal vein. Wound clips are used liberally because there are many arterial branches and occasional accessory venous branches as well. Meticulous use of both coagulation and wound clips is advisable.

The dissection proceeds until the main adrenal vein is identified, and two clips are placed on the vena caval side and one on the specimen side. The adrenal vein is transected, and the adrenal gland containing its tumor is resected. The specimen is held with Babcock forceps and a retrieval pouch is inserted via one of the port sites. The specimen is inserted into the retrieval pouch, which is then pulled up to the port site. It is necessary to slightly enlarge the port site to facilitate retrieval because the specimen is invariably larger than the port site. This is accomplished by slightly enlarging the skin incision and carefully inserting a Kelly clamp into the port site and dilating the fascia. Before removing the tumor, the retroperitoneum is inspected for hemostasis and irrigation is performed. Once the tumor has been removed, the pneumoperitoneum will be lost through the dilated port site, so it is important to visualize the retroperitoneum before specimen removal. The specimen is then extirpated and carefully inspected to make sure that the entire tumor has been removed; it is then sent for pathologic analysis. The port sites, fascia, and skin are closed.

The approach to the left adrenal gland is slightly more difficult. When the tumor is small, such as in aldosteronomas, visualization by intraoperative US can be extremely useful. Again, the patient is placed in the lateral decubitus position, and the ports are placed on the left side (Fig 2). It is often necessary to mobilize the left colon, especially along its attachments to the spleen. The spleen is then mobilized from the retroperitoneum by approaching it laterally. This allows the spleen to fall in a medial position. It is important to pay special attention to the tail of the pancreas and the splenic vessels to avoid injury. If the adrenal gland is not noted as a bulge superior to the left kidney or if it is not visualized, intraoperative US is used. Ultrasonography is particularly useful because it establishes the position of the left kidney and then by proceeding superiorly and medially the left adrenal gland is readily identified. Ultrasound is also useful for identifying the renal hilum and its vasculature. Occasionally, the adrenal gland is located by tracing the left renal vein into which the left adrenal vein invariably drains. The adrenal gland is mobilized along Gerota's fascia with the liberal use of clips and cautery. The adrenal gland is also approached medially and the adrenal vein carefully identified and doubly clipped to ensure that no injury occurs to the left renal vein. The adrenal gland is then mobilized, and the entire gland containing the tumor is excised. Retrieval is identical to that for the right side. We have not used a drain in any of our patients, although other groups routinely do so.

The combination of two experienced endoscopic surgeons is particularly advantageous in these cases. As in all procedures, there is a significant learning curve associated with the technical aspects of laparoscopic adrenalectomy.

POSTOPERATIVE CARE

After surgery, patients are admitted to the postoperative recovery room. We have reserved postoperative intensive unit care for patients with severe endocrinopathies, particularly patients with poorly controlled pheochromocytomas and fragile cushingoid patients. Most patients begin a clear liquid diet the evening of surgery and are fed a regular diet the following morning. Patients are strongly encouraged to ambulate with assistance the night of surgery and independently as tolerated beginning on postoperative day 1. The majority of our patients undergoing laparoscopic adrenalectomy are discharged on postoperative day 1.

RESULTS FROM REPORTED SERIES

Since Gagner and associates' initial description,[1] over 50 reports have described the indications, applications, and modifications of laparoscopic adrenalectomy. Since 1995, 7 major studies have examined laparoscopic adrenalectomy for a variety of adrenal disorders, in addition to descriptions of alternative methods for laparoscopic approaches to these tumors.[2-4, 15, 19, 21, 22] These reviews collectively examined 334 patients and characterized tumor type and location, postoperative length of stay, operative times, surgical complications, and intraoperative blood loss (Table 3). Two studies also examined postoperative analgesia requirements.[3, 4]

Patients undergoing adrenalectomy in these series ranged from 5 to 78 years of age. In agreement with previously published open reports, females present with adrenal disease more frequently than men. Aldosterone-producing adenomas were the most commonly reported adrenal tumor in these series (35%). Pheochromocytomas represented 25% of the tumors, followed by cortisol-producing tumors of all types (11%). Ten percent of the tumors removed were nonfunctioning "incidentalomas," and the remaining 11% consisted of tumors not falling into the aforementioned categories. The average length of stay for laparoscopic adrenalectomy ranged from 1.5 to 3.4 days, as compared with 5.5 to 9 days in patients undergoing an open procedure. Mean operative times ranged from 109 to 228 minutes for laparoscopic adrenalectomy vs. 136 to 174 minutes for open procedures.

TABLE 3.
Incidence of Adrenal Tumors in Selected Series of Laparoscopic Adrenalectomy

Author	N	Age	Sex		APA	Pheochromocytoma	Cortisol-Producing Tumors	Nonfunctioning Tumors (Incidentalomas)	Other Tumors
Guazzoni, 1995	40	18–65	M:15	F:25	17	17	6	0	0
Prinz, 1995	34	28–78	M:13	F:21	0	4	1	3	2
Miccoli, 1995	24	23–72	M:11	F:13	8	3	2	9	2
Rutherford, 1995	67	NR	M:37	F:30	52	6	1	8	0
Gagner, 1996	67	44*	M:24	F:43	9	19	13	11	15
Duh, 1996	36	5–78	M:15	F:21	18	4	6	3	5
Brunt, 1996	66	19–85	M:29	F:37	14	30	9	0	13
Total	334				118 (35%)	83 (25%)	38 (11%)	34 (10%)	37 (11%)

*Mean Age
Abbreviations: APA, aldosterone-producing adenoma; NR, not reported.

The instrumentation requirements for laparoscopic adrenalectomy incur additional patient costs. Brunt et al. examined total patient charges for laparoscopic and open adrenalectomy to determine whether laparoscopic instrumentation costs were offset by decreased length of stay.[4] The overall costs for laparoscopic adrenalectomy were not significantly different from those for open adrenalectomy.

Mean intraoperative blood loss was decreased in patients undergoing laparoscopic (range, 100 to 228 mL) vs. open adrenalectomy (range, 300 to 450 mL). Postoperative complications similarly appeared to be decreased in patients undergoing laparoscopic procedures. Finally, in the studies examining postoperative analgesia requirements, it appears that patients undergoing open adrenalectomy required threefold to fourfold higher doses of narcotic analgesia in one study[4] and nearly tenfold higher cumulative total doses,[3] as shown in Table 4

The results of laparoscopic adrenalectomy in 14 consecutive patients at the Johns Hopkins Hospital compare favorably with those of previously published results. The mean length of stay and blood loss were significantly decreased in the laparoscopic adrenalectomy group. Our operative times were not significantly different between the two groups. Finally, the time required for resumption of a regular diet and independent activity were significantly reduced in the laparoscopic group, as summarized in Figure 4.

FUTURE DIRECTIONS

The advent of more sophisticated endoscopic cameras, as well as the development of three-dimensional simulation using array-type camera devices, will improve the "view" provided to endoscopic surgeons. Combined with these advances in imaging technology are more sophisticated robotics for control of laparoscopic cameras and instruments. Investigators at our institution have already begun trials of distant "telesurgery" using robotic controls and transmission of endoscopic video images to remote locations. Application of "telesurgery" may provide training and backup support to surgeons skilled in open adrenal surgery and further broaden the application of this technology. Although laparoscopic adrenalectomy is becoming more widely accepted in the surgical community, the principles of adrenal surgery are paramount: first, each patient must be evaluated to ascertain whether surgery is indicated and whether clinically apparent or occult endocrinopathies are present. Next, surgery should be performed by surgeons with significant experi-

TABLE 4.
Results of Laparoscopic Adrenalectomy in Published Series

Author	N	Length of Stay, Days		Operative Time, min		Complications, Total		Analgesia		Blood Loss, ml	
		Open	Lap	Open	Lap	Open	Lap	Open	Lap	Open	Lap
Guazzoni, 1995	40	9	3.4	145	170	35%	5.0%	NR	NR	450	100
Prinz, 1995	34	6.4/5.5*	2.1	174/139*	212	NR	NR	15.8/14.7†	1.4	391/288*	228
Miccoli, 1995	24	NR	3	NR	109	NR	0.0%	NR	NR	NR	0
Rutherford, 1995	67	9.8	5.1	NR	124	NR	7.5%	NR	NR	NR	NR
Gagner, 1996	67	NR	3	NR	126	NR	19.4%	NR	5.5	NR	NR
Duh, 1996	36	NR	2.2/1.5‡	NR	228/204‡	NR	2.8%	NR	NR	NR	0
Brunt, 1996	66	8.7/6.2*	3.2	142/136*	183	21%/0	0.0%	142/54§	15.9	408/366*	104

*Anterior vs. posterior approach.
†Number of doses.
‡Transabdominal vs. posterior retroperitoneal approach.
§Total dosage (milligrams).
Abbreviations: Lap, laparoscopy; *NR,* not reported.

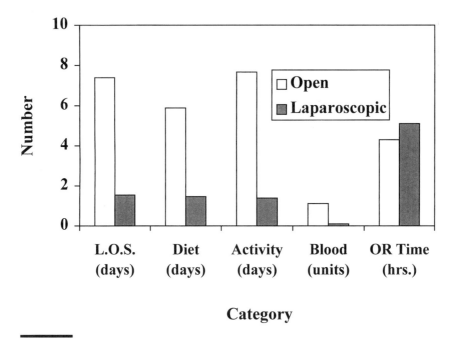

FIGURE 4.
The Johns Hopkins laparoscopic adrenalectomy outcome comparison. The results of laparoscopic adrenalectomy in 14 consecutive patients are compared with the results of open adrenalectomy in 16 consecutive patients. *Abbreviations: L.O.S.,* length of stay; *Diet,* days until resumption of a regular diet; *Activity,* days to resumption of independent activity; *Blood,* blood transfusion requirement (U); *OR Time,* hours of operating room time. One patient who underwent bilateral laparoscopic adrenalectomy for life-threatening refractory Cushing's disease died on postoperative day 58 of severe manifestations of Cushing's syndrome and is excluded from this analysis.

ence in both open and laparoscopic surgery. Finally, the surgeon must be willing and able to convert to open adrenalectomy when necessary.

REFERENCES

1. Gagner M, Lacroix A, Bolte E: Laparoscopic adrenalectomy in Cushing's syndrome and pheochromocytoma (letter). *N Engl J Med* 327:1033, 1992.
2. Gagner M: Laparoscopic adrenalectomy. *Surg Clin North Am* 76:523–537, 1996.
3. Prinz RA: A comparison of laparoscopic and open adrenalectomies. *Arch Surg* 130:489–494, 1995.
4. Brunt LM, Doherty GM, Norton JA, et al: Laparoscopic adrenalectomy

compared to open adrenalectomy for benign adrenal neoplasms (see comments). *J Am Coll Surg* 183:1–10, 1996.

5. Mercan S, Seven R, Ozarmagan S, et al: Endoscopic retroperitoneal adrenalectomy. *Surgery* 118:1071–1076, 1995.

6. Staren ED, Prinz RA: Adrenalectomy in the era of laparoscopy. *Surgery* 120:706–711, 1996.

7. Go H, Takeda M, Takahashi H, et al: Laparoscopic adrenalectomy for primary aldosteronism: A new operative method. *J Laparoendosc Surg* 3:455–459, 1993.

8. Takeda M, Go H, Imai T, et al: Laparoscopic adrenalectomy for primary aldosteronism: Report of initial ten cases. *Surgery* 115:621–625, 1994.

9. Sardi A, McKinnon WM: Laparoscopic adrenalectomy in patients with primary aldosteronism. *Surg Laparosc Endosc* 4:86–91, 1994.

10. Go H, Takeda M, Imai T, et al: Laparoscopic adrenalectomy for Cushing's syndrome: Comparison with primary aldosteronism. *Surgery* 117:11–17, 1995.

11. Gagner M, Lacroix A, Prinz RA, et al: Early experience with laparoscopic approach for adrenalectomy. *Surgery* 114:1120–1125, 1993.

12. Fletcher DR, Beiles CB, Hardy KJ: Laparoscopic adrenalectomy. *Aust N Z J Surg* 64:427–430, 1994.

13. Takeda M, Go H, Imai T, et al: Experience with 17 cases of laparoscopic adrenalectomy: Use of ultrasonic aspirator and argon beam coagulator. *J Urol* 152:902–905, 1994.

14. Udelsman R, Mersey JH: A clinical moment with endocrinology and metabolism: Laparoscopic adrenalectomy. *Md Med J* 44:611–612, 1995.

15. Duh QY, Siperstein AE, Clark OH, et al: Laparoscopic adrenalectomy. Comparison of the lateral and posterior approaches. *Arch Surg* 131:870–876, 1996.

16. Proye CA, Huart JY, Cuvillier XD, et al: Safety of the posterior approach in adrenal surgery: Experience in 105 cases. *Surgery* 114:1126–1131, 1993.

17. Gagner M, Lacroix A, Bolte E, et al: Laparoscopic adrenalectomy. The importance of a flank approach in the lateral decubitus position. *Surg Endosc* 8:135–138, 1994.

18. Guazzoni G, Montorsi F, Bergamaschi F, et al: Effectiveness and safety of laparoscopic adrenalectomy. *J Urol* 152:1375–1378, 1994.

19. Guazzoni G, Montorsi F, Bocciardi A, et al: Transperitoneal laparoscopic versus open adrenalectomy for benign hyperfunctioning adrenal tumors: A comparative study (see comments). *J Urol* 153:1597–1600, 1995.

20. Meurisse M, Joris J, Hamoir E, et al: Laparoscopic adrenalectomy in pheochromocytoma and Cushing's syndrome. Reflections about two case reports. *Acta Chir Belg* 94:301–306, 1994.

21. Miccoli P, Iacconi P, Conte M, et al: Laparoscopic adrenalectomy. *J Laparoendosc Surg* 5:221–226, 1995.

22. Rutherford JC, Gordon RD, Stowasser M, et al: Laparoscopic adrenalectomy for adrenal tumours causing hypertension and for 'incidentalomas' of the adrenal on computerized tomography scanning. *Clin Exp Pharmacol Physiol* 22:490–492, 1995.

23. Stoker ME, Patwardhan N, Maini BS: Laparoscopic adrenal surgery. *Surg Endosc* 9:387–391, 1995.

24. Stuart RC, Chung SC, Lau JY, et al: Laparoscopic adrenalectomy. *Br J Surg* 82:1498–1499, 1995.

25. Suzuki K, Kageyama S, Ueda D, et al: Laparoscopic adrenalectomy: Clinical experience with 12 cases (see comments). *J Urol* 150:1099–1102, 1993.

26. Meurisse M, Joris J, Hamoir E, et al: Laparoscopic removal of pheochromocytoma. Why? When? and Who? (reflections on one case report). *Surg Endosc* 9:431–436, 1995.

CHAPTER 16

Outcome of Surgical Therapy for Metastatic Cancer to the Brain

Rajesh K. Bindal, M.D.
Department Resident/Neurological Surgery, Indiana University School of Medicine, Indianapolis, Indiana

Ajay K. Bindal, M.D.
Staff Surgeon, Section of Neurosurgery, Saint Joseph's Hospital, Houston, Texas

Raymond Sawaya, M.D.
Chairman, Department of Neurosurgery, M.D. Anderson Cancer Center, Houston, Texas

B rain metastasis, the most common type of intracranial tumor, has an estimated incidence of over 100,000 per year.[1] This may be rising with the increasing incidence of cancer, improved survival of patients with metastatic disease, and use of chemotherapy that does not penetrate the blood-brain barrier.[2] In contrast, the incidence of primary brain tumors is estimated at 17,000 per year.[3] Overall, 20% to 25% of patients dying of cancer have brain metastasis at autopsy.[4] The incidence of brain metastasis varies dramatically according to the type of primary tumor. By far, the most common primary tumors in patients with brain metastasis are lung, breast, melanoma, renal cell, and colon cancers in declining order. Brain metastasis from other types of cancer such as sarcoma,[5] ovarian,[6] prostate,[7] and bladder[8, 9] cancer is less common.

Approximately one third of the patients with lung cancer have brain metastasis on autopsy.[1] This incidence is higher with small-cell carcinoma and adenocarcinoma. Lung cancer metastasizes to the brain relatively early in its clinical course, with the median interval from the initial diagnosis of cancer to a diagnosis of brain metastasis being only 6 months. Between 20% and 30% of patients dying of breast cancer have brain metastasis,[10] and there is a median interval of 2 to 3 years from the initial diagnosis to the development of brain metastasis. This interval is similar to that of melanoma. However, half of the patients dying of melanoma have brain metastasis.[11] The incidence of brain metastasis with renal cell carcinoma is 10% to 11%,[12] whereas for colon cancer it is 6% to 11%.[13]

Two thirds of all patients with brain metastasis on autopsy are symptomatic during life.[14, 15] Symptoms of brain metastasis are similar to those of any intracranial mass lesion,[16] the most common symptom being headache. Also common are focal weakness, mental or behavioral changes, seizures, ataxia, aphasia, visual field defect, and sensory deficit. The symptoms are related to the location of the tumor in the brain and associated mass effect from both the lesion itself and surrounding edema.

SURGICAL DECISION MAKING

The major treatment modalities for brain metastasis are steroids, whole-brain radiation therapy (WBRT), surgery, and radiosurgery. Chemotherapy has not been proved to be of much value except in selected cases of patients with germ cell tumors or small-cell lung cancer.[17–20] Brain metastases are often surrounded by an impressive amount of vasogenic edema relative to the size of the lesion, which results in increased mass effect (Fig 1). Steroids serve to reduce this edema and thereby reduce associated symptoms. In older series, the median survival in untreated patients was 1 month[21] but was increased to 2 months in patients treated with steroids alone.[22]

A large percentage of patients with brain metastasis have widespread, uncontrolled systemic cancer. In these patients the brain metastasis is not likely to be a substantial survival-limiting factor, and the goal of treatment in these patients is palliation. The treatment of choice in this setting is WBRT, which is associated with symptomatic response rates of 70% to 93%, depending on the individual symptoms.[23–26] Many investigators have examined the optimal dose of WBRT. The use of 30 Gy in ten fractions has become standard at many institutions.[27] Despite numerous studies, there is limited evidence that the use of higher radiation doses results in improved palliation or survival.[28] Unfortunately, palliation with WBRT is only temporary, and studies show that metastases will begin to enlarge a median of 21 weeks after treatment.[29] In a study of patients with a controlled or absent primary tumor, Karnofsky Performance Score *KPS) of 70 to 100, no evidence of metastasis elsewhere, and age less than 60 years, median survival with WBRT

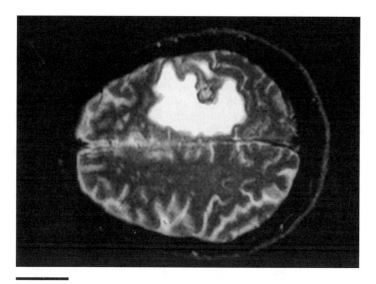

FIGURE 1.

T2-weighted image of a 1-cm left parietal renal carcinoma metastasis surrounded by an extensive zone of edema.

alone was only 7.4 months.[30] This group represented the most favorable subset of 87 patients from a group of 780. Thus WBRT is only indicated for patients not expected to survive for a prolonged period with respect to their systemic disease.

Brain metastasis in a certain percentage of patients will develop in the setting of absent, limited, or controlled systemic disease. Up to 50% of patients with lung cancer[31] and 44% to 65% of patients with breast cancer[32–34] are in this category. In these patients the brain metastasis is likely to be the survival limiting factor. In this setting, aggressive local control of the brain metastasis via surgery can be expected to result in improved survival and quality of life.

In evaluating a patient for surgery, the number of brain metastases is important. At autopsy, 58% to 85% of patients will have multiple lesions.[35–37] This varies with the type of primary tumor. In approximate numbers, the percentage of multiple lesions with lung cancer is 60%,[38] with breast cancer it is 50% to 60%,[39] with melanoma it is 75%,[40] with renal cell carcinoma it is 50%,[41] and with colon cancer it is 20%.[42] On CT, 50% to 56% of patients will have multiple lesions.[43, 44] Magnetic resonance imaging is more sensitive than CT scanning in detecting brain metastasis.[45] The percentage of multiple lesions detected by MRI is unknown but is probably somewhere between that of CT scan and autopsy. Historically, patients with multiple brain metastases have been considered surgical candidates only in rare instances.[46] However, recent data suggest that patients with a limited number of brain metastases in whom all lesions can be removed can benefit from surgery.[47] Thus patients with up to three lesions or rarely four may be considered surgical candidates if all lesions are surgically accessible.

Surgical accessibility has already been referred to and is an important consideration. A lesion is considered accessible if it can be resected with an acceptable risk of morbidity. The definition is therefore dependent on the definition of acceptable risk. Small lesions deep within the brain and lesions in the motor cortex, speech centers, internal capsule, thalamus, basal ganglia, and the brain stem are generally considered unresectable. However, with modern surgical techniques such as intraoperative US, stereotactic guidance, cortical mapping, and image-guided surgery, some lesions that had previously been considered unresectable can now be safely removed[48–50] (see Fig 2). Thus each lesion must be carefully evaluated to determine accessibility.

SURGERY FOR A SINGLE BRAIN METASTASIS

RANDOMIZED TRIALS

In a landmark study, Patchell and colleagues firmly established the role of surgery in the treatment of brain metastasis.[29] In a controlled, randomized trial they compared surgery followed by WBRT with needle biopsy followed by WBRT in patients with a known history of cancer and a KPS of 70 or greater. Six patients (11%) were found to have nonmetastatic disease, including primary brain tumors and abscesses, and were excluded from the trial. It is interesting to note that 30 of the 48 patients in this trial had either an unresected primary tumor or disseminated metastases at the time of randomization. Patients in the surgical arm had a longer median survival (40 vs. 15 weeks) and functionally independent survival (38 vs. 8 weeks) than those treated by irradiation alone. In addition, recurrence at the site of the original metastasis was lower with surgery (20% vs. 52%). When the length of time to death from neurologic causes was compared, patients in the surgical arm again had a longer survival (median of 62 vs. 26 weeks). Thirty-day mortality in both arms was 4%. Thirty-day morbidity rates in the surgical and radiation arms were 8% and 17%, respectively. From this trial it was definitively proved that surgery along with WBRT was superior to WBRT alone in selected patients with a single brain metastasis.

A second controlled, randomized trial from Europe has corroborated these findings.[50] In this trial, survival in the surgical group was 10 months vs. 6 months with WBRT alone. Progressive extracranial disease and age older than 60 years were negative prognostic indicators. Patients with active extracranial disease had a median survival of 6 months in each arm of the trial. The authors concluded that surgery was indicated for patients with a single lesion in the face of stable systemic disease, especially if they were less than 60 years of age.

SURVIVAL AND PROGNOSTIC FACTORS

Recent studies indicate that the median survival after resection of a brain metastasis is 11 to 16 months, depending on various prognostic factors.[47, 51-53] Larger series in the literature have also consistently demonstrated a 5-year survival rate of 10% to 15%. By far the most important prognostic factors are the extent of systemic disease and performance status. In addition, location of the tumor and age play a role in postoperative survival. Other possible factors that have not been definitively proved include time to development of brain metastasis, tumor histology, and failure of prior WBRT.

Study after study has repeatedly shown that the extent of systemic disease and performance status are the most important factors in postoperative survival. In a study of 125 patients with a single brain metastasis from tumors of various histologic types, the median survival of patients with systemic disease was 6 months whereas that for patients without systemic disease was 22 months with a greater than 25% 5-year survival rate.[53] Survival was also stratified by neurologic status. Survival was 22 months for patients with no or minimal deficit, 10 months for those with moderate deficit, and 6 months for those with severe deficit. A special subset of patients may be those with a single brain metastasis and a lung primary that can both be resected and no other evidence of disease. The prognosis for this subset of patients is relatively good. In one study, the 4-year survival rate was 56%,[54] whereas in another the 5-year survival rate was 45%.[55]

Location of the tumor is important in that patients with infratentorial lesions tend to have a poorer survival rate. Patients with supratentorial lesions survived 12 months as compared with 7 months for patients with infratentorial lesions in a large series.[53] This finding had been supported by multivariate analysis.[54, 56] Patients with infratentorial lesions have a much higher incidence of carcinomatous meningitis after surgery, which is an ominous development. It has been found that meningeal relapse after surgery develops in 30% to 38% of the patients with cerebellar metastasis as compared with 4.7% of those with supratentorial tumors.[57, 58] This may be one factor resulting in the poorer overall survival in these patients.

Age has been shown to be a prognostic indicator in multiple studies, including two randomized trials.[29, 50] In a study by Noordijk et al., patients over 60 years old treated with surgery survived 6 months as compared with 19 months for younger patients.[50] Multivariate analysis in retrospective studies also supports the prognostic value of age.[54, 57]

Time to development of brain metastasis may also be a prognostic indicator. Multivariate analysis in some studies has indicated that the development of brain metastasis soon after a diagnosis of cancer may be an independent negative prognostic indicator. In the randomized trial of Patchell et al., a longer time between diagnosis of the primary cancer and the brain metastasis was a significant prognostic indicator by multivariate analysis.[29] In a study of patients with lung cancer, patients with brain metastasis diagnosed synchronously with the lung primary survived a median of 9.2 months as compared with 13 months for patients in whom the cancers were diagnosed metachronously.[54] However, with multivariate analysis to correct for differences in other prognostic factors, the time of onset of brain metastasis no longer had any influence on survival. Results in other studies are similarly mixed.[47, 53, 57]

Minimal data in the literature suggest a role of tumor histology on survival. Very few studies on tumors of varying histologic type have found significant differences in survival by tumor histology.[47, 53] In one study on 229 patients operated on largely in the 1970s, lung, gastrointestinal, and genitourinary primaries were associated with longer survival by multivariate analysis.[57] However, with the many recent advances in oncology, the relevance of these data in the modern era is unclear. From examining the many studies on survival after resection of brain metastasis, it does appear that patients with renal primaries may have a superior prognosis and those with melanoma may have a poorer prognosis.[1] However, this is far from definite.

Some data suggest that male gender is associated with poorer outcome. In studies from the Mayo Clinic and Memorial Sloan-Kettering Cancer Center, multivariate analysis indicated that male gender was an independent negative prognostic indicator.[54, 57] The reasons for this are unclear, and additional confirmation of these findings is necessary.

COMPLICATIONS OF SURGERY

Brain metastases tend to be located subcortically, at the junction between the gray and white matter, and tend to be well demarcated from surrounding, healthy brain. It is mainly these characteristics that account for the low morbidity and mortality of surgery for brain metastases as compared with other brain tumors. In recent large series, operative morbidity is estimated at 5% or less and 30-day mortality is in the range of 3%.[47, 53, 54] The complication rates are dependent on factors such as tumor location. Lesions in eloquent cortex such as the motor strip will have a higher incidence of morbidity, whereas lesions in the posterior fossa may also be associated with increased 30-day mortality. Tools such as stereotactic localization and cortical mapping can be useful in reducing morbidity. Uniformly, studies indicate that the large majority of patients will be improved neurologically after surgery. Postoperative hospital stays are short, with one study reporting that patients were discharged a median of 3 days after surgery.[47]

POSTOPERATIVE WHOLE-BRAIN RADIOTHERAPY

The use of postoperative WBRT is standard at most institutions, and a number of studies have examined its efficacy.[58–63] The first such study, from the Mayo Clinic, examined a series of 85 patients operated on between 1972 and 1982.[63] In this study, patients receiving postoperative WBRT had a 21% rate of recurrence in the brain as compared with 85% for those not receiving WBRT. Patients receiving WBRT also had a significantly improved survival rate. This study has been cited as proof of the efficacy of WBRT, and the 85% relapse figure without WBRT has been widely quoted. Unfortunately, the figures from this study may not be applicable to patients being treated currently. Given the years in which the patients were treated, it is clear that some patients did not receive CT scans before surgery. In the absence of such imaging, many patients with multiple metastases may have been thought to have only a single lesion at the time of surgery. Certainly these patients would be more likely to have rapid enlargement of their previously undiagnosed lesions without WBRT. The 85% relapse figure is much higher than that reported in a number of other studies. Four more recent studies have been reported in the literature, and three of these showed a decrease in recurrence rates with WBRT.[58, 60, 62]

Only one study, on patients with melanoma, showed increased survival with WBRT.[64] However, multivariate analysis was not performed, which makes it impossible to know whether this survival advantage was simply due to a difference in prognostic factors. There have been numerous reports of neurotoxicity from WBRT, including radiation necrosis and dementia.[64, 65] In one study, dementia attributable to WBRT developed in 11% of the 1-year survivors, whereas in another study, 50% of the 2-year survivors were thus affected. Many of the patients in these studies were treated with doses greater than the 30 Gy in ten fractions that is currently widely used. However, even in patients receiving 30 Gy in ten fractions, leukoencephalopathy not attributable to other causes is frequently found.[66] Data on detailed neuropsychological testing in longer-term survivors after WBRT are limited, but studies suggest that deterioration does occur in these patients.[67, 68] Although only a minority of patients with brain metastasis will survive longer term, toxicity in this subgroup is very important because these survivors are the greatest beneficiaries of surgery and the group with the greatest need for aggressive treatment. In summary, the preponderance of evidence indicates that WBRT probably decreases recurrence rates in the brain and is associated with definite but unquantified toxicity. A survival benefit with WBRT in modern neurosurgical practice has not been proved. Despite this, WBRT is considered standard treatment at most institutions, including our own. Further studies are required to settle this controversial issue.

SURGERY FOR MULTIPLE BRAIN METASTASES

Historically, patients with multiple brain metastases were not considered surgical candidates except in rare instances, despite the fact that no study had ever carefully examined the role of surgery in such patients. Eventually, isolated reports of patients with multiple brain metastases treated with surgery began to appear in the literature.[1]

We recently examined the role of surgery in the treatment of patients with multiple brain metastases at M. D. Anderson Cancer Center.[47] We examined 56 patients with multiple brain metastases who underwent surgical resection of one or more lesions. The patients were divided into two groups: those who did not undergo resection of all known lesions (group A, n = 30) and those who had all lesions removed (group B, n = 26). In group A, 12 patients had one lesion removed, 6 patients had two lesions removed, and 2 patients had three lesions removed in one or more craniotomies.

In group B, 23 patients had two lesions removed and 3 patients had three lesions removed in one or more craniotomies. Multiple craniotomies, if required, were generally performed in a single operation. Prognostic indicators of groups A and B, including the type of primary cancer, length of time from the first diagnosis of cancer to the diagnosis of brain metastases, KPS, the percentage of patients with systemic disease, and age, were statistically compared and found to be homogeneous. Patients in group B were matched with 26 patients (group C) undergoing surgery for a single metastasis by the following criteria: type of primary cancer, onset interval, KPS, and presence or absence of systemic disease.

Median survival for all patients with multiple brain metastases was 10 months. Survival data for groups A, B, and C are shown in Figure 2. The median life spans were 6 months for patients in group A, 14 months for patients in group B, and 14 months for patients in group C. Two-year survival rates for groups A, B, and C were 0%, 32%, and 30%, respectively. Five-year survival rates for groups B and C were 11% and 16%, respectively. Survival duration differed significantly between groups A and B and between

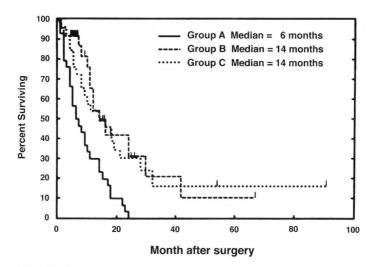

FIGURE 2.

Survival of patients with multiple metastases treated surgically. Group A, patients with multiple metastases in whom one or more lesions were left unresected; group B, patients with multiple metastases in whom all the lesions were resected; group C, patients with solitary, completely resected metastases. (Courtesy of Bindal RK, Sawaya R, Leavens ME, et al: Surgical treatment of multiple brain metastases. *J Neurosurg* 79:210, 1993.)

groups A and C, but not between groups B and C. Multivariate analysis was performed to determine what variables were significantly correlated with a difference in survival under the Cox regression model. The following variables were examined: patient group (A, B, or C), presence or absence of systemic disease, onset interval, histologic type of the primary, and recurrence of brain metastasis. The only variables significantly affecting survival were the patient group and the presence or absence of systemic disease.

Groups B and C had total brain recurrent rates of 31% and 35%, respectively. No significant difference in recurrence rate was detected between these groups by Kaplan-Meier analysis. Because patients in group A already had one or more lesions remaining in the brain after surgery, recurrence data were not deemed relevant.

Complication and mortality rates were low in all three groups. Complication rates in groups A, B, and C were 8%, 9%, and 8%, respectively. Thirty-day mortality rates in each group were 3%, 4%, and 0%, respectively. Multiple craniotomies were also well tolerated. The complication rate for patients undergoing multiple craniotomies was 7%, and the 30-day mortality rate was 0%.

Most patients were neurologically improved after surgery. In group A, 65% of the symptomatic patients improved postoperatively, 22% remained neurologically stable, 13% had progressive worsening of symptoms, and 8% were asymptomatic preoperatively and postoperatively. In group B, 83% of the patients improved, 11% were stable, 6% were worse, and 10% were asymptomatic preoperatively and postoperatively. In group C, 84% improved, 16% stabilized, 0% worsened, and 0% were asymptomatic preoperatively. A comparison of the improvement rates of patients in group A with those in groups B and C resulted in a difference approaching but not reaching significance.

Recent studies from Memorial Sloan-Kettering Cancer Center have reported similar results. In a study on patients with lung cancer, the presence of multiple brain metastases was not a negative prognostic indicator by multivariate analysis.[54] In a study of 670 patients with various tumor histologic types, 49 of whom had multiple lesions, multivariate analysis again failed to demonstrate multiple brain metastases as a prognostic factor inasmuch as patients with a single lesion survived 9.2 months vs. 9 months for those with multiple lesions.[69]

A study from the University of Colorado appeared to present a different conclusion.[70] Forty-six patients undergoing surgery for brain metastasis were evaluated. Of these, 28 had a single lesion and 18 had two or more metastases. They found that patients with multiple metastases had a median survival of 5 months as compared with 12 months for those with a single lesion, a difference that was significant by univariate analysis. However, only 1 of the patients with multiple lesions underwent excision of all lesions. This patient survived 46 months after surgery. The 5-month median survival rate for those patients who did not have all known lesions removed is very consistent with the 6-month survival rate that we had previously reported for such patients. Thus although this paper at first glance seems to contradict the previously mentioned studies, their data actually corroborate our conclusion that patients with multiple lesions who do not have all lesions removed have a poorer prognosis.

From these studies it appears that surgery for multiple brain metastases is warranted in selected cases, especially if all known brain metastases can be removed. Complication rates are low, and multiple craniotomies to achieve the goal of complete resection are well tolerated. Survival appears to be similar to that of patients with a single brain metastasis, and a significant percentage of patients can enjoy prolonged survival. However, only a limited number of studies have dealt with this controversial issue, and further research is needed to more clearly define the role of surgery for these patients.

RECURRENCE AFTER SURGERY

Unfortunately, tumors will recur in the brain in 31% to 51% of surgically treated patients.[29, 53, 71] Treatment options for such patients are limited. Many have already received WBRT, and the results of retreatment with this modality are mixed.[72, 73] Chemotherapy, as previously discussed, generally gives poor results.

We recently studied a group of 44 patients with recurrence to determine the characteristics of such lesions. The median time from initial surgery to recurrence was 6 months. Recurrence was local in 20, distant in 18, and both local and distant in 6 patients. Twenty-nine patients (66%) had a single lesion at time of diagnosis of recurrence, 8 (18%) had two lesions, 3 (7%) had three lesions, and 4 (9%) had four or more lesions. Thirty patients had known systemic disease at recurrence. The median survival for all patients after recurrence was 8.7 months. A total of 29 (66%) patients, including 3 with multiple lesions, underwent reoperation. Of the 15 patients not undergoing surgery, 10 received chemotherapy. The median survival for patients undergoing reoperation was 11 months as compared with 3 months for those without reoperation. Patients undergoing reoperation were more likely to have local recurrence, a single metastasis, and a better KPS and less likely to have systemic disease. Multivariate analysis was performed to correct for these differences in patient population and still found reoperation to be a positive independent prognostic factor.

Another study evaluated 109 patients with recurrent brain metastasis from non–small-cell lung cancer.[72] The median time to recurrence was 5 months. In 48.5%, recurrence was only local, in 13.5% it was both local and distant, 30% had one or more distant recurrences, and meningeal carcinomatosis developed in 8%. Of all 109 patients, multiple lesions appeared to develop at recurrence in 28.5%. Thirty-two patients (30%) underwent reoperation and will be discussed in the next section. The survival after recurrence for patients not undergoing reoperation is not stated. In the entire group of 109 patients, reoperation, histology of the adenocarcinoma, complete resection of the primary tumor, and female sex were found to be positive independent prognostic indicators.

These studies indicate that the majority of patients in whom lesions recur have only a single lesion. A significant percentage of patients may be treated with reoperation. Reoperation has a positive independent influence on survival, and survival is very dismal for patients who are not candidates for reoperation.

REOPERATION FOR RECURRENCE

A study by Sundaresan et al. in 1988 examined the role of reoperation for brain metastasis in 21 patients.[74] Radiation necrosis was found in 3 patients. Neurologically, 13 patients were improved after surgery whereas a new deficit developed in 1 patient. There was no surgical mortality. Wound-related complications resulting in loss of the bone flap developed in 2 patients, and in 1 patient a CSF leak and infection developed. The overall median survival after reoperation was 9 months.

In a recent study we evaluated the results of reoperation for brain metastasis at M. D. Anderson Cancer Center in 48 patients.[75] The median interval from the initial craniotomy to the diagnosis of recurrence in the brain was 6.7 months. At the time of recurrence, 6 (12.5%) patients had two lesions. Five of the 6 patients with two tumors required two craniotomies to allow resection of both lesions. Recurrence was local in 30 (62.5%) patients, distant in 16 (33.3%) patients, and both local and distant in 2 (4.2%) patients. The median prereoperative KPS was 80. Systemic disease was present at the time of reoperation in 23 (47.9%) patients. As determined by KPS evaluation at the time of reoperation and 30 days later, 33 (75.0%) of the 44 symptomatic patients improved after reoperation, and 11 (25.0%) stabilized. There was no operative mortality. No patients suffered wound infections, dehiscence, or CSF leaks after reoperation. As determined by neurologic examination, new or increased neurologic deficits after surgery developed in 5 patients (10.4%). In 3 of these patients, the deficits completely resolved within 30 days of surgery. The median hospital stay after surgery for all patients was 5 days.

Survival after reoperation was 11.5 months, and the 5-year survival rate was 17%. Multivariate analysis was performed to determine which variables correlated with survival. Systemic disease status, KPS, time to recurrence, age, and type of primary tumor significantly influenced survival.

A model was developed to predict patient survival according to the five prognostic factors determined by multivariate analysis. In this system, a patient was first assigned a score by adding together the number of negative prognostic indicators as presented in Table 1. This score was then converted to a grade (Table 2). For example, after initial craniotomy 9 months previously, a 65-year-old man who has a recurrent brain metastasis from lung cancer, no evidence of systemic disease, and a KPS of 70 has a score of 2 and therefore has grade II disease. Nine patients had grade I, 19 had grade II, 14 had grade III, and six had grade IV disease. Figure 3 presents survival as a function of grade. The median survival for patients with grade I disease was not reached. Patients with grades II, III, and IV survived a median of 13.4, 6.8, and 3.4 months, respectively. Patients with grade I disease had a 5-year survival rate of 57%. Patients with grade II had 3- and 5-year survival rates of 23% and 11%, respectively. Patients with grade III and IV lesions had 1-year survival rates of 17% and 0%, respectively.

Location of recurrence was not found to correlate with the risk of development of a second recurrence. Overall, a second recurrence developed in 26 patients. Eighteen of these patients had only a single lesion at the second recurrence. Seventeen of the 26 patients underwent a second reoperation. These patients had a median survival of 8.9 months after the second recurrence, which was significantly longer than the 2.8-month survival for patients not receiving a second reoperation.

Another study from Memorial Sloan-Kettering Cancer Center supports our results.[72] In this study, 32 patients with non–small-cell lung cancer underwent reoperation for recurrent brain metas-

TABLE 1.
Method of Calculating Score
to Determine a Patient's Grade

Factor Evaluated	Score
Status of systemic disease	
Present	1
Absent	0
Prereoperative KPS	
≤70	1
>70	0
Time to recurrence	
<4 mo	1
≥4 mo	0
Age	
≥40 yr	1
<40 yr	0
Type of primary tumor	
Melanoma or breast	1
Lung or other	0

Abbreviation: KPS, Karnofsky Performance Score.

tasis. The median time from initial surgery to recurrence was 5 months. The mean KPS before reoperation was 77.1. Of this group, 84.4% had a single brain metastasis. Median survival from the time of reoperation was 10 months. Eight of these 32 patients underwent a second reoperation and survived an additional 10.5 months. Reir-

TABLE 2.
Conversion of
Score to Grade

Score	Grade
0–1	I
2	II
3	III
4–5	IV

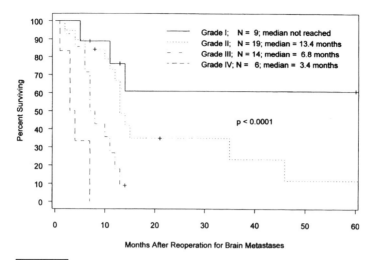

FIGURE 3.

Reoperation for recurrent brain metastases. The graph illustrates survival after reoperation for recurrent metastases according to grade. (See Tables 1 and 2 for prognostic factors and the scoring system used to determine the grade of patients with recurrent metastases.) (Courtesy of Bindal RK, Sawaya R, Leavens ME, et al: Reoperation for recurrent metastatic brain tumors. *J Neurosurg* 83:600, 1995.)

radiation did not increase survival. Multivariate analysis of the entire group of 109 patients with recurrent brain metastasis on whom this study was based revealed that reoperation was an independent factor associated with increased survival.

These studies indicate that reoperation plays a role in managing recurrent brain metastasis, especially in patients with lower-grade disease. Reoperation is well tolerated and appeared to prolong life. Given the limited treatment options for patients with recurrence in the brain, reoperation must be strongly considered in selected cases.

THE ROLE OF RADIOSURGERY

Stereotactic radiosurgery is a relatively new treatment modality increasingly being used to treat brain metastases. It refers to the use of small well-collimated beams of ionizing radiation to ablate intracranial lesions. All stereotactic systems have the ability to (1) accurately locate and immobilize an intracranial target in three-dimensional space, (2) produce sharply collimated beams of radiation with a steep dose gradient at the beam edge, and (3) target the beams accurately to minimize radiation exposure to surrounding brain tissue. The radiation dose is usually delivered in a single fraction. Hypofractionation has a more lethal effect on tissue than is possible by delivery of the same dose of radiation in many fractions. The use of numerous beams of radiation converging on the target site results in a high dose of radiation delivery to the tumor site. This dose rapidly falls off distally to the target in a ratio dependent on the size of the target. With a small target, surrounding brain tissue receives a smaller radiation dose than with a large target.

The main advantage of stereotactic radiosurgery with regard to brain metastasis lies primarily in its ability to treat lesions that are not amenable to surgical resection and secondarily in its noninvasive nature with fewer attendant risks and a shorter hospital stay. Brain metastases are particularly well suited for treatment by stereotactic radiosurgery because (1) metastases are often spherical with enhancing margins on MRI or CT; (2) they are generally small (<3 cm) when first detected; (3) normal brain parenchyma is circumferentially displaced by the lesion, thus reducing the chance of damaging normal brain tissue; and (4) brain metastases tend to be well demarcated and minimally invasive. Even so, because of the developing nature of radiosurgery, rarely are lesions that would otherwise be surgically resected being treated by this modality. Recurrent brain metastases and lesions located in unreachable regions of the brain are the ones that are often selected for radiosurgical procedures.

Studies have shown that radiosurgery is effective in treating brain metastasis and appears to be superior to WBRT alone.[76, 77] Some authors have even suggested that radiosurgery is effective enough to replace surgery as the treatment of choice in patients with a limited number of lesions and controlled systemic disease.[78] However, this concept is very controversial and not endorsed by the authors.

SURGERY VS. RADIOSURGERY FOR BRAIN METASTASES

We recently performed a study comparing surgery with radiosurgery for brain metastases.[79] We evaluated 31 consecutive patients with brain metastasis treated by radiosurgery who were monitored prospectively. The median size of the treated lesions and the median radiation dose at the isocenter and at the tumor margin were all similar to what has recently been reported from other institutions.[78] Each radiosurgical patient was matched with two patients from a pool of over 500 who underwent surgery for brain metastasis. Patients were matched by the following criteria: histologic type of primary tumor, extent of systemic disease, preoperative Karnofsky score, time to brain metastasis, number of brain metastases, and patient age and sex. Retrospective analysis of the tumors treated with radiosurgery demonstrated that 80.5% were surgically resectable with minimal or no morbidity.

The median survival of the surgical group was 16.4 months, whereas that of the radiosurgical group was 7.5 months, which was a statistically significant difference (Fig 4). The cause of death differed significantly between the two groups, with neurologic causes accounting for 50% of the deaths in the radiosurgical group but only 19% of the deaths in the surgical group. There was no statistically significant difference in survival by systemic cause of death, thus indicating that the extent of systemic disease was similar in both groups. However, radiosurgically treated patients had significantly shorter neurologic survival by both univariate and multivariate analysis. This indicated a greater mortality from progressive brain metastasis.

In the surgical group, 5 (8.1%) patients had local recurrence, 13 (21.0%) had distant recurrence, and 3 (4.8%) had both local and

Overall survival

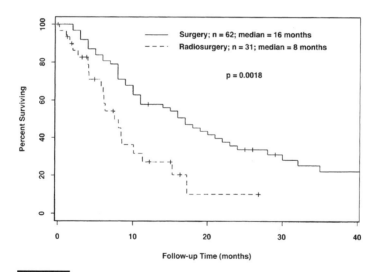

FIGURE 4.

Graph depicting a comparison of survival periods in surgically and radiosurgically treated patients. Radiosurgically treated patients had a shorter overall survival period according to both univariate analyses. (Courtesy of Bindal AK, Bindal RK, Hess KR, et al: Surgery versus radiosurgery in the treatment of brain metastasis. *J Neurosurg* 84:748, 1996.)

distant recurrences. In the radiosurgical group, 12 (38.7%) patients had local progression of disease, 3 (9.7%) had distant recurrence, and 0 (0%) had both local and distant recurrences. The median time from the last MRI to death or the last follow-up was 2 months each. There was no statistically significant difference in distant recurrence rates between the two groups. However, control of the treated lesion was significantly poorer in the radiosurgical group by both univariate and multivariate analysis.

Complications in the radiosurgery group included symptomatic radiation necrosis in four (12.9%) patients. Spontaneous intratumoral hemorrhage occurred in three (9.7%) patients and resulted in death for one. Three patients underwent craniotomy for tumor resection after radiosurgery failed to control the lesion size; one of these patients had significant radiation necrosis in addition to local tumor recurrence, the second had recurrent tumor, and the third had significant spontaneous intratumoral hemorrhage. Significant deep-vein thrombosis developed in four patients within 30 days after radiation treatment and necessitated anticoagulation therapy or placement of a Greenfield filter. Radiosurgery patients generally remained in the hospital overnight and left the next day. Complications in the surgery group included postoperative hematomas in two patients, neither requiring additional surgery. One patient had a postoperative wound infection that was treated with antibiotics. The median hospital stay for the surgical group was 4 days. This length of stay was significantly longer than the 1-day stay for radiosurgery patients.

From this study we conclude that surgery is superior to radiosurgery in the treatment of brain metastasis. Patients who undergo surgical treatment survive longer and have better local tumor control. Our data suggest that the indications for radiosurgery are limited to surgically inaccessible metastatic tumors or patients in poor medical condition. Surgery should remain the treatment of choice whenever possible. However, because radiosurgery is a noninvasive treatment, it can be used to treat patients who are not surgical candidates because of either advanced systemic disease or poor medical condition. Radiosurgery is more effective at local control than WBRT is and may therefore be used as an adjunct to or even in lieu of WBRT for patients in poor medical condition. Thus radiosurgery remains an important and powerful tool in the treatment of brain metastasis.

CONCLUSIONS

Brain metastasis is a deadly disease and portends a very poor overall prognosis. Most patients have widespread, disseminated disease. The goal of treatment in these patients is palliation, and surgery very rarely plays a role. However, in a significant subset of patients, an aggressive surgical approach can extend survival, reduce symptoms, and improve quality of life. Combined-modality treatment with surgery, fractionated radiation, and radiosurgery can prevent a significant number of patients from dying of their brain metastasis and improve the prognosis of this otherwise dismal disease.

REFERENCES

1. Sawaya R, Bindal RK: Brain metastasis, in Kaye AH, Laws ER (eds): *Brain Tumors: An Encyclopedic Approach.* New York, Churchill Livingstone, 1995, pp 923–946.
2. Posner JB, Chernik NL: Intracranial metastases from systemic cancer. *Adv Neurol* 579–592, 1978.
3. Walker AE, Robins M, Weinfeld FD: Epidemiology of brain tumors: The national survey of intracranial neoplasms. *Neurology* 35:219–226, 1985.
4. Takakura K, Sano K, Hojo S, et al: *Metastatic Tumors of the Nervous System.* New York, Igaku-Shoin, 1982.
5. Bindal RK, Sawaya R, Leavens ME, et al: Brain metastasis from sarcoma: Results of surgical treatment. *Neurosurgery* 35:185–191, 1994.
6. Stein M, Steiner M, Klein B, et al: Involvement of the central nervous system by ovarian carcinoma. *Cancer* 58:2066–2069, 1986.
7. Castaldo J, Bernat J, Meier F, et al: Intracranial metastases due to prostatic carcinoma. *Cancer* 52:1739–1747, 1983.
8. Anderson R, El-Mahdi A, Kuban D, et al: Brain metastases from transitional cell carcinoma of urinary bladder. *Urology* 39:17–20, 1992.
9. Bloch J, Nieh P, Walzak M: Brain metastases from transitional cell carcinoma. *J Urol* 137:97–99, 1987.
10. Lee YT: Breast carcinoma: Pattern of metastasis at autopsy. *J Surg Oncol* 23:175–180, 1983.
11. Patel JK, Didolkar MS, Pickren JW: Metastatic pattern of malignant melanoma: A study of 216 autopsy cases. *Am J Surg* 135:807–810, 1978.
12. Weiss L, Harlos JP, Torhorst J, et al: Metastatic patterns of renal carcinoma: An analysis of 687 necropsies. *J Cancer Res Clin Oncol* 114:605–612, 1988.
13. Weiss L, Grundmann E, Torhorst J, et al: Haematogenous metastatic patterns in colonic carcinoma: An analysis of 1541 necropsies. *J Pathol* 150:195–203, 1986.
14. Cairncross J, Posner J: The management of brain metastases, in Walker M (ed): *Oncology of the Nervous System.* Boston, Martinus Nijhoff, 1983, pp 341–377.
15. Hirsch FR, Paulson OB, Hansen HH, et al: Intracranial metastases in small cell carcinoma of the lung: Correlation of clinical and autopsy findings. *Cancer* 50:2433–2437, 1982.

16. Posner JB: Diagnosis and treatment of metastases to the brain. *Clin Bull* 4:47–57, 1974.
17. Buckner J: The role of chemotherapy in the treatment of patients with brain metastases from solid tumors. *Cancer Metastasis Rev* 10:335–341, 1991.
18. Giannone L, Johnson D, Hande K, et al: Favorable prognosis of brain metastases in small cell lung cancer. *Ann Intern Med* 106:386–389, 1987.
19. Greig N: Chemotherapy of brain metastases: Current status. *Cancer Treat Rev* 11:157–186, 1984.
20. Lee JS, Murphy WK, Glisson BS, et al: Primary chemotherapy of brain metastasis in small-cell lung cancer. *J Clin Oncol* 7:916–922, 1989.
21. Markesbery WR, Brooks WH, Gupta GD, et al: Treatment for patients with cerebral metastases. *Arch Neurol* 35:754–756, 1978.
22. Ruderman NB, Hall TC: Use of glucocorticoids in the palliative treatment of metastatic brain tumors. *Cancer* 18:298–306, 1965.
23. Borgelt B, Gelber R, Kramer S, et al: The palliation of brain metastases: Final results of the first two studies by the Radiation Therapy Oncology Group. *Int J Radiat Oncol Biol Phys* 6:1–9, 1980.
24. Cairncross JG, Kim JH, Posner JB: Radiation therapy for brain metastases. *Ann Neurol* 7:529–541, 1980.
25. Hendrickson F: The optimum schedule for palliative radiotherapy for metastatic brain cancer. *Int J Radiat Oncol Biol Phys* 2:165–168, 1977.
26. Hoskin P, Crow J, Ford H: The influence of extent and local management on the outcome of radiotherapy for brain metastases. *Int J Radiat Oncol Biol Phys* 19:111–115, 1990.
27. Sheline GE, Brady LW: Radiation therapy for brain metastases. *J Neurooncol* 4:219–225, 1987.
28. Gelber R, Larson M, Borgelt B, et al: Equivalence of radiation schedules for the palliative treatment of brain metastases in patients with favorable prognosis. *Cancer* 48:1749–1753, 1981.
29. Patchell R, Tibbs P, Walsh J, et al: A randomized trial of surgery in the treatment of single metastases to the brain. *N Engl J Med* 322:494–500, 1990.
30. Diener-West M, Dobbins TW, Phillips TL, et al: Identification of an optimal subgroup for treatment evaluation of patients with brain metastases using RTOG study 7916. *Int J Radiat Oncol Biol Phys* 16:669–673, 1989.
31. Patchell RA, Cirrincione C, Thaler HT, et al: Single brain metastases: Surgery plus radiation or radiation alone. *Neurology* 36:447–453, 1986.
32. Boogerd W, Vos VW, Hart AAM, et al: Brain metastases in breast cancer: Natural history, prognostic factors, and outcome. *J Neurooncol* 15:165–174, 1993.
33. Dethy S, Piccart MJ, Paesmans M, et al: History of brain and epidural metastases from breast cancer in relation with the disease evolution outside the central nervous system. *Eur Neurol* 35:38–42, 1995.

34. DiStefano A, Yap HY, Hortobagyi GN, et al: The natural history of breast cancer patients with brain metastases. *Cancer* 44:1913–1918, 1979.

35. Ask-Upmark E: Metastatic tumours of the brain and their localization. *Acta Med Scand* 154:1–9, 1956.

36. Chason J, Walker F, Landers J: Metastatic carcinoma in the central nervous system and dorsal root ganglia. *Cancer* 16:781–787, 1963.

37. Graf A, Buchberger W, Langmayr H, et al: Site preference of metastatic tumours of the brain. *Virchows Arch* 412:493–498, 1988.

38. Galluzzi S, Payne P: Brain metastases from primary bronchial carcinoma: A statistical study of 741 necropsies. *Cancer* 10:408–414, 1956.

39. Tsukada Y, Fouad A, Pickren J: Central nervous system metastasis from breast carcinoma. *Cancer* 52:2349–2354, 1983.

40. Patel J, Didolkar M, Pickren J, et al: Metastatic pattern of malignant melanoma. A study of 216 autopsy cases. *Am J Surg* 135:807–810, 1978.

41. Decker D, Decker V, Herskovic A, et al: Brain metastases in patients with renal cell carcinoma: Prognosis and treatment. *J Clin Oncol* 2:169–173, 1984.

42. Cascino T, Leavengood M, Kemeny N, et al: Brain metastases from colon cancer. *J Neurooncol* 1:203–209, 1983.

43. Delattre J, Krol G, Thaler H, et al: Distribution of brain metastases. *Arch Neurol* 45:741–744, 1988.

44. Swift PS, Phillips T, Martz K, et al: CT characteristics of patients with brain metastases treated in RTOG study 79-16. *Int J Radiat Oncol Biol Phys* 25:209–214, 1993.

45. Sze G, Milano E, Johnson C, et al: Detection of brain metastases: Comparison of contrast-enhanced MR with unenhanced MR and enhanced CT. *AJNR Am J Neuroradiol* 11:785–791, 1990.

46. Patchell R: Brain metastases. *Neurol Clin* 9:817–824, 1991.

47. Bindal RK, Sawaya R, Leavens ME, et al: Surgical treatment of multiple brain metastases. *J Neurosurg* 79:210–216, 1993.

48. Pillay PK, Hassenbusch SJ, Sawaya R: Minimally invasive brain surgery. *Ann Acad Med Singapore* 459–463, 1993.

49. Kelly PK, Kall BA, Goerss SJ: Results of computed tomography–based computer-assisted stereotactic resection of metastatic intracranial tumors. *Neurosurgery* 22:7–17, 1988.

50. Noordijk EM, Vecht CJ, Haaxma-Reiche H, et al: The choice of treatment of single brain metastasis should be based on extracranial tumor activity and age. *Int J Radiat Oncol Biol Phys* 29:711–717, 1994.

51. Ferrara M, Bizzozzero F, Talamonti G, et al: Surgical treatment of 100 single brain metastases. *J Neurosurg Sci* 34:303–308, 1990.

52. Sundaresan N, Galicich JH: Surgical treatment of brain metastases: Clinical and computerized tomography evaluation of the results of treatment. *Cancer* 55:1382–1388, 1985.

53. Wronski M, Arbit E, But M, et al: Survival after surgical treatment of

brain metastasis from lung cancer: A follow-up study of 231 patients treated between 1976 and 1991. *J Neurosurg* 83:605–616, 1995.

54. Catinella F, Kittle F, Milloy F, et al: Surgical treatment of primary lung cancer and solitary intracranial metastasis. *Chest* 95:972–975, 1989.

55. Hankins J, Miller J, Salchman M, et al: Surgical management of lung cancer with solitary cerebral metastasis. *Ann Thorac Surg* 46:24–28, 1988.

56. Smalley SR, Laws ER, O'Fallon JR, et al: Resection for solitary brain metastasis: Role of adjuvant radiation and prognostic variables in 229 patients. *J Neurosurg* 77:531–540, 1992.

57. Kitaoka K, Abe H, Aida T, et al: Follow-up study on metastatic cerebellar tumor surgery: Characteristic problems of surgical treatment. *Neurol Med Chir* 30:591–598, 1990.

58. Armstrong JG, Wronski M, Galicich J, et al: Post-operative radiation for lung cancer metastatic to the brain. *J Clin Oncol* 12:2340–2344, 1994.

59. DeAngelis LM, Mandell LR, Thaler H, et al: The role of postoperative radiotherapy after resection of single brain metastases. *Neurosurgery* 24:798–805, 1989.

60. Dorsoretz DE, Blitzer PH, Russell AH, et al: Management of solitary metastasis to the brain: The role of elective brain irradiation following complete surgical resection. *Int J Radiat Oncol Biol Phys* 6:1727–1730, 1980.

61. Hagen NA, Cirrincione C, Thaler HT, et al: The role of radiation therapy following resection of single brain metastasis from melanoma. *Neurology* 40:158–160, 1990.

62. Smalley SR, Schray MF, Laws ER, et al: Adjuvant radiation therapy after surgical resection of solitary brain metastasis: Association with pattern of failure and survival. *Int J Radiat Oncol Biol Phys* 13:1611–1616, 1987.

63. Skibber JM, Soong SJ, Austin L, et al: Cranial irradiation after surgical excision of brain metastases in melanoma patients. *Ann Surg Oncol* 3:118–123, 1996.

64. DeAngelis LA, Delattre J, Posner J: Radiation-induced dementia in patients cured of brain metastases. *Neurology* 39:789–796, 1989.

65. Sundaresan N, Galicich JH, Deck MD, et al: Radiation necrosis after treatment of solitary intracranial metastases. *Neurosurgery* 8:329–333, 1981.

66. Lee YY, Nauert C, Glass JP: Treatment related white matter changes in cancer patients. *Cancer* 57:1473–1482, 1986.

67. Laukkanen E, Klonoff H, Allan B, et al: The role of prophylactic brain irradiation in limited stage small cell lung cancer: Clinical, neuropsychologic, and CT sequelae. *Int J Radiat Oncol Biol Phys* 14:1109–1117, 1988.

68. Johnson B, Patronas N, Hayes W: Neurologic, computed cranial tomographic, and magnetic resonance imaging abnormalities in patients

with small-cell lung cancer: Further follow-up of 6- to 13-year survivors. *J Clin Oncol* 8:48–56, 1990.

69. Arbit E, Wronski M, Galicich JH: Surgical resection of brain metastasis in 670 patients: The Memorial Sloan-Kettering Cancer Center experience, 1972–1992. *J Neurosurg* 80:386A, 1994.

70. Hazuka MB, Burleson WD, Stroud DN, et al: Multiple brain metastases are associated with poor survival in patients treated with surgery and radiotherapy. *J Clin Oncol* 11:369–373, 1993.

71. Arbit E, Wronski M, Burt M, et al: The treatment of patients with recurrent brain metastases: A retrospective analysis of 109 patients with nonsmall cell lung cancer. *Cancer* 76:765–773, 1995.

72. Kurup P, Reddy S, Hendrickson FR: Results of re-irradiation for cerebral metastases. *Cancer* 46:2587–2589, 1980.

73. Shehata WM, Hendrickson FR, Hindo W: Rapid fraction technique and retreatment of cerebral metastases by irradiation. *Cancer* 34:257–261, 1974.

74. Sundaresan N, Sachdev VP, DiGiacinto GV, et al: Reoperation for brain metastases. *J Clin Oncol* 6:1625–1629, 1988.

75. Bindal RK, Sawaya R, Leavens ME, et al: Reoperation for recurrent metastatic brain tumors. *J Neurosurg* 83:600–604, 1995.

76. Flecklinger JC, Kondziolka D, Lundsford LD, et al: A prospective multicenter report on radiosurgery for the treatment of brain metastases. *Int J Radiat Oncol Biol Phys* 28:797–802, 1994.

77. Loeffler JS, Alexander E: Radiosurgery for the treatment of intracranial metastases, in Alexander E, Loeffler JS, Lundsford LD (eds): *Stereotactic Radiosurgery.* New York, McGraw-Hill, 1993, pp 197–206.

78. Mehta MP, Rozental JM, Levin AB, et al: Defining the role of radiosurgery in the management of brain metastases. *Int J Radiat Oncol Biol Phys* 24:619–625, 1992.

79. Bindal AK, Bindal RK, Hess KR, et al: Surgery versus radiosurgery in the treatment of brain metastasis. *J Neurosurg* 84:748–754, 1996.

CHAPTER 17

Portal Vein Involvement in Pancreatic Cancer: A Sign of Unresectability?

Lawrence E. Harrison, M.D.

Assistant Professor of Surgery, Department of Surgery, University of Medicine and Dentistry of New Jersey/New Jersey Medical School, Newark, New Jersey

Murray F. Brennan, M.D.

Professor, Chairman, Department of Surgery, Memorial Sloan-Kettering Cancer Center, New York, New York

A lthough surgical resection remains the only potential curative treatment for adenocarcinoma of the pancreas, only 10% to 20% of all patients are candidates for pancreatic resection.[1, 2] This low resectability rate reflects the advanced stage of disease at the time of diagnosis. When first seen, almost 50% of patients have distant spread of tumor and 35% manifest locally advanced disease. Although distant metastases constitute an absolute contraindication for resection, locally advanced disease may also preclude curative resection. An inability to separate the pancreas from the portal vein (PV) has historically been a locoregional contraindication for resection in patients with adenocarcinoma of the pancreas, and not infrequently, isolated local invasion of the PV is the only obstacle to curative resection.

Although described as early as the 1950s,[3] the technique of portal vein resection (PVR) was popularized by Fortner in the 1970s. In an attempt to improve resectability rates, he proposed excision of the pancreatic tumor combined with resection of the PV and hepatic/superior mesenteric artery (SMA).[4] Even though this extended resection lead to an improved resectability rate, high morbidity and mortality rates and failure to convincingly improve long-term survival dissuaded most surgeons from pursuing the "regional" pancreatectomy.[5] Since Fortner's original report, this procedure has undergone considerable evolution and refinement with acceptable morbidity and mortality.[6]

Technically, PVR with reconstruction is feasible, and for isolated PV involvement, pancreatectomy with PVR can render patients free of gross tumor. However, the central issues concerning PVR for isolated involvement in pancreatic adenocarcinoma are (1) whether PVR can be performed safely and (2) to what extent isolated PV involvement affects overall survival for patients undergoing pancreatic resection. Many groups around the world continue to resect the PV or superior mesenteric vein (SMV) for clinical suspicion of tumor involvement. This chapter summarizes recent data regarding PVR as it pertains to technique and outcome measures, including operative morbidity and mortality, as well as overall survival.

DIAGNOSTIC IMAGING OF THE PORTAL VEIN

In the absence of distant metastatic disease, patients with suspected PV involvement are considered candidates for resection. Preoperative evaluation of the mesenteric vasculature is an important step before exploration. Historically, surgeons have relied on angiography to determine vascular involvement by tumor. During the venous phase of a mesenteric angiogram, the PV can be visualized and tumor invasion is suggested by narrowing of the vessel. Using angiography in a series of patients undergoing PVR, Ishikawa et al. developed a grading system to classify tumor invasion of the PV/SMV based on the mesenteric angiogram. By retrospective analysis, they suggested that patients whose angiogram showed less than semicircular encroachment or invasion less than 1.2 cm in length benefited from PVR.[7] Similar grading systems have also been used to predict resectability and outcome after PVR.[8]

Many surgeons have abandoned the use of mesenteric angiography for preoperative evaluation of patients with peripancreatic masses because a high-quality CT scan evaluates tumor invasion of the PV as well if not better than angiography. A contrast-enhanced helical CT scan of the abdomen with 5-mm cuts through the pancreas allows very accurate evaluation of the SMV-PV complex, as well as arterial involvement by the tumor. We have found that the CT scan has supplanted the use of angiography to determine vascular involvement of peripancreatic tumors. At the present time, a quality CT scan should be considered the standard of care for evaluation of tumor involvement of the PV.

Ultrasonography also plays a role in imaging the PV and may have clinical application. Transabdominal or endoscopic US may detect PV invasion and thrombosis. More recently, laparoscopic US has been used to stage patients with peripancreatic masses and has been found to be a useful method to detect tumor involvement of the PV.[9, 10] A novel method of PV evaluation entails intraportal endovascular US (IPEUS) performed either by a percutaneous transhepatic route or intraoperatively by cannulation of a branch of the SMV. In a recent study, findings of IPEUS were confirmed by pathologic examination of resected PV specimens, and the results were compared with angiography and CT scan. The authors reported that the sensitivity and specificity of IPEUS was 100% and 93.3%, respectively, for predicting histologic invasion of the PV, which was superior to both angiography and CT scanning.[11] This technique, although interesting and technically challenging, would seem unlikely to gain acceptance as a routine test.

By whatever imaging modality, evaluation of the PV, SMV, and mesenteric arterial vessels is necessary before exploration. Although our philosophy is that isolated PV involvement is not a contraindication to resection, we are reluctant to resect patients with evidence of PV thrombosis either by clinical signs or by radiographic evidence of PV clot or associated varices. Tumors involving the SMA or celiac axis are considered an absolute contraindication to resection.

TECHNIQUE OF PORTAL VEIN RESECTION

For patients with otherwise resectable lesions, a standard pancreatic resection is performed. in most cases, intraoperative assessment will reveal adherence of the tumor to the PV or SMV, often on the lateral aspect of the vein after the gland has been divided. At this point, the dissection is nearly complete, and the final step before removal of the specimen is segmental resection of the PV.

The first step in PVR is proximal and distal control of the PV. Clamp placement and approach to the splenic vein will depend on tumor location. For SMV lesions, the splenic vein is spared by placing the proximal clamp at or just distal to the splenic-portal vein confluence (Fig 1). For low PV lesions, the splenic vein can be maintained by placing the proximal clamp at an angle as shown in Figure 2. For mid or high PV involvement, we routinely ligate and divide the splenic vein for mobility (Fig 3).

After transection of the PV segment and removal of the specimen, a primary anastomosis with monofilament suture is almost always possible with elevation of the small-bowel mesentery. Although others have used interposition grafts, this is rarely needed. If a conduit is required, autologous (internal jugular, renal, or sa-

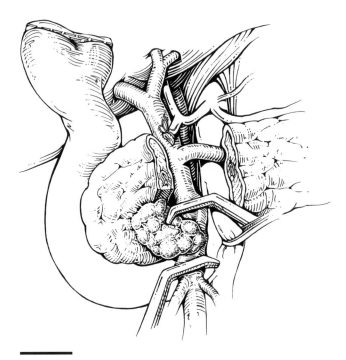

FIGURE 1.

Technique of portal vein resection: tumor involving the superior mesenteric vein. Proximal and distal control of the portal vein can be accomplished without sacrificing the splenic vein.

phenous vein) tissue is preferred over synthetic material because of higher patency rates.[12]

A lateral venorrhaphy for adequate tumor clearance may also be used. This is usually accomplished by placing a vascular clamp on the lateral aspect of the PV after the pancreas is divided (Fig 4). With lateral venorrhaphy, a word of caution must be given regarding narrowing the PV. If too much of the lateral wall is resected, PV congestion and thrombosis will occur. Revision after a lateral venorrhaphy for narrowing often requires segmental resection. This will result in a much longer segment of resected vein than would originally be required if a segmental resection were attempted primarily. This increases PV clamp and operative time and almost always requires an interposition graft.

ISOLATED PORTAL VEIN INVOLVEMENT: A CONTRAINDICATION FOR RESECTION?

The rationale for performing PVR is based on the fact that patients with adenocarcinoma of the pancreas who undergo pancreatic re-

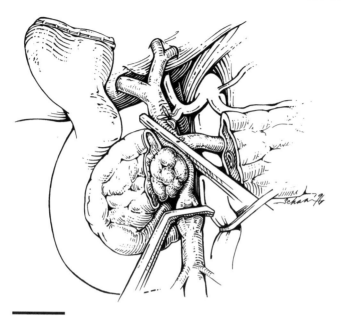

FIGURE 2.

Technique of portal vein resection: tumor involving the distal portal vein. By placing the proximal vascular clamp at an angle, the splenic vein can be maintained.

section have a significantly longer survival duration than those patients who undergo palliative bypass or no surgery[1] (Fig 5). In addition, some groups have proposed that locally advanced disease not be a contraindication to resection inasmuch as resection provides the best palliation.[13] Therefore, if patients have an improved survival and better palliation after pancreatic resection and PVR allows an increase in resectability, patients should benefit from pancreatic resection with PVR.

However, before PVR is recommended for isolated PV involvement, issues of safety and survival need to be addressed. For PVR to be of benefit, survival after pancreatic resection with PVR should approach that of those resections without PVR and should surpass that of either palliative bypass or nonoperative supportive care. In addition, PVR should be able to be performed with little added in the way of postoperative mortality and morbidity over a standard pancreatic resection.

To address these issues regarding PVR, we evaluated the morbidity, mortality, and overall survival of patients undergoing PVR for adenocarcinoma of the pancreas at Memorial Sloan-Kettering Cancer Center (MSKCC) over an 11-year period. These results of

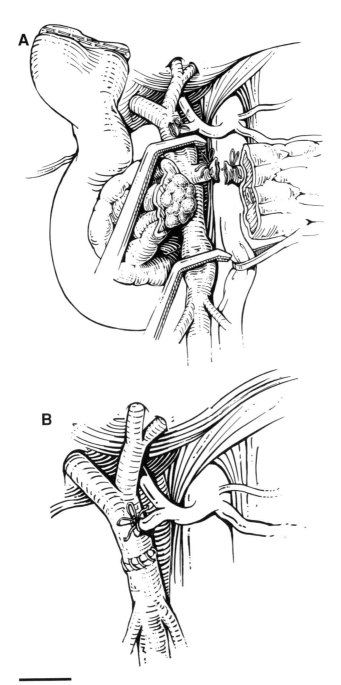

FIGURE 3.
Technique of portal vein resection: tumor involving the proximal portal vein. **A,** Ligation of the splenic vein is necessary for tumors involving the proximal portal vein. **B,** primary reconstruction of the portal vein.

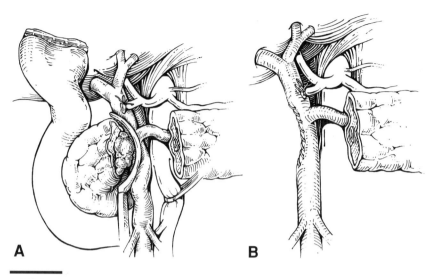

FIGURE 4.

Technique of portal vein resection. For minimal tumor invasion of the lateral wall, a side-biting vascular clamp is used to perform a lateral venorrhaphy. Care must be used to not narrow the portal vein. **B,** primary reconstruction of the portal vein.

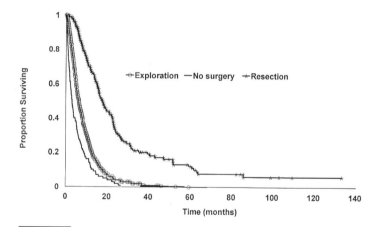

FIGURE 5.

Survival of patients with adenocarcinoma of the pancreas at Memorial Sloan-Kettering Cancer Center. Patients able to undergo resection have a significantly longer survival than those undergoing bypass or no surgery.

this evaluation are summarized in the following sections and compared with recent data from other series.

MEMORIAL SLOAN-KETTERING CANCER CENTER EXPERIENCE WITH PORTAL VEIN RESECTION

A review of the prospective pancreatic database at MSKCC between October 1983 and August 1995 identified 727 patients who underwent pancreatic resection. During this time period, 332 patients underwent resection for histologically confirmed adenocarcinoma of the pancreas. Fifty-eight of the 332 (17%) were identified as having isolated clinical involvement of the PV and underwent pancreatic resection with PVR. Patients undergoing pancreatic resection with curative intent without PVR over this same time period constituted the control group.

The following data were analyzed: (1) demographics; (2) intraoperative factors, including operative time, blood loss, and transfusion requirements; (3) tumor characteristics, including tumor size, margin and lymph node status, and grade; and (4) outcome, including reoperative rate, length of hospital stay, operative mortality, and overall survival. Data are presented as median values (range).

Operative procedures included pancreaticoduodenectomy (n = 42 with PVR, n = 231 without PVR), total pancreatectomy (n = 8 with PVR, n = 18 without PVR), or distal subtotal pancreatectomy (n = 8 with PVR, n = 25 without PVR). Of the 58 patients who underwent PVR, 38 had a primary end-to-end anastomosis and 20 patients underwent lateral venorrhaphy of the PV. Total anesthesia time was significantly longer for those patients undergoing PVR (7.4 hours [2.8 to 14.5]) than for those in the control group (5.8 hours [2 to 11.3], $P < 0.01$). Estimated intraoperative blood/fluid loss and transfusion requirements were also significantly increased in the PVR group (1,900 mL [350 to 8,500], 3 U [0 to 13]) as compared with those patients undergoing pancreatic resection without vascular excision (1,200 mL [130 to 7,600], 1 U [0 to 13], ($P < 0.01$) (Table 1).

Median tumor size was significantly larger in those patients undergoing PVR (4 cm [1.1 to 12]) than in the control group (3.5 cm [0.5 to 16], $P < 0.01$). Microscopic surgical margins were found to be histologically positive in 15 (27%) patients requiring PVR as compared with 65 (24%) of the controls. Metastatic lymph node involvement was identified pathologically in 30 (52%) PVR patients and 152 (55%) controls. Tumor grade was not significantly different between the two groups (Table 1).

TABLE 1.
Memorial Sloan-Kettering Cancer Center Experience With Portal Vein Resection

Characteristic	PD		DP		TP		Overall	
	PVR (42)	No PVR (231)	PVR (8)	No PVR (25)	PVR (8)	No PVR (18)	PVR (58)	No PVR (274)
Operative factors								
EBL, mL	2,050 (550–8,500)*	1,200 (130–4,500)	1,700 (350–3,500)	1,400 (400–5,500)	1,950 (900–4,500)	3,200 (350–7,600)	1,900 (350–8,500)*	1,200 (130–7,600)
Transfusion (U PRBC)	2.5 (0–13)*	1 (0–9)	2 (0–6)	2 (0–9)	3.5 (0–7)	5 (0–13)	3 (0–13)*	1 (0–13)
Operative time, hr	8 (3–14.5)*	5.8 (2.0–11)	5 (2.8–10.4)	3.6 (2–7.7)	7.8 (6–11)	8.5 (4.5–11.3)	7.4 (2.8–14.5)*	5.8 (2–11.3)
Tumor Characteristics								
Tumor size, cm	3.5 (1.1–7)	3.2 (0.5–16)	6.5 (4–8.2)	4.5 (1–10)	5 (3.5–12)	3.5 (2–10)	4 (1.1–12)*	3.5 (0.5–16)
No. with margin positivity (%)	10 (24)	51 (22)	3 (38)	7 (28)	2 (25)	4 (22)	15 (27)	65 (24)
No. with LN positivity (%)	24 (59)	132 (57)	4 (50)	11 (44)	2 (25)	9 (41)	30 (52)	152 (55)
Differentiation, (%)								
Well	17	17	25	20	25	23	20	18
Moderate	57	55	12	44	38	29	47	53
Poor	26	28	63	36	37	48	33	29
Outcome								
LOS, days	22 (8–58)*	15 (6–88)	14.5 (8–29)	12 (5–88)	29 (23–125)*	25 (13–37)	22 (8–125)*	15 (5–88)
Reoperative rate (%)	6 (14)	28 (12)	1 (13)	5 (20)	3 (38)	3 (17)	10 (17)	36 (13)
Operative mortality (%)	1 (2)	8 (3)	0 (0)	0 (0)	2 (25)	1 (6)	3 (5)	9 (3)

Note: Data are expressed as median values (range).
*$P < 0.01$.

Abbreviations: PD, pancreaticoduodenectomy; *DP*, distal subtotal pancreatectomy; *TP*, total pancreatectomy; *PVR*, portal vein resection; *EBL*, estimated blood loss; *PRBC*, peripheral red blood cells; *LN*, lymph node; *LOS*, length of hospital stay.

TABLE 2.
Memorial Sloan-Kettering Cancer Center
Experience With Portal Vein Resection:
Reoperation for Pancreatic Resection

Reason for Reoperation	No PVR	PVR
Bleeding	15	2
Abscess	11	2
Wound	2	1
Portal vein obstruction	0	1
Other*	4	1
Total	32 (12%)	7 (12%)

*Include colonic perforation (n = 3), hepatic artery thrombosis (n = 1), and gastric outlet obstruction (n = 1).
Abbreviation: PVR, portal vein resection.

The in-hospital reoperative rate was similar between the two groups: 7 of 58 patients (12%) undergoing PVR required surgical re-exploration as compared with 32 of 274 controls (12%). Importantly, PVR did not alter the cause for re-exploration (Table 2). By contrast, the length of hospital stay was significantly longer for those patients undergoing PVR (22 days [8 to 125] and 15 days [5 to 88] in the PVR and control groups, respectively, $P < 0.01$). There were 3 postoperative deaths in the PVR group for an in-hospital mortality rate of 5%. However, this was not significantly different from the operative mortality rate seen in those patients not undergoing PVR (9 patients [3%]). The overall median survival for the PVR group was 13 months (<1 to 109 months), which was not statistically different from those patients undergoing pancreatic resection without PVR (17 months [<1 to 132]). No difference in survival was detected when the patients were stratified according to operative procedure[14] (Fig 6, A–D).

SAFETY OF PORTAL VEIN RESECTION

At the present time, most surgeons do not perform vascular resections for tumor invasion because of earlier reports of high morbidity and mortality without obvious benefit to the patient.[5] However, before deeming all patients unresectable because of vascular involvement, it is important to distinguish PVR for isolated PV in-

Overall

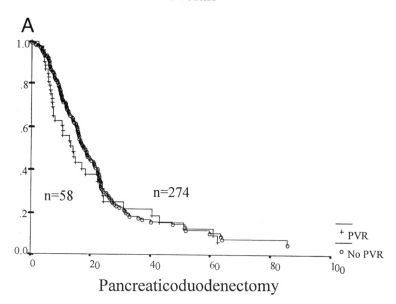

Pancreaticoduodenectomy

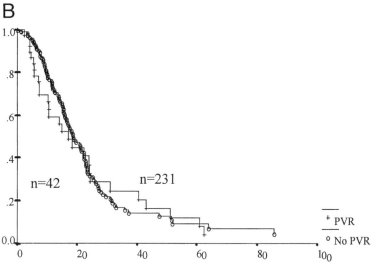

FIGURE 6.

Memorial Sloan-Kettering Cancer Center experience with portal vein re-section *(PVR):* survival after PVR vs. no PVR. **A,** overall survival **B,** pan-creaticoduodenectomy.   *(Continued.)*

Distal Pancreatectomy

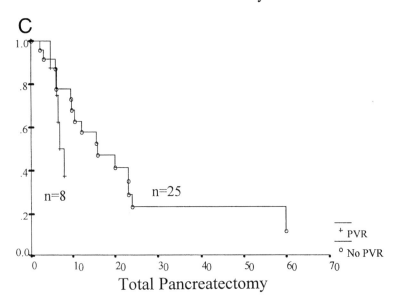

Total Pancreatectomy

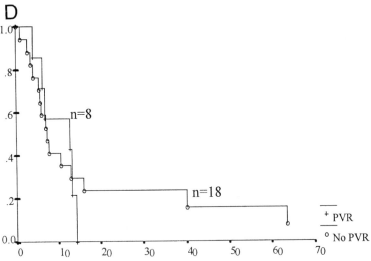

FIGURE 6. (cont.)
C, distal subtotal pancreatectomy; **D,** total pancreatectomy. There was no significant difference in survival in any group.

volvement from resections involving arterial reconstruction. The high morbidity and mortality rates originally reported by Fortner were associated with major arterial reconstruction (type II resection). Although select groups continue to perform arterial resection for tumor invasion, high postoperative death and complication rates are still reported.[15] For Fortner's type I resection (PV only), acceptable mortality rates are reached and recent data support the contention that isolated PVR in the absence of arterial resection is well tolerated.

Data from our series demonstrate that patients undergoing pancreatic resection with PVR require a longer operation with increased blood loss and have an increased transfusion requirement and a longer postoperative hospital stay. However, the reoperative rate and postoperative mortality are similar to those associated with pancreatic resection without PVR. In addition, the number and distribution of complications leading to reoperation are similar between those patients undergoing PVR and no PVR. Only one patient undergoing PVR required reoperation for PV thrombosis. During our more recent experience with PVR, we have not documented any evidence of delayed PV thrombosis, including clinical ascites or bleeding varicies.

These data are similar to those of other recent reports evaluating the safety of PVR. Allema et al. evaluated 20 patients with pancreatic adenocarcinoma requiring PVR for suspicion of macroscopic tumor involvement. They reported that minor and major morbidity, as well as operative mortality, were similar between those patients undergoing PVR and those undergoing pancreatic resection without PV reconstruction.[16] The experience at M. D. Anderson with PVR also demonstrates that resection of the PVR can be performed safely. Similar to the MSKCC results, Fuhrman et al. noted an increase in operative time, blood loss, and transfusion requirement for patients undergoing PVR. They reported a similar median hospital stay and complication rate between the two procedures (28% for standard pancreatectomy vs. 30% for PVR). A low operative mortality after PVR (4%) was also achieved.[17]

In those centers performing a significant number of pancreatic resections annually, the postoperative mortality rate after standard resection ranges from 1% to 5%.[18] Similar postoperative mortality rates have been achieved after PVR. The technical safety of PVR is well documented, and in the absence of arterial resection, PVR is well tolerated. Therefore, PVR for isolated involvement of the PV should not be a contraindication to resection based on a prohibitive morbidity or mortality.

SURVIVAL AFTER PORTAL VEIN RESECTION FOR PANCREATIC ADENOCARCINOMA

Although Fortner introduced the concept that PVR is technically feasible and recent reports confirm the safety of the procedure, the question of whether PVR for clinically apparent PV involvement has an impact on survival needs to be evaluated. Even though some groups have reported that extended pancreatic resections improve overall survival for patients with pancreatic carcinoma,[19, 20] these results have not been consistently reproduced. Although it is doubtful that PVR by itself will improve survival, equivalent survival to that of resected patients not requiring PVR suggests that isolated PV involvement should not be deterrent to resection.

In a comparison of known prognostic factors for adenocarcinoma of the pancreas,[21–23] the percentage of patients in our series with positive lymph nodes, tumor differentiation, and microscopically positive margins was similar in those patients undergoing PVR and those undergoing standard pancreatectomy. A similar distribution of prognostic determinants between no PVR and PVR has been noted by others.[16, 17] The only negative prognostic factor associated with PVR in our series was a larger tumor size. Thirty-four percent of the patients undergoing standard pancreatic resection had tumors less than or equal to 2.5 cm as compared with only 17% of the patients requiring PVR. Although some have noted this size discrepancy after pancreatectomy with PVR,[16] others have reported similar tumor sizes.[17]

Even though large tumor size is a negative prognostic factor for adenocarcinoma of the pancreas,[21, 22, 24] the overall survival of patients undergoing pancreatic resection with PVR in our series was similar to that of those patients undergoing standard pancreatectomy. Importantly, both techniques have an outcome superior to that of palliative bypass or nonoperative treatment.[21]

Other groups have reported similar survival after PVR. Takahashi and Tsuzuki, reported on 63 patients requiring PVR for pancreatic adenocarcinoma, observed that those patients with negative margins after resection had a 5-year survival rate of 14%. They also demonstrated no difference in survival in patients undergoing pancreatic resection with or without PVR.[15] Ishikawa et al. reported a 29% 3-year and 18% 5-year survival rate after pancreatectomy with PVR.[7] Similar survival data have been reported by others.[20]

Not all series report equivalent survival for patients undergoing PVR and those undergoing a standard pancreatic resection. Roder et al. compared 22 patients undergoing pancreaticoduodenectomy and PVR with 89 patients undergoing pancreaticoduode-nectomy without PVR. Of the patients undergoing PVR, none sur-vived longer than 16 months, and the overall survival (median sur-vival, 8 months) was statistically less than that of those undergoing standard resection. They report similar results with distal common bile duct adenocarcinoma. However, interpretation of their survival data must be tempered by the fact that the median survival after a standard pancreatic resection was only 12 months.[25] Lanouis et al., reporting their experience with total pancreatectomy for adenocar-cinoma of the pancreas, noted that the mean survival for those pa-tients undergoing PVR (n = 9) was 6.1 months vs. 18 months for those treated by standard total pancreatectomy.[26] However, conclu-sions regarding poor survival after PVR are limited by the small number of PVRs in this series.

Although agreement is not unanimous in the literature, recent data emerging from large series evaluating PVR for isolated tumor invasion suggest that survival is similar to that of patients under-going standard pancreatic resection. The reason for this similar overall survival between patients undergoing PVR and those requiring only pancreatic resection may be multifactorial. One may rationalize that because the overall prognosis for adenocarcinoma of the pancreas is so dismal, it is difficult to detect small differ-ences in survival after any intervention. Although patients requir-ing PVR may in fact do worse, any difference may be overshad-owed by the overall poor outcome.

Beyond this nihilistic approach, another reason for similar sur-vival may be based on the fact that the need for PVR is not a pre-dictor of aggressive tumor biology, but rather a reflection of tumor size and location. In our series and others, tumors were larger in those patients requiring PVR and, by sheer mass effect, may involve the PV. Importantly, these patients are self-selected by virtue of having locally advanced disease without evidence of arterial involvement and distant tumor spread.

A third rationale for the similar survivorship is that the resec-tions reported in all series are performed for clinical suspicion of PV involvement. Multivariate analysis evaluating prognostic fac-tors for survival after resection for adenocarcinoma of the pancreas demonstrates that although PVR itself is not a negative prognostic indicator, PV invasion is a predictor of poor outcome.[21–23] True vas-cular invasion is difficult to differentiate from inflammatory adhe-sions by preoperative imaging and conventional surgical explora-tion. Up to 50% of the tumors thought to have vascular invasion intraoperatively are subsequently found to only have inflammatory adhesions to the PV after histologic examination (Table 3). Tashiro et al. noted that 35% of the 17 patients undergoing PVR for adenocarcinoma of the pancreas had no true histologic invasion of the PV, although macroscopic invasion of the PV was suspected during surgery. Of the 17 patients resected, 11 patients had involvement of the adventitia and media and only 2 patients had histologic tumor involvement of the intima.[27]

The difference in survival in patients with adhesion only vs. those with true invasion is well documented. In a series of 31 patients undergoing PV/SMV resection for suspected tumor invasion, only 19 (61%) had histologic confirmation of true tumor invasion. Those patients without histologic invasion had significantly improved survival when compared with those with invasion[25] (Fig 7). In addition to the presence and absence of invasion, the degree of invasion correlates with survival. Nakao et al. performed 89 PV and/or SMV resections for clinical suspicion of tumor involvement during exploration. By histologic examination, the degree of carcinoma invasion into the PV or SMV was subsequently classified into one of the following three grades: grade 0, no carcinoma into the wall of the vein; grade I, invasion of tumor into the tunica adven-

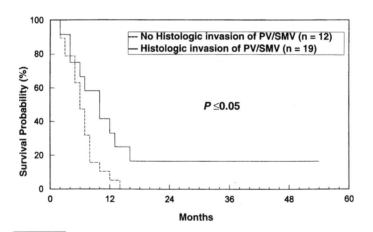

FIGURE 7.
Histologic invasion of the portal vein/superior mesenteric vein: comparison of survival. Patients without pathologic documentation of invasion did statistically better than those with true histologic involvement. (Reprinted by permission of the publisher from Roder JD, Stein HJ, Siewert JR: Carcinoma of the periampullary region: Who benefits from portal vein resection? *Am J Surg* 171:170–176. Copyright 1996 by Excerpta Medica Inc.)

TABLE 3.
Portal Vein Resection for Suspected Clinical Involvement: Summary of the Literature

Author	Country	N	Operative Mortality	LOS, Days	EBL, mL	Node Positivity	Positive Margins	Percent Histologic Invasion of PV/SMV	Survival
Harrison[14]	USA	58	3 (5%)	15	1,200	30 (52%)	15 (27%)		13 mo*
Fuhrman[17]	USA	23	1 (4%)	17	1,700	9 (39%)	4 (17%)		
Roder[25]	Germany	22	0 (0%)	28		17 (77.3%)	15 (68%)	61.3	8 mo*
Allema[16]	Netherlands	20	3 (15%)			14 (70%)	17 (85%)	50	7 mo*
Launois[26]	France	9	0 (0%)	30.5					6.1 mo*
Tashiro[27]	Japan	17	1 (5.9%)			9 (53%)		25.9	
Ishikawa[7]	Japan	30	1 (3.3%)			28 (93%)		85.7	18%+
Takahashi[15]	Japan	63	6 (9.5%)				24 (38%)	61	14%+

*Median survival.
+Five-year survival.
Abbreviations: LOS, length of hospital stay; *EBL,* estimated blood loss; *PV,* portal vein; *SMV,* superior mesenteric vein.

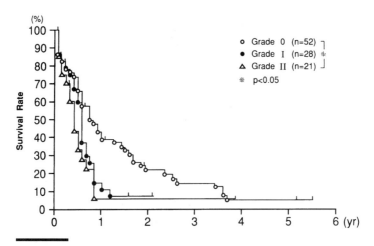

FIGURE 8.
Survival according to the degree of histologic invasion of the portal vein/ superior mesenteric vein. Grade 0, no carcinoma into the wall of the vein; grade I, invasion of tumor into the tunica adventitia or media; grade II, invasion into the tunica intima. (Courtesy of Nakao A, Harada A, Nonami T, et al: Clinical significance of portal invasion by pancreatic head carcinoma. *Surgery* 117:50–55, 1995.)

titia or media; and grade II, invasion into the tunica intima. The survival rate associated with no histologic invasion (grade 0) was significantly higher than that associated with invasion into the intima (grade II)[8] (Fig 8). The relationship between depth of cancer invasion of the PV and survival has been confirmed by others.[15] Most likely, a combination of the aforementioned arguments contribute to the similar survival between patients undergoing PVR and those requiring standard pancreatic resection. Regardless of the rationale, the data are compelling that PVR can be performed safely and that patients requiring PVR for isolated clinical involvement by tumor have an outcome similar to those without PVR.

SUMMARY

Although the prognosis remains poor, surgical exploration with complete resection provides the only potential cure for patients with adenocarcinoma of the pancreas. However, only 15% to 20% of patients are candidates for resection because of the presence of distant tumor outside the confines of resection or because of locally advanced disease. Even though isolated portal vein involvement has classically been a contraindication for resection, PVR can be performed safely with a low perioperative mortality rate.

Besides PV involvement and size, the distribution of histopathologic prognostic factors is no different between patients undergoing PVR and those undergoing standard pancreatic resection. Importantly, overall survival is similar between both groups. Therefore, suspected isolated PV involvement frequently does not preclude operability and, by itself, should not be a contraindication to pancreatic resection.

REFERENCES

1. Brennan MF, Kinsella TJ, Casper ES: Cancer of the pancreas, in DeVita VT, Hellman S, Rosenberg SA (eds): *Cancer: Principles & Practice of Oncology.* Philadelphia, JB Lippincott, 1993, pp 849–882.
2. Brennan MF, Moccia RD, Klimstra D: Management of adenocarcinoma of the body and tail of the pancreas. *Ann Surg* 223:506–512, 1996.
3. Child CG, Gore AL, O'Neill EA: Pancreaticoduodenectomy with resection of the portal vein in the Macaca mulatta monkey and in man. *Surg Gynecol Obstet* 94:31–45, 1952.
4. Fortner JG: Regional resection of cancer of the pancreas: A new surgical approach. *Surgery* 73:307–320, 1973.
5. Sindelar W: Clinical experience with regional pancreatectomy for adenocarcinoma of the pancreas. *Arch Surg* 124:127–132, 1989.
6. Fortner JG: Technique of regional subtotal and total pancreatectomy. *Am J Surg* 150:593–600, 1985.
7. Ishikawa O, Ohigashi H, Imaoka S, et al: Preoperative indications for extended pancreatectomy for locally advanced pancreas cancer involving the portal vein. *Ann Surg* 215:231–236, 1992.
8. Nakao A, Harada A, Nonami T, et al: Clinical significance of portal invasion by pancreatic head carcinoma. *Surgery* 117:50–55, 1995.
9. Conlon KC, Dougherty E, Klimstra DS, et al: The value of minimal access surgery in the staging of patients with potentially resectable peripancreatic malignancy. *Ann Surg* 223:134–140, 1996.
10. John TG, Greig JD, Carter DC, et al: Carcinoma of the pancreatic head and periampullary region: Tumor staging with laparoscopy and laparoscopic ultrasonography. *Ann Surg* 221:156–164, 1995.
11. Kaneko T, Nakao A, Inoue S, et al: Intraportal endovascular ultrasonography in the diagnosis of portal vein invasion by pancreatobiliary carcinoma. *Ann Surg* 222:711–718, 1995.
12. Leach SD, Lowry AM, Fuhrman GM, et al: Pancreatic malignancy involving the superior mesenteric-portal vein confluence is not a contraindication to pancreaticoduodenectomy. *Gastroenterology* 108:1228A, 1995.
13. Lillemoe KD, Cameron JL, Yeo CJ, et al: Pancreaticoduodenectomy: Does it have a role in the palliation of pancreatic cancer? *Ann Surg* 223:718–728, 1996.
14. Harrison LE, Klimstra D, Brennan MF: Portal vein resection for ad-

enocarcinoma of the pancreas: A contraindication for resection? *Ann Surg* 224:342–349, 1996.

15. Takahashi S, Tsuzuki T: Combined resection of the pancreas and portal vein for pancreatic cancer. *Br J Surg* 81:1190–1193, 1994.

16. Allema JH, Reinder ME, van Gulik TM, et al: Portal vein resection in patients undergoing pancreaticoduodenectomy for carcinoma of the pancreatic head. *Br J Surg* 81:1642–1646, 1994.

17. Fuhrman GM, Leach SD, Staley CA, et al: Rationale for *en bloc* vein resection in the treatment of pancreatic adenocarcinoma adherent to the superior mesenteric-portal vein confluence. *Ann Surg* 223:154–162, 1996.

18. Lieberman MD, Kilburn H, Lindsey M, et al: Relation of perioperative deaths to hospital volume among patients undergoing pancreatic resection for malignancy. Ann Surg 222:638–645, 1995.

19. Satake K, Nishiwaki H, Yokomatsu H, et al: Surgical curability and prognosis for standard versus extended resection for T1 carcinoma of the pancreas. *Surg Gynecol Obstet* 175:259–265, 1992.

20. Manabe T, Ohsio G, Baba N: Radical pancreatectomy for ductal cell carcinoma of the head of the pancreas. *Cancer* 64:1132–1137, 1989.

21. Geer RJ, Brennan MF: Prognostic indicators for survival after resection of pancreatic adenocarcinoma. *Am J Surg* 165:68–73, 1993.

22. Cameron JL, Crist DW, Sitzman JV, et al: Factors influencing survival after pancreaticoduodenectomy for pancreatic resection. *Am J Surg* 161:120–125, 1991.

23. Allema JH, Reinders ME, van Gulik TM, et al: Prognostic factors for survival after pancreaticoduodenectomy for patients with carcinoma of the pancreatic head region. *Cancer* 75:2069–2076, 1994.

24. Fortner JG, Klimstra DS, Senie RT, et al: Tumor size is the primary prognosticator for pancreatic cancer after regional pancreatectomy. *Ann Surg* 223:147–153, 1996.

25. Roder JD, Stein HJ, Siewert JR: Carcinoma of the periampullary region: Who benefits from portal vein resection? *Am J Surg* 171:170–175, 1996.

26. Launois B, Franci J, Bardaxoglou E, et al: Total pancreatectomy for ductal adenocarcinoma of the pancreas with special reference to resection of the portal vein and multicentric cancer. *World J Surg* 17:122–127, 1993.

27. Tashiro S, Uchino R, Hiraoka T, et al: Surgical indications and significance of portal vein resection in biliary and pancreatic cancer. *Surgery* 109:481–487, 1991.

CHAPTER 18

Surgical Management of Soft-tissue Sarcoma

Samuel Singer, M.D.

Surgical Director, Sarcoma Program, Dana Farber Cancer Institute, Boston, Massachusetts Surgeon, Brigham & Women's Hospital, Boston, Massachusetts; Assistant Professor of Surgery, Harvard Medical School, Boston, Massachusetts

Timothy J. Eberlein, M.D.

Chief, Division of Surgical Oncology, Brigham and Women's Hospital, Boston, Massachusetts; Richard E. Wilson Professor of Surgery, Harvard Medical School, Boston, Massachusetts

S oft-tissue sarcomas of the extremity, trunk, and retroperitoneum continue to provide therapeutic challenges for surgeons who treat these tumors. In the 1970s, 50% of the patients with extremity sarcoma underwent amputation, and the patients treated with wide excision alone and limb preservation had a 30% local recurrence rate. In the 1980s, with the application of radiotherapy, the amputation rate dropped to under 10% and the local recurrence rate in those patients undergoing limb preservation was reduced to 10% to 15%. It is now well accepted that carefully planned conservative surgery combined with radiotherapy has improved functional preservation with excellent local control and no measurable decline in overall survival when compared with amputation. Recent randomized trials[1, 2] have demonstrated that adjuvant chemotherapy has had a significant impact on local control as well, without a demonstrable effect on overall survival.

Although surgery remains the principal modality of therapy in soft-tissue sarcoma management, the extent of surgery required along with the optimal combination of radiotherapy and chemotherapy remains controversial. Advances in diagnostic pathology permitting a precise diagnosis of sarcoma histology and grade, as well as advances in noninvasive imaging, have provided for a more accurate staging of patients. With these important clinical and pathologic prognostic variables, a multidisciplinary team consisting of surgical oncologists, radiation oncologists, medical oncologists, and plastic surgeons try to design the most effective treatment plan for the patient with the major goals of minimizing local recurrence, maximizing function, and improving overall survival. Progress in soft-tissue sarcoma has evolved by judicious combinations of available modalities of therapy (surgery, radiation therapy, and chemotherapy). With the advent of advanced reconstructive techniques, large soft-tissue defects may be filled and thus permit complete tumor eradication with limb preservation. Such combined therapy has improved local tumor control, and we are now able to salvage many limbs with sarcoma that previously required amputation.

DEMOGRAPHICS

Soft-tissue sarcomas account for only 1% of all cancers, with roughly 7,500 cases diagnosed each year in this country.[3] They occur in almost every anatomical site and are found in all age groups. The most common clinical finding is a mass with or without pain. Extremity and truncal sarcomas tend to metastasize initially to lung. Visceral and retroperitoneal sarcomas tend to metastasize to liver. High-grade soft tissue sarcomas are prone to distant metastasis in over 50% of patients. In contrast in only 10% to 15% of the patients with low-grade sarcomas are distant metastases found or subsequently develop.[4, 5]

About 50% of sarcomas occur in the extremities, with about 75% of these confined to the lower extremity and originating at or above the knee (Table 1). The site of origin of the sarcoma is an important factor to consider when a treatment plan is designed. The location of the sarcoma influences both the type of resection

---

TABLE 1.
Location of Sarcoma

Extremity	52%
Retroperitoneum/ intra-abdominal	25%
Trunk	15%
Head and neck	4%
Breast	4%

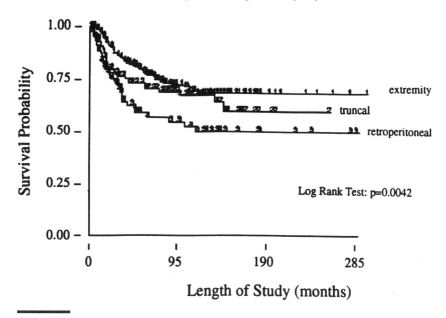

FIGURE 1.
Overall survival by location of the sarcoma.

performed and the surgical margin obtainable. Lesions in the trunk and retroperitoneum may grow to a large size and involve vital structures before causing clinical symptoms. Thus the location of the soft-tissue sarcoma may influence both local control and survival[5] (Fig 1).

PATHOLOGY

Soft-tissue sarcoma is not a single disease, but a collection of over 35 different types of neoplasms related only by a common histogenetic origin. These neoplasms are grouped together because they share similar principles of diagnosis, staging, and treatment. The clinical behavior of a given sarcoma is determined largely by its tissue of origin, degree of differentiation, grade, size, and anatomical site.[6, 7] The skill and experience of the pathologist are key to the proper classification and grading of these tumors. Even among experienced pathologists, recent studies suggest a 30% to 40% discordance rate in the grading of soft-tissue sarcoma.[8, 9] Liposarcoma is the single most common soft tissue sarcoma and accounts for at least 20% of all sarcomas in adulthood. Leiomyosarcoma, liposarcoma, and malignant peripheral nerve sheath tumor are the most common histologic types seen in the retroperitoneal location[5] (Fig 2). Lipo-sarcoma and malignant fibrous histiocytoma (MFH) are the most common histologic types found in extremity sarcoma[4] (Fig 3).

Grade is determined by several factors, including histologic cell type, necrosis, cellularity, mitotic activity, differentiation, and pleomorphism.[10] For some sarcomas the histologic cell type is used as the sole determinant of the grade. For example, rhab-domyosarcoma and Ewing's sarcoma are always considered to be high-grade sarcomas. Two-, three-, and four-grade staging systems have been used at various institutions.[6, 8, 10, 11] In our institution we have classified sarcomas as low, intermediate, and high grade. The reproducibility of these grading systems remains to be studied, and the development of new methods for grading sar-coma would be important for improving the accuracy of prognos-tication.

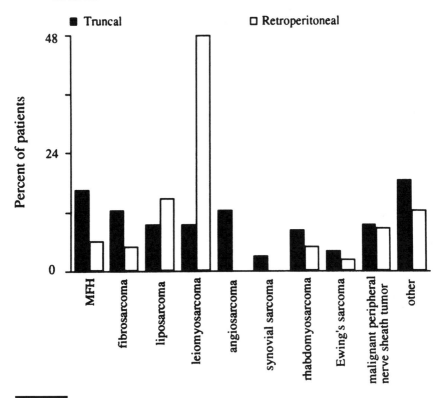

FIGURE 2.

Distribution of truncal and retroperitoneal sarcoma by histology. *Abbreviation: MFH,* malignant fibrous histiocytoma.

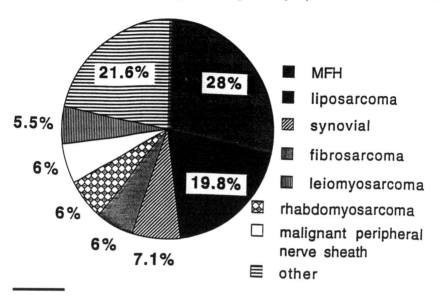

FIGURE 3.

Distribution of extremity sarcoma by histology. *Abbreviation: MFH,* malignant fibrous histiocytoma.

PROGNOSIS

The two most important prognostic factors for survival that have been identified in most studies of patients with soft-tissue sarcoma are grade and size. The American Joint Committee staging system for soft tissue sarcoma is based on four parameters: T (primary tumor size), G (histologic grade), N (regional lymph nodes), and M (distant metastasis, Table 2). In this system the histologic grade is the most important determinant of stage, with a primary of low-, intermediate-, and high-grade sarcoma staged as stage I, stage II, and stage III, respectively.

Site-specific factors prognostic for survival in sarcoma have been identified by several institutions. For extremity sarcoma, high grade, size greater than 10 cm, mean mitotic activity greater than 19 mitoses per 10 high-power field (hpf), and histologic subtype of either Ewing's sarcoma, synovial sarcoma, or angiosarcoma were all associated with a particularly poor prognosis for survival.[4] The mean mitotic activity of the extremity sarcoma was found to be prognostic for survival even if one adjusts for other prognostic factors such as grade, size, and histologic cell type. Figure 4. shows overall survival by mean mitotic activity for extremity sarcoma. Thus the mean mitotic activity may serve as a measure of the sar-

TABLE 2.
American Joint Committee Staging of Soft-Tissue Sarcoma

G	Histologic grade	G1	Low grade
		G2	Intermediate grade
		G3	High grade
T	Primary tumor size	T1	<5 cm diameter
		T2	≥5 cm diameter
N	Regional lymph node status	N0	No regional lymph node metastasis
		N1	Regional lymph node metastasis
M	Distant metastasis	M0	No distant metastasis
		M1	Distant metastasis
Stage I*	Low	IA	G1T1N0M0
		IB	G1T2N0M0
Stage II	Intermediate	IIA	G2T1N0M0
		IIB	G2T2N0M0
Stage III	High	IIIA	G3T1N0M0
		IIIB	G3T2N0M0
Stage IV	Metastasis to regional node	IVA	G3T2N1M0
	Metastasis to distant sites	IVB	G3T2N1M1

*The 5-year survival rate for patients with stage I disease is 79%, for stage II disease it is 65%, for stage III disease it is 45%, and for stage IV disease it is 10%.

coma's growth rate, which if carefully performed may be used as a reproducible quantitative prognostic factor for extremity sarcoma. Other extremity studies have identified the surgical margin as an important prognostic variable for overall survival in extremity sarcoma even if one adjusts for tumor size and grade.[12]

Grade and size were found to be important prognostic factors for survival in truncal sarcoma as well. The presence of a positive gross or microscopic margin of resection for truncal sarcoma was associated with an increase risk of death when compared with a clean margin of resection.[5] This may be explained in part by the observation that the presence of a positive margin after resection of a truncal sarcoma increases the risk of local recurrence. Central location of a truncal sarcoma may make the subsequent salvage of

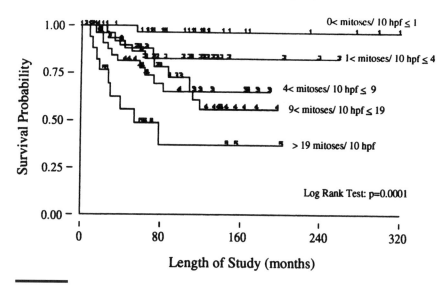

FIGURE 4.

Overall survival of extremity sarcoma by the mean number of mitoses per 10 high-power field.

a local recurrence extremely difficult, thus leading to a direct adverse impact on survival. For truncal sarcoma, the overall survival rate was 67% at 12 years if microscopically clean margins were obtained at resection vs. 49% for microscopically positive margins and 33% for grossly positive margins (Fig 5).

Both grade and margin of resection were found to be prognostic for survival in retroperitoneal sarcoma.[5] Unlike truncal or extremity sarcoma, size was not found to be an important independent prognostic factor for overall survival on multivariate analysis for retroperitoneal sarcoma. Figure 6 shows overall survival by margin of resection for retroperitoneal sarcoma. Thus a complete, clean-margin excision of retroperitoneal sarcoma is extremely important for optimizing survival, thus stressing the importance of aggressive surgical management of retroperitoneal sarcomas.

CLINICAL EVALUATION

Two of the most important factors in the surgical management of soft-tissue sarcoma are whether the sarcoma is confined to an anatomical compartment and the sarcoma's relation to major neurovascular structures. Both physical examination and radiographic evaluation are crucial to surgical planning, with the main goals being local control and maximizing preservation of function. Mag-

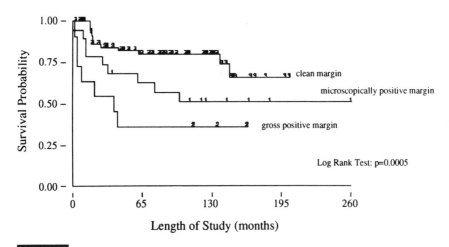

FIGURE 5.
Overall survival by margin of resection for truncal sarcoma.

netic resonance imaging is the radiographic method of choice for extremity and retroperitoneal sarcoma. It has greater versatility than CT in delineating soft-tissue tumors from adjacent normal tissue such as normal muscle and fat. T1-weighted images delineate tumor from fat and bone marrow; T2-weighted images delineate tu-

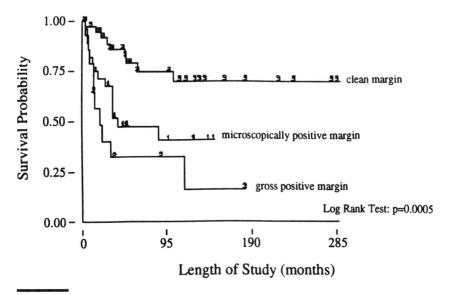

FIGURE 6.
Overall survival by margin of resection for retroperitoneal sarcoma.

mor from muscle. The administration of gadolinium contrast along with dynamic imaging improves sarcoma localization and is often helpful in distinguishing tumor from edema. Extremity images produced by MRI are usually superior to those produced by CT. Important relationships to fascial layers, bone, and blood vessels are better displayed by MRI than by CT examination with contrast. However, spiral CT is preferable in many instances for examining sarcomas of the chest and abdomen because the air/tissue interface and motion artifacts in these cavities often degrade the resolution of MR imaging associated with these locations.

BIOPSY OF SOFT-TISSUE SARCOMA

The purpose of biopsy is to determine the specific histologic type of sarcoma and grade of malignancy so that a plan can be designed for treatment. For example, in the case of a large (>5 cm), high-grade liposarcoma, synovial sarcoma, rhabdomyosarcoma, or Ewing's sarcoma, treatment with preoperative chemotherapy followed by definitive surgery/radiotherapy may be the preferred approach. Neoadjuvant therapy may convert the large high-grade sarcoma to a more easily resectable lesion, preserve more function, reduce the rate of local recurrence, and in responders, improve survival.

Biopsy of a soft-tissue sarcoma can be performed by fine-needle aspiration, core-needle biopsy, incisional biopsy, or excisional biopsy. Given the heterogeneity of these tumors, a large enough sample from a viable area of sarcoma is often required for definitive diagnosis (for incisional biopsy, a 1-cm cube of tissue is usually required). The fresh sarcoma tissue obtained should be partitioned by the pathologist for special studies such as cytogenetics, electron microscopy, and immunohistochemistry.

Fine-needle Aspiration

Fine-needle aspiration is used at some centers with considerable expertise in the cytopathologic diagnosis of malignancy; however, definitive grading is extremely difficult if not impossible with such small samples of malignant cells. Given these limitations, we in general recommend this approach for evaluating recurrent disease or if open incisional biopsy is difficult or hazardous.

Core-needle Biopsy

The advantages of core-needle biopsy include minimal contamination of tissue planes and the availability of tissue architecture. This technique is especially useful for large deep-seated tumors in the pelvis or paraspinal area, which then avoids an open surgical biopsy. Drawbacks include a small sample size that may not be representative of the entire tumor and may miss high-grade areas of the tumor that are not sampled with a core biopsy.

Excisional Biopsy

Excisional biopsy is only used for *small superficial* tumors less than 3 cm in size. The surgeon should avoid contamination of surrounding tissue planes as well as obtain meticulous hemostasis.

Incisional Biopsy

Incisional biopsy provides a small (1 cm^3), yet representative piece of tissue with minimal violation of normal surrounding tissue. The incisional biopsy should be performed through a longitudinal incision for extremity masses so that one can completely and easily excise the entire biopsy tissue tract on definitive resection with a 2-cm surrounding cuff of normal fat and skin.

SURGICAL APPROACH TO SOFT-TISSUE SARCOMA
GENERAL CONSIDERATIONS

The main treatment plan goals for a patient with soft-tissue sarcoma include avoiding local recurrence, maximizing function, reducing morbidity, and improving survival. To design the best surgical approach to a given sarcoma, the surgeon needs to consider these main treatment goals and the optimal combination of radiotherapy and chemotherapy to achieve these goals. In general, the scope of the excision is dictated by the size and anatomical relationship of tumor to normal structures such as major neurovascular bundles and the amount of function that will be sacrificed after an excision. If excessive functional loss is contemplated, can this be minimized by the use of neoadjuvant chemotherapy or radiotherapy?

Sarcomas tend to grow along muscle bundles and along fascial septa well beyond the boundaries of the palpable tumor mass, and this explains the high frequency of local tumor recurrence after limited or even wide excision of soft-tissue sarcomas. Two clinical/pathologic features of soft-tissue sarcoma determine the likelihood of local control with surgery alone or with surgery and adjuvant therapy. The first is the anatomical extent of the sarcoma and the second is whether the sarcoma was primary or recurrent. A sarcoma confined to soft tissues away from major skeletal, neurovascular, or organ structures can be excised with a wide margin (2 to 3 cm) of normal uninvolved tissues. However, a sarcoma that abuts or invades a major neurovascular structure may require sacrifice of this structure to achieve an adequate margin of excision with the risk of serious functional loss. If structure is preserved in the interest of function, one may increase the risk of local recurrence. This recurrence risk may be diminished by the addition of appropriate adjuvant therapy. Sarcomas involving the axial skeleton, shoulder, or pelvic girdle are difficult to treat because if local recurrence occurs, salvage therapy by high amputation may not be feasible.

Locally recurrent sarcomas are more difficult to treat and are more likely to recur. Resection must encompass all palpable tumor and all microscopic foci present in adjacent tissues traversed in previous surgical procedures (fascial planes opened up in dissection, skin flaps, and drain tracks). It may be possible for the surgeon to remove the entire recurrent tumor by dissecting it off nerve, artery, and vein. This usually fails to control tumor unless adjuvant radiation therapy is administered either by external-beam or brachytherapy techniques or unless neoadjuvant chemotherapy is given before tumor excision. Of greater concern is that locally recurrent sarcomas frequently appear more poorly differentiated and of higher grade than the primary sarcoma. For example, when a well-differentiated liposarcoma recurs, it may recur as a dedifferentiated liposarcoma with a significant risk of subsequent distant metastasis. There is general agreement that having a local recurrence is a significant risk factor for the development of a subsequent local recurrence; however, the influence of a local recurrence on overall survival remains controversial. Recent randomized brachytherapy trials[13] have demonstrated marked differences in local recurrence rates without any observable difference in overall survival, thus suggesting that local recurrence for extremity lesions does not have an impact on overall survival.

TYPES OF RESECTION

The size and anatomical relation to neurovascular bundles dictate the minimal scope of resection. Three basic types of resection are performed.

Marginal Excision (Excisional Biopsy)

Marginal excision is used for tumor abutting a major nerve, vascular bundle, or organ. This type of excision can only be used as part of multimodality therapy (usually in the neoadjuvant setting) if carefully planned. If marginal excision is used, placement of interstitial radiotherapy with or without external-beam radiotherapy will often be required.

Wide-margin Excision

Wide-margin excision can effectively control many superficial lesions of the limb or low-grade sarcomas if the margin achieved is widely negative. In addition, wide-margin excision can be used in a sarcoma adjacent to a major neurovascular structure or organ when combined with adjuvant radiation therapy. Often the margin achieved is dictated by important adjacent structures.

Compartmental Resection or Muscle Group Resection

This type of resection is suitable for wide resection of a sarcoma located within muscle bundles and the fleshy part of the limb (e.g., thigh). Provided that ample margins of uninvolved tissue are obtained and the tumor is well within the fascial compartment, such a resection should have a local recurrence rate equivalent to that of amputation. When compartmental resections are performed, two options are available if the sarcoma lies partly within and partly outside a defined compartment.

1. If important to achieve a wide margin, the surgeon may resect not only the muscle groups directly involved but also adjacent muscle groups and the neurovascular bundle or bone involved. The vessels can be repaired with vascular grafts of autogenous vein, but the patient will have major sensory or motor deficits after resection of a major nerve (such as the sciatic nerve). Smaller nerves (such as the ulnar and radial nerves) may be reconstructed with nerve grafts with varying success rates depending on the age of the patient and the length of nerve resected. Bone may be replaced with cadaver allografts or vascularized autogenous bone grafts by using microvascular techniques (for example, fibular free flap).

2. A narrower margin may be accepted to preserve function (tumor is dissected from major nerves, vessels, or bone unless already destroyed by tumor). If the surgeon chooses to preserve these structures, one is left with three possible outcomes: a narrower but tumor-free margin is attained, a microscopically positive margin is left, or gross fragments of sarcoma are left beside preserved structures. For high-grade sarcomas, both clean but close margins (>0.1 cm to <0.5 cm) and microscopically positive margins definitely require adjuvant radiotherapy for local control. With gross tumor left behind, even the addition of adjuvant radiotherapy may not result in effective local sarcoma cell eradication and high local failure rates are common. Thus the local anatomical setting, size, and grade of the sarcoma determine the scope of resection, the need for adjuvant radiation therapy, and the resulting functional deficit. All these characteristics also affect local control.

To avoid amputation and local recurrence, many sarcoma centers have administered adjuvant radiotherapy to all patients undergoing limb preservation. Radiotherapy is not without significant morbidity as far as wound complications, joint stiffness/diminished range of motion, and the generation of secondary tumors are concerned. A prospective selected series of 70 patients with subcutaneous and intramuscular sarcoma were all treated by local surgery.[14] For subcutaneous sarcomas, a wide margin cuff of fat around the tumor and inclusion of an intact layer of deep fascia beneath the tumor were achieved. A wide margin for an intramuscular tumor consisted of an unbroken muscle fascia or thick muscle cuff around the tumor (removing the entire length of the involved muscle). In 56 patients, Rydholm et al. were able to obtain a wide-margin excision and not give radiotherapy. With a median follow-up of 5 years, only 4 of 56 patients had local recurrence, which corresponds to a local recurrence rate of less than 10%. Forty-seven of the 56 patients had high-grade sarcomas. Thus if the surgery is carefully performed, wide-excision limb-sparing surgery may be applied to selected patients with extremity soft tissue sarcoma without the need for adjuvant radiotherapy.

Illustrative Case 1: Wide Excision Alone

A 45-year-old female was evaluated for a 4.5 × 4 × 4-cm anterior thigh mass that on incisional biopsy at an outside institution was found to be a high-grade malignant peripheral nerve sheath tumor. The metastatic workup was negative, and the patient was treated by wide-margin excision (2.5-cm excision) to include a surrounding fat cuff and the deep fascia with a superficial layer of vastus medialis. The wound was closed primarily (Fig 7). Given the wide margins achieved and intact fascia serving as a deep margin barrier to sarcoma cell spread, no adjuvant radiotherapy was given.

ADJUVANT RADIOTHERAPY FOR EXTREMITY SARCOMA

A prospective randomized study at the National Cancer Institute (NCI)[15] validated the concept that in carefully selected patients, limb-sparing resectional surgery combined with adjuvant radiation therapy can offer local control and survival rates equivalent to those obtainable by amputation.

EXTERNAL-BEAM RADIATION THERAPY

Most studies of surgery and adjuvant external-beam irradiation show local control rates for high-grade extremity sarcomas of greater than 90% and local control rates for low-grade sarcomas of

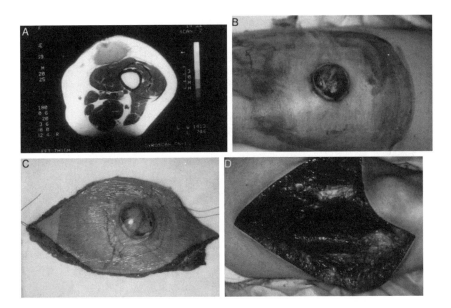

FIGURE 7.
Illustrative case 1: surgery alone.

90% to 100%, depending on the size of the sarcoma.[4, 15–19] The role of radiotherapy is to eradicate any residual microscopic sarcoma cells after wide-margin surgical excision of the sarcoma. To kill these residual tumor cells, doses in the range of 50 to 60 Gy are required. The combination of conservative surgery with radiotherapy has reduced the amputation rate to 5% in most major sarcoma treatment centers and has improved functional results for many patients. External-beam radiotherapy may be given before or after definitive surgery, with advantages to each approach. The advantages of postoperative radiotherapy are (1) availability of the entire nonirradiated pathologic specimen for accurate evaluation of sarcoma grade and histologic cell type, as well as an accurate evaluation of disease extent; (2) incorporation of all tumor by radiotherapy; (3) fewer wound healing complications; and (4) complete evaluation of the resected specimen so as to permit selective application of radiotherapy depending on surgical margins and whether the sarcoma is subcutaneous or intramuscular.

Illustrative Case 2: Wide Excision plus Postoperative Radiotherapy
A 35-year-old man had a 5 × 6-cm mass in the biceps femoris of the distal posterior aspect of the left thigh. Magnetic resonance im-

aging revealed a mass confined to the biceps femoris muscle immediately adjacent to the sciatic nerve. An incisional biopsy revealed a low-grade myxoid liposarcoma. The patient underwent wide-margin excision of the biceps femoris with skeletinization of the sciatic nerve as well as a portion of the tibial and peroneal nerve trunks (Fig 8). The final pathologic examination of the resected specimen revealed a close but clean (1 to 2 mm) margin of excision along the sciatic nerve with 1- to 2-cm margins elsewhere. Twenty-five percent of the sarcoma was found to contain round cell areas, and thus after resection this tumor was reclassified as high grade, thus implying a 50% risk of subsequent distant recurrence. The patient was treated with 6,300 cGY of postoperative radiotherapy 6 weeks after surgery and, 2 months after therapy, ran in the Boston marathon with full range of motion about the knee.

Adjuvant radiotherapy may be given before surgery, which has the advantages of (1) reducing radiotherapy treatment volume, (2) presumably reducing the viability of tumor cells in case the surgeon violates the sarcoma pseudocapsule during excision, and (3) reducing the size of the sarcoma before surgery and thus permit-

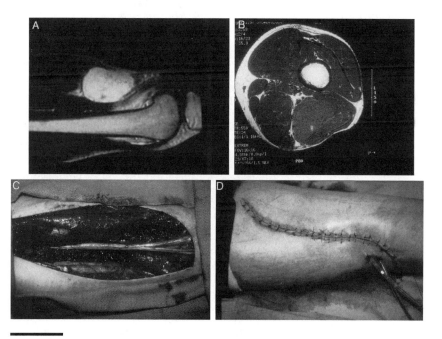

FIGURE 8.
Illustrative case 2: wide excision plus postoperative radiotherapy.

ting more conservative resection. The major disadvantages of pre-operative radiotherapy include delayed wound healing, an in-creased wound complication rate, and the complete sarcoma is not available for grading and prognostication prior to treatment.

Preoperative and postoperative radiotherapy have never been compared in a *randomized prospective* trial. In a retrospective se-ries[20] by Suit et al., 220 patients with extremity and truncal sar-coma were treated with limb-sparing surgery and adjuvant radio-therapy. In this nonrandomized study, 131 patients were treated with surgery plus postoperative radiotherapy and had a 5-year lo-cal control rate of 85%, and 89 patients were treated with preop-erative radiotherapy plus surgery and had a 5-year local control rate of 90%. The improved local control was largely observed for sar-comas larger than 15 cm with the preoperative radiotherapy ap-proach. However, preoperative radiotherapy has been associated with significant and serious wound complications. A recent study of 202 patients with extremity and truncal sarcomas treated with preoperative radiotherapy reported a 37% wound complication rate. One patient died of necrotizing fasciitis, 33 patients (16.5%) required a second operation, and 6 of these 33 patients required an amputation.

Illustrative Case 3: Preoperative Radiation Therapy

An example of the application of preoperative radiotherapy to a difficult limb salvage situation is depicted in Figure 9. The patient shown is a 65-year-old man with a $24 \times 14 \times 13$-cm mass with occasional numbness and paresthesia in the foot. Magnetic reso-nance imaging demonstrated a large fat-containing mass com-pletely surrounding the sciatic nerve as well as the distal popliteal vessels and abutting the distal superficial femoral vessels. Inci-sional biopsy revealed a well-differentiated liposarcoma. This pa-tient refused amputation under any circumstance and was treated with preoperative radiotherapy to a dose of 60 Gy. Four weeks af-ter radiotherapy the patient's tumor was resected along with the posterior compartment of the thigh. The tumor was bivalved around the sciatic nerve and its tibial and peroneal branches (Fig-ure 9, C). The tumor was dissected off the distal superficial femo-ral vessels and distal popliteal vessels, and all gross tumor was re-moved. However, a microscopically positive margin of hopefully nonviable irradiated cells remains along the popliteal vessels and perhaps the sciatic nerve. The patient ambulates well with full sci-atic nerve function and remains without evidence of disease on follow-up MRI.

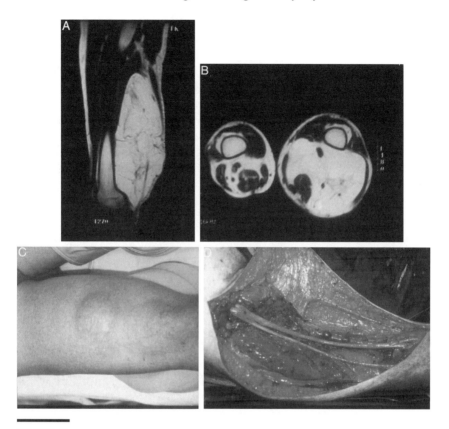

FIGURE 9.
Illustrative case 3: preoperative radiotherapy plus wide excision.

BRACHYTHERAPY ALONE

Brachytherapy is generally administered by placing afterloading catheters in a target area of the tumor operative bed defined by the surgeon. The afterloading catheters are inserted percutaneously through the skin and are placed on the tumor bed and spaced at 1-cm intervals to cover the entire area of risk. The catheters are sewn in place with chronic catgut, and a tension-free wound closer over drains is established. On postoperative day 2, localization films are taken and computerized dosimetry calculated. A loading plan is then designed to deliver 45 Gy over a 4- to 6-day period depending on the strength of the iridium seeds used. Typically, the catheters are loaded with iridium seeds on postoperative day 5, with the seeds and catheters removed on postoperative day 9 to 11, at which time the patient is discharged from the hospital.

The Memorial Sloan-Kettering Cancer Center (MSKCC)[13, 21] implemented a prospective randomized trial between 1982 and 1987 for patients with extremity soft tissue sarcomas who underwent complete gross resection and compared these patients with patients intraoperatively randomized to receive adjuvant brachytherapy. The total dose of radiotherapy for those patients randomized to receive adjuvant brachytherapy was 42 to 45 Gy. Patients were stratified by grade, size, site, and depth of the sarcoma. Treatment arms were balanced with respect to prognostic factors. The 5-year local control of soft tissues sarcoma at MSKCC in patients receiving or not receiving adjuvant brachytherapy was as follows:

Tumor	Brachytherapy	No Brachytherapy −BRT	Significance
High grade	90%	65%	$P = 0.01$
Low grade	65%	65%	NS

No difference in overall survival was found between the brachytherapy and control groups. This series demonstrates that brachytherapy was effective in improving local control for high-grade sarcoma; however, brachytherapy failed to improve local control for low-grade tumors. This may be due to the slow kinetics of a low-grade tumor in relation to relatively short (5 day) exposure to the radiotherapy implant. Thus brachytherapy alone is not thought to be effective for low-grade tumors. Adjuvant brachytherapy has been demonstrated to be effective in improving local control for high-grade sarcoma of the extremity in randomized trials and has the advantage of minimizing radiation doses to the surrounding normal tissues (such as joints to avoid radiation-induced contractures) while maximizing delivery to the tumor bed at risk for residual microscopic disease. Brachytherapy has the additional advantage of shortening the treatment time when compared with external-beam radiotherapy and achieving definitive therapy in a single hospitalization.

ROLE FOR ADJUVANT/NEOADJUVANT CHEMOTHERAPY

In addition to radiation therapy, adjuvant chemotherapy has been reported to decrease the local recurrence rate in extremity but not truncal sarcoma[2] or in truncal but not extremity sarcoma.[1] The only two randomized prospective trials to show a survival benefit of adjuvant chemotherapy were conducted at the Rizzoli Institute in Italy[22] and in Brodeaux, France.[23] The NCI trial demonstrated a significant difference in disease-free survival but not overall for extremity lesions.[2] However, in that study the control group (no chemotherapy) did extremely poorly. The treated patients also experienced significant cardiotoxicity secondary to doxorubicin administration. The NCI trial actually reported a statistically significant decreased survival for patients with retroperitoneal sarcomas treated with the same chemotherapy regimen used for the extremity lesions. No group has shown that chemotherapy is beneficial in truncal or retroperitoneal sarcoma. In addition, three recent studies have shown no benefit from doxorubicin chemotherapy in overall survival.[24–27] The largest randomized trial of extremity and truncal sarcoma using CYVADIC chemotherapy (cyclophosphamide, vincristine, Adriamycin [doxorubicin], DIC [dacarbazine]) was reported in 1994 after having successfully randomized 317 patients from 1977 to 1988.[1] With a median follow-up of 80 months, Bramwell et al. reported an improved relapse-free survival rate for CYVADIC-treated patients, 56% vs. 43% ($P = 0.007$), and a reduced local recurrence rate in the CYVADIC arm, 17% vs. 31% ($P = 0.004$). However, the rate of distant metastasis and overall survival rates were not statistically different. Thus until better drugs are introduced, adjuvant chemotherapy in sarcoma should be offered in protocol settings only. Given the lack of proven benefit for adjuvant chemotherapy on survival, we have restricted the use of chemotherapy to high-risk patients with measurable disease.

Neoadjuvant chemotherapy has the advantage of permitting direct measurement of chemotherapy effect by using serial MRI and physical examination. For most sarcoma histologic types we continue to use a combination of doxorubicin (60 mg/m^2 IV over a 4-day period), ifosfamide (7.5 g/m^2 IV over a period of 3 days), dacarbazine (1 g/m^2 IV over a period of 4 days), and mesna (10 g/m^2 IV over a 4-day period). In patients whose primary sarcoma responds to two cycles of chemotherapy, an additional two cycles of chemotherapy may be given to maximize response. After four cycles of chemotherapy, local control is obtained with surgery with or without adjuvant radiotherapy by using the same criteria as previously discussed. In those patients whose disease progresses while undergoing chemotherapy, no further cycles of chemotherapy are given and the patient undergoes surgery followed by adjuvant radiotherapy if indicated. This approach thus reduces the toxicity of chemotherapy in patients who are unlikely to benefit from prolonged chemotherapy administration. The aforementioned approach is particularly useful for patients with high-grade, greater than 5-cm sarcomas that closely abut major neurovascular bundles.

In responders, neoadjuvant chemotherapy reduces tumor size and eradicates infiltrating tumor cells at the periphery of the tumor. This in turn improves the surgeon's ability to achieve a clean-margin resection without sacrificing neurovascular bundles that are critical to limb function. Neoadjuvant chemotherapy does not significantly impair wound healing or produce local tissue fibrosis as is the case with preoperative external-beam radiotherapy.

ILLUSTRATIVE CASE 4: NEOADJUVANT CHEMOTHERAPY PLUS WIDE EXCISION AND POSTOPERATIVE RADIOTHERAPY

A 58-year-old female with a rapidly growing, 8-cm, proximal thigh mass had the MRI shown in Figure 10, A. An incisional biopsy revealed a high-grade leiomyosarcoma with a mean mitotic activity of 16 mitoses per 10 hpf. The patient was treated with two cycles of MAID chemotherapy (mesna, Adriamycin [doxorubicin], ifosfamide, dacarbazine) with a reduction in tumor size, so a total of four cycles of neoadjuvant MAID chemotherapy were given. A 30% reduction in tumor volume was achieved and the patient was treated with wide excision of the vastus lateralis and vastus intermedius

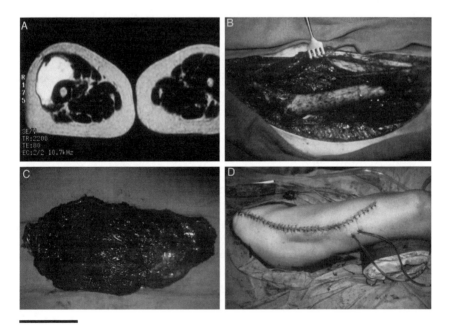

FIGURE 10.

Illustrative case 4: neoadjuvant chemotherapy, wide excision, and postoperative radiotherapy.

with preservation of the rectus femoris and vastus medialis. An intact clean-margin (1 to 1.5 cm) muscle cuff around the tumor was obtained, and the patient was treated with 6,300 rad of postoperative external-beam radiotherapy.

PRESENT RECOMMENDATIONS FOR EXTREMITY OR TRUNCAL SARCOMAS

For subcutaneous or intramuscular sarcomas smaller than 5 cm, high-grade sarcoma, or any size low-grade sarcoma, surgery *alone* should be considered if adequate wide-margin excision with a good 2-cm cuff of surrounding fat and muscle can be achieved. However, if the excision margin is close or extramuscular involvement is present, adjuvant radiotherapy should be added to the surgical resection to reduce the probability of local failure. For high-grade sarcomas greater than 5 cm in size, neoadjuvant chemotherapy should be considered, followed by definitive surgery after four cycles in responders and two cycles in nonresponders. Most of these patients will require the addition of either postoperative external-beam radiation therapy, brachytherapy, or a combination of both techniques after definitive surgery.

RETROPERITONEAL SOFT-TISSUE SARCOMAS

By virtue of their location, large size, and tendency to invade adjacent organs, retroperitoneal sarcomas are associated with a 20% to 40% reduction in survival rate when compared with extremity sarcomas.[5] The most important aspect in terms of survival is the resectability of these tumors. In most series of patients who have no prior surgery, only about 50% can be completely resected, 40% are partially resected, and about 10% are unresectable. Chemotherapy and radiation therapy have little to offer if the tumor is not completely resectable. Thus surgical resection is of primary importance in determining outcome.[5, 28-32] A recent analysis of our retroperitoneal sarcoma experience demonstrated that the most important prognostic factors for survival were the completeness of resection and the histologic grade of the sarcoma.[5] These data support the need for performing aggressive surgical procedures in an attempt to eradicate tumor. The surgeon who performs the first definitive resection must obtain the widest possible resection, and there should be little hesitation to excise and remove adjacent organs to obtain clear margins. Despite this aggressive approach, local recurrence is still a major problem, with multiple, unresectable tumors recurring in many patients. In some patients they may recur at a single site, and these can be dealt with at a subsequent operation and be re-resected for long-term benefit. The role of external-beam radiation therapy in these sarcomas is under investigation in high-risk patients, but it is often difficult to treat the tumor bed area with sufficient dose for local tumor control and at the same time avoid toxic effects on the surrounding bowel. Placement of interstitial implants on a polyglactin 910 (Vicryl) mesh at the time of resection may be used to treat a localized area where margins are microscopically positive and further surgical excision is not possible without significant morbidity.

ILLUSTRATIVE CASE 5: WIDE-EXCISION RETROPERITONEAL SARCOMA

A 60-year-old man had a 1-year history of increasing abdominal girth and decreased appetite. An abdominal/pelvic CT scan revealed a large mass of fat density occupying the entire right half of the abdomen and displacing the right kidney anteromedially such that it lay anterior to the abdominal aorta (Fig 11, A). The mass extended from the region of the right lobe of the liver inferiorly to surround the displaced right kidney and continued caudally to the level of the bladder. Figure 11, B shows the appearance of the mass at surgery. The mass was resected in an en bloc resection that included the right kidney/adrenal, right colon, and a 12 × 6-cm segment of diaphragm. The closest margin was abutting the vena cava and undersurface of the duodenal/pancreatic head, and this area was implanted with radioactive ^{125}I seeds sewn in place on a Vicryl mesh 14 × 7 cm. Final pathologic examination revealed a low-grade liposarcoma, mixed adipocytic and sclerosing types (0 mitoses/10 hpf; cytogenetics: 48–50,XY,del(16)(q23),+2-4rings), with focal myxoid areas measuring 42 cm in greatest dimension and within 0.2 cm of the posterior margin. The tumor encased the kidney and adrenal and invaded the right colon mesentery.

FUTURE DIRECTIONS

Advances in the multidisciplinary management of soft-tissue sarcoma have reduced amputation rates dramatically and continue to improve the functional results of limb-sparing procedures. Further randomized trials that critically examine the role of adjuvant radiotherapy and neoadjuvant chemotherapy are needed to determine the sarcoma patient population most likely to benefit from such therapy. An improved understanding of the molecular, cytogenetic, and biochemical factors that are predictive of local or distant relapse will further improve the treating physician's ability to

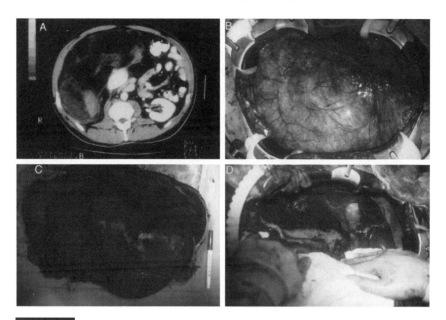

FIGURE 11.
Illustrative case 5: en bloc resection of a large retroperitoneal liposarcoma.

design an effective treatment plan for an individual patient and avoid potentially toxic therapy in those patients who are either unlikely to respond or will not require adjuvant treatment. Recent identification of specific chromosomal translocations in liposarcoma, Ewing's sarcoma, synovial sarcoma, and alveolar rhabdomyosarcoma will provide for a more accurate diagnosis and classification of soft-tissue tumors and may have significant prognostic and therapeutic value in the future. The development of new molecular and biochemical predictors of sarcoma response to chemotherapy and radiotherapy would represent a dramatic step forward in patient management. In addition, new cytotoxic drugs and novel nontoxic treatment strategies such as sarcoma-specific differentiation agents will probably be added to our standard antisarcoma therapy in the future, with the expectation of improved patient survival.

REFERENCES

1. Bramwell V, Rouesse J, Steward W, et al: Adjuvant CYVADIC chemotherapy for adult soft tissue sarcoma—reduced local recurrence but no improvement in survival: A study of the European Organization

for Research and Treatment of Cancer Soft Tissue and Bone Sarcoma Group. *J Clin Oncol* 12:1137–1149, 1994.

2. Chang AE, Kinsella T, Glatstein E, et al: Adjuvant chemotherapy for patients with high-grade soft-tissue sarcomas of the extremity. *J Clin Oncol* 6:1491–1500, 1988.

3. Boring C, Squires T, Montgomery S, et al: Cancer statistics. *CA Cancer J Clin* 44:7–26, 1994.

4. Singer S, Corson JM, Gonin R, et al: Prognostic factors predictive of survival and local recurrence for extremity soft tissue sarcoma [see comments]. *Ann Surg* 219:165–173, 1994.

5. Singer S, Corson JM, Demetri GD, et al: Prognostic factors predictive of survival for truncal and retroperitoneal soft-tissue sarcoma. *Ann Surg* 221:185–195, 1995.

6. Trojani M, Contesso G, Coindre JM, et al: Soft-tissue sarcomas of adults; study of pathological prognostic variables and definition of a histopathological grading system. *Int J Cancer* 33:37–42, 1984.

7. Suit H, Russell W, Martin R: Sarcoma of soft tissue, clinical and histopathologic parameters and response to treatment. *Cancer* 35:1478–1483, 1975.

8. Alvegård TA, Berg NO: Histopathology peer review of high-grade soft tissue sarcoma: The Scandinavian Sarcoma Group experience. *J Clin Oncol* 7:1845–1851, 1989.

9. Presant CA, Russell WO, Alexander RW, et al: Soft-tissue and bone sarcoma histopathology peer review: The frequency of disagreement in diagnosis and the need for second pathology opinions. The Southwestern Cancer Study Group experience. *J Clin Oncol* 4:1658–1661, 1986.

10. Russell W, Cohen J, Enzinger F, et al: A clinical and pathological staging system for soft-tissue sarcomas. *Cancer* 40:1562–1570, 1977.

11. Gaynor JJ, Tan CC, Casper ES, et al: Refinement of clinicopathologic staging for localized soft tissue sarcoma of the extremity: A study of 423 adults. *J Clin Oncol* 10:1317–1329, 1992.

12. Pisters PW, Leung DH, Woodruff J, et al: Analysis of prognostic factors in 1,041 patients with localized soft tissue sarcomas of the extremities. *J Clin Oncol* 14:1679–1689, 1996.

13. Pisters PW, Harrison LB, Leung DH, et al: Long-term results of a prospective randomized trial of adjuvant brachytherapy in soft tissue sarcoma. *J Clin Oncol* 14;859–868, 1996.

14. Rydholm A, Gustafson P, Rööser B, et al: Limb-sparing surgery without radiotherapy based on anatomic location of soft tissue sarcoma. *J Clin Oncol* 9:1757–1765, 1991.

15. Rosenberg SA, Tepper J, Glatstein E, et al: The treatment of soft-tissue sarcomas of the extremities: Prospective randomized evaluations of (1) limb-sparing surgery plus radiation therapy compared with amputation and (2) the role of adjuvant chemotherapy. *Ann Surg* 196:305–315, 1982.

16. Robinson M, Barr L, Fisher C, et al: Treatment of extremity soft tissue sarcomas with surgery and radiotherapy. *Radiother Oncol* 18:221–233, 1990.
17. Suit HD, Poppe KH, Mankin HJ, et al: Preoperative radiation therapy for sarcoma of soft tissue. *Cancer* 47:2269–2274, 1981.
18. Donohue JH, Collin C, Friedrich C, et al: Low-grade soft tissue sarcomas of the extremities. Analysis of risk factors for metastasis. *Cancer* 62:184–193, 1988.
19. Antognoni P, Cerizza L, Vavassori V, et al: Postoperative radiation therapy for adult soft tissue sarcomas: A retrospective study. *Ann Oncol* 3 suppl 2:S103–S106, 1992.
20. Suit HD, Mankin HJ, Wood WC, et al: Treatment of the patient with stage M0 soft tissue sarcoma. *J Clin Oncol* 6:854–862, 1988.
21. Brennan MF, Hilaris B, Shiu MH, et al: Local recurrence in adult soft-tissue sarcoma. A randomized trial of brachytherapy. *Arch Surg* 122(11):1289–1293, 1987.
22. Picci P, Bacci G, Gherlinzoni F, et al: Results of a randomized trial for the treatment of localized soft tissue tumors (sts) of the extremities in adult patients. *Dev Oncol* 55:144–148, 1988.
23. Ravaud A, Nguyen B, Coindre J: Adjuvant chemotherapy with CyVADIC in high-risk soft tissue sarcoma: A randomized prospective trial, in Salmon S (ed): *Adjuvant Therapy of Cancer VI.* Philadelphia, WB Saunders, 1990, pp 556–566.
24. Alvegård TA, Sigurdsson H, Mouridsen H, et al: Adjuvant chemotherapy with doxorubicin in high-grade soft tissue sarcoma: A randomized trial of the Scandinavian Sarcoma Group. *J Clin Oncol* 7:1504–1513, 1989.
25. Antman K, Suit H, Amato D, et al: Preliminary results of a randomized trial of adjuvant doxorubicin for sarcomas: Lack of apparent difference between treatment groups. *J Clin Oncol* 2:601–608, 1984.
26. Antman K, Amato D, Pilepich M, et al: A randomized intergroup soft tissue sarcoma (sts) adjuvant trial of doxorubicin (dox) versus observation (obs) (abstract). Presented at the Fifth International Conference on the Adjuvant Therapy of Cancer, March 1987.
27. Antman K, Ryan L, Borden E: Pooled results from three randomized adjuvant studies of doxorubicin versus observation in soft tissue sarcoma: 10-Year results and review of the literature, in Salmon SE (ed): *Adjuvant Therapy of Cancer,* vol VI, Philadelphia, WB Saunders, 1990, pp 529–43.
28. Bevilacqua RG, Rogatko A, Hajdu SI, et al: Prognostic factors in primary retroperitoneal soft-tissue sarcomas. *Arch Surg* 126:328–334, 1991.
29. Shiloni E, Szold A, White DE, et al: High-grade retroperitoneal sarcomas: Role of an aggressive palliative approach. *J Surg Oncol* 53:197–203, 1993.
30. Sondak VK, Economou JS, Eilber FR: Soft tissue sarcomas of the ex-

tremity and retroperitoneum: Advances in management. *Adv Surg* 24:333–359, 1991.
31. Storm FK, Eilber FR, Mirra J, et al: Retroperitoneal sarcomas: A reappraisal of treatment. *J Surg Oncol* 17:1–7, 1981.
32. Storm FK, Mahvi DM: Diagnosis and management of retroperitoneal soft-tissue sarcoma. *Ann Surg* 214:2–10, 1991.

Index

E

ECCO₂R, intravascular oxygenator and, 209–211

Echinococcal hepatic cysts, 133–136
clinical manifestations, 136–138
treatment, 138–142

Echinococcus granulosus, 134–136

Eck's fistula, 106

ECLS (*see* Extracorporeal life support for cardiorespiratory failure)

ECMO, 189, 190–191 (*see also* Extracorporeal life support for cardiorespiratory failure)

Economics, of shunts for portal hypertension, 118–119

Edema, pulmonary, in acute respiratory distress syndrome, 168, 170, 182

Encephalopathy, with shunts for portal hypertension, 115–117, 120–121

Endoscopic retrograde cholangioportography, of hepatic cysts, 136, 137, 138

Enteral diet, to decrease sepsis after trauma, 53–78
blunt or penetrating trauma, 55–57, 63–64
conflicting studies, 60–61
specialty diets, 61–63
supportive studies, 54, 58–59
gastrointestinal tract and, 54
indications for direct small-bowel cannulation, 73–75
severe head injuries, 69–73
thermal trauma, 68–69
enteral vs. parenteral nutrition, 64–67
specialty diets, 68
timing and protein content, 67–68

Enteritis, radiation, small-bowel obstruction from, management, 25–26

Enteroclysis study, in small-bowel obstruction, 20–21

Enterococcus faecium, vancomycin-resistant, 322

Epstein-Barr virus, in transplant recipients, 308

Esophageal varices, bleeding, history of surgical management of, 106–107 (*see also* Shunts for portal hypertension)

Estrogen replacement therapy, ductal carcinoma in situ and, 42

External-beam radiation therapy, for soft-tissue sarcomas, 407–411

Extracorporeal life support for cardiorespiratory failure, 189–215
centers performing, 208
historical perspective, 189–191
innovations, 208–211
patient selection, 201–204
results, 204–208
technique and management, 191–201

Extracorporeal membrane oxygenation, 189, 190–191 (*see also* Extracorporeal life support for cardiorespiratory failure)

Extrapleural pneumonectomy, for malignant pleural mesothelioma, 255
adjuvant therapy, 264
left-sided procedure, 262–263
patient selection, 255
postoperative management, 263–264
results and discussion, 264–269
right-sided procedure, 255–262

F

Familial hypocalciuric hypercalcemia, in primary hyperparathyroidism, 279

Fatigue, in primary hyperparathyroidism, 275, 276

Feeding tubes, in trauma, 73–75

Fine-needle aspiration biopsy, of soft-tissue sarcomas, 403